DID YOU KNOW?

That a baby born between March 21 and April 20 is destined to be a dynamic leader? A complete horoscope for your baby is just one of the many unique features contained in NAME YOUR BABY.

DID YOU KNOW?

That every name has a special meaning? For example: Anne means "graceful," Emily means "flattering," Alan means "handsome." You can find the meanings of all the different names in NAME YOUR BABY.

DID YOU KNOW?

That there are more than two dozen separate nicknames for Elizabeth? Nicknames are another of the many special features in NAME YOUR BABY.

NAME YOUR BABY

**THE MOST COMPLETE BOOK
OF ITS KIND
AND
THE WORLD'S BESTSELLER
. . . NOW, BIGGER THAN EVER!**

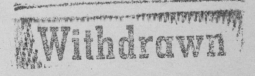

NAME
YOUR BABY

•

LAREINA RULE

•

REVISED EDITION

BANTAM BOOKS
NEW YORK · TORONTO · LONDON · SYDNEY · AUCKLAND

NAME YOUR BABY
A Bantam Book / June 1963
48 printings through July 1985
Bantam revised edition / May 1986
5 printings through March 1988

ISBN 0-553-25599-1

Published simultaneously in the United States and Canada

Bantam Books are published by Bantam Books, a division of Bantam
Doubleday Dell Publishing Group, Inc. Its trademark, consisting of the
words "Bantam Books" and the portrayal of a rooster, is Registered in
U.S. Patent and Trademark Office and in other countries. Marca
Registrada. Bantam Books, 666 Fifth Avenue, New York, New York
10103.

PRINTED IN THE UNITED STATES OF AMERICA

O   14   13   12   11   10   9   8   7

Contents

•

Introduction

•

Names we give our children come from all over the world. Although the United States is an English-speaking nation, we are made up of many cultures and races whose names, except for native Americans', have roots in other countries. Interpreting the meaning of names takes us into the archives of the world history and reflects the times we live in. Many names popular today come from the movies and television; others are as old as the Bible, or older, coming from Greece and Egypt, from the Near and Far East and from other early civilizations.

Names may reflect our cultural heritage, or present information about our ancestors' occupations, environments, or geographic locations, or they may stand for some physical characteristic or specific achievement. They may honor a respected family member or other significant person, or they may be totally new to us, chosen just because we like the way they sound.

Naming your baby is an important responsibility. Psychologists find that if people are happy with their names, they will be happy with themselves. Time spent considering the best, most fitting, and the most pleasant name for your baby is time well spent.

THE ORIGIN OF NAMES

Many first names we use today are derived from root words of Hebrew, English, German, French, Spanish, and Dutch. These words may stand for attributes such as beauty, stature, coloring, or for such virtues as courage and kindness. The first Russell was probably red-headed, and Charity was most likely a person who did good deeds for others.

Some names came from the work that people did. Taylor originated with a person who practiced that profession. Other names tell us where our ancestors lived, in certain forests or fields, villages or countries. Others identified a person's clan or tribe, or their religion or beliefs. People were named after flowers, trees, or plants, as in Rosemary, and for animals. Leo and Leotine stand for the bravery of the lion. In earlier times, people were often named after months, or holidays, for their places in the family (Septimus would be the seventh son), or for ancient gods and goddesses.

Over the years, names have evolved gradually and have come in and out of fashion. Many old ones are seldom used today, with the exception of religious names which are still very popular. The titles of current songs, novels, or movies, and those who create them often influence names, as do national heroes and leaders. Some parents, inspired by the French heroine, Joan of Arc, choose the name Joan, others name their babies Martin Luther after Dr. King, the civil rights leader and Nobel peace prize winner.

The use of surnames as given names has increased through the centuries. A large percentage of boys' given names, and some girls' names, owe their origin to family names. This book includes many of these names, especially those of English, Irish, and Scottish origin which are widely used by people of every ethnic heritage. These names usually came from the mother's birth name or are from her side of the family. Today they are often chosen at random for their distinction and dignity.

ABOUT THIS BOOK

The meanings of names are presented in modern phraseology, and whenever possible root words in English, German, and French are cited in early source spellings to demonstrate evolution of the name. In cases where authorities disagree widely on the meaning of a name, both sources and meanings are included.

Nicknames that are widely used as independent names are listed alphabetically among the given names. Otherwise they are included below the given name from which they are derived.

This book includes names from African, North American Indian, Arabic, Japanese, Hawaiian, and other non-European cultures.

SUGGESTIONS FOR NAMING YOUR BABY

1. Consider your last name when selecting a given name
   for your baby. The name you choose should combine,
   visually and vocally, with your family name. A short first
   name coupled with a short last name may sound harsh or
   insignificant. If you have a short surname such as Smith,
   Brown, or Hill, perhaps you should choose a longer,
   more distinguishing first name. If your family name is
   two syllables or more, a short given name may be more
   harmonious. Thus, John Westermore and Meredith
   Brown.

2. Consider the sound and rhythm. To evaluate the sound
   and rhythm of a name, repeat it and listen carefully.

3. Consider a first name distinct from your surname. It is
   best to avoid names which run together when spoken, as
   in Ralph Forbes or Sheri Yeets. If these names are
   spoken rapidly the distinctive sounds of the separate
   names disappear.

4. Consider the spelling. A striking variation in the spelling of a name may be bothersome for your child, as in
   Jyssica spelled with a "y" instead of an "e."

5. Adding a middle name. Two given names make identifi-
   cation easier in our ever-growing population. The giving
   of middle names is a relatively recent custom, but one
   which is increasing in popularity. Many parents choose
   a name from the mother's family for a middle name.
   Yet, whatever you decide, be sure the name sounds
   agreeable with the first name you have selected and
   your family name. Then check the initials you have
   created, discarding names that spell awkward or embar-
   rassing words.

6. Unisex names. There is a growing trend toward giving
   children names like Alex, Toby, Page, Kelly, and Jamie,
   names that can be used by girls or boys. In general,
   giving a girl a unisex name may not cause a problem,
   whereas giving a boy such a name may. A boy named
   Shirley or Carroll is likely to suffer teasing. Therefore,
   think carefully before giving your child a unisex name.

7. Nicknames. They are widely used as given names today
   and are often spelled with an "i" instead of a "y", as
   Toni or Terri. Also, be sure to consider the nickname

for the given name you choose. If you like the name Margaret but dislike the nickname Maggie, you will probably want to consider another given name.

In the end, the best name for your baby is one that you love and feel your child will be happy with. A well-chosen name is one of the most important gifts you give your baby. Peruse the pages of names in this book, and somewhere in this wealth of names, in this roll call of history both recent and long-past, is the perfect name for your child.

Astrology and Your Baby

•

THE ARIES CHILD

is one born between March 21 and April 20.

The birthstone is the diamond.
The flower is the daisy.
The color is deep red.

April was the second month of the old Roman calendar and was named from the Latin word "aperire" meaning "to open," because it ushers in the astrological new year.

The symbol of the Sign of Aries is the Ram. The ruling planet of Aries is Mars.

Personality characteristics:

If your child is born under the Sign of Aries, he or she has the qualities that make a leader. Aries is a positive sign, giving much force and active energy. Those born in Aries are pioneers. These people love to lead as well as to govern others. They are aggressive and enthusiastic, yet inclined to be impulsive and quick in action. Persons born in this sign are extremely impatient and inclined to be very headstrong and self-willed. Aries children attract many admirers. Aries children dislike to work for others; they welcome changes in occupation, home location, and friends. The changes, however, are from a desire to progress in life, as well as to eliminate monotony. This sign is one of great strength of character. When challenged, the Aries person is a formidable opponent who is both bold and firm. Aries children must learn to curb their natural determination to have their own way. He or she must learn to yield and to give in, to admit when they are wrong. Their pioneer instincts and attributes should not be discouraged. Their dreams and plans for the future should be given attention and understanding. Physically this child has a strong constitution and good recuperative powers. They suffer most when they are frustrated in obtaining their objectives.

Talents and attributes:

Aries children are always thinking up new enterprises, new schemes and ideas. Some of their remarkable ideas are so advanced that they are often misunderstood and laughed at. However, the Aries person is noted for the unusual ability to plan the future. Aries excel in a position of authority, for they are not at their best with others over them. They can achieve great things if they can direct others to carry out their original ideas. In their life's work they do best managing enterprises, businesses, or corporations. They also do well in exploring new or unknown fields.

The Aries child will usually find Sagittarius and Leo, and to a lesser degree Aquarius and Gemini people the most compatible.

Among great political leaders born in the Sign of Aries are:

Margreth II, Queen of Denmark, April 16.
Thomas Jefferson, 3rd U.S. President, April 2.
Robert the Bruce, King of Scotland, March 21.
Henry Clay, U.S. Senator, April 12.
Cesar Chavez, farm labor leader, March 31.

Other internationally known persons born in the Sign of Aries are:

Booker T. Washington, educator, April 18.
Gloria Steinem, editor and author, March 25.
Sandra Day O'Connor, Supreme Court Justice, March 26.
James Watson, Nobel scientist, April 6.
Eudora Welty, novelist, April 13.

Outstanding entertainment personalities:

Gregory Peck, April 3.   Billy Dee Williams, April 6.
Warren Beatty, March 30.   Andre Previn, April 6.
Pearl Bailey, March 29.   Jessica Lange, April 20.
Stephen Sondheim, March 22.   Omar Sharif, April 9.
Loretta Lynn, April 14.   Diana Ross, March 26.

THE TAURUS CHILD

is one born between April 21 and May 20.

The birthstone is the emerald.
The flower is the lily-of-the-valley.
The color is deep yellow.

May was the third month of the old Roman calendar. Its name source was the Roman goddess Maia, the wife of Vulcan.

The symbol of the Sign of Taurus which rules May is the Bull. The ruling planet of Taurus is Venus.

Personality characteristics:

If your child is born in Taurus he or she is resolute, practical, matter-of-fact, obstinate, patient, and overly conservative. He or she is reliable and is careful in speech and action. The Taurus child has reserve energies and desires, often hidden and held in check until provocation releases them. Then the pent-up energy and emotion of Taurus erupts like water over a broken dam. The child's apparently good nature loses its complacency, and he or she is transfixed with rage. Taurus children are like mad bulls, ungovernable while the anger lasts. The Taurus child can also be peaceful, forgiving, and loving. Thought and feeling are blended in these children, though their desires are often hard to understand.

Taurus children who are helped to control their emotional storms can develop into sensitive, intuitive persons.

The Taurus child is a lover of beauty and harmony and dislikes discord. He or she generally has a happy mien unless he or she becomes a martyr seeking sympathy. Taurus children are generous, kindhearted, and trustworthy, intensely strong-willed, dogmatic, and forceful. They can be molded by the ones they love. They are usually sensible and prudent until crossed. Taurus children have excellent memories, are well informed, energetic, artistic, and musical. They are usually affable and pleasant but tend to be opinionated without reason. Their strong likes, dislikes, and prejudices often offend others. These children will act from preconceived motives, either for good or selfish purposes. They are fond of luxury, never overexpressive in speech.

Taurus children are usually strong and have great physical

endurance, but they are liable to suffer from overexertion and overindulgence in physical pleasures such as eating. Ruled by Venus, they take great pride in their looks, bodies, and general appearance and in their environment.

The Taurus child is inclined to fits of jealousy, envy, and hatred and should be left when making a scene, then made to understand why he or she was doing wrong. This child should be given responsibility.

Talents and attributes:

This child's wish is for personal success and attainment, and a Taurus will be gifted with many talents. He or she will be good in executive work in charge of others. Things to do with the earth, such as real estate, mining, and oil fields may attract this child. Taurus will be competent in positions of trust and confidence. This child can qualify as a doctor, nurse, lawyer, electrician, financier, or company director. Many artists, designers, and interior decorators are found in Taurus, working with colors, happy and satisfied with their beautiful creations. Even though practical ability is there and can always be utilized, they can become the most eccentric of artists. Taurus people can also excel as entertainers, actors, and models.

The Taurus child will usually find Capricorn and Virgo, and to a lesser degree Pisces and Cancer people the most compatible.

Among great political leaders born in the Sign of Taurus are:

Queen Elizabeth II of England, April 21.

Harry S. Truman, 33rd U.S. President, May 8.

Emperor Hirohito of Japan, April 29.

Pope John Paul II, May 18.

Golda Meir, Prime Minister of Israel, May 3.

Other internationally known persons born in the Sign of Taurus are:

William Shakespeare, April 23.

Jeanne Suavé, Canadian Governor-General, April 26.

Kurt Gödel, mathematician, April 28.

Willie Mays, baseball player, May 6.

Mary Wollstonecraft, political philosopher, April 27.

Outstanding entertainment personalities:

Fred Astaire, May 10.   Duke Ellington, April 30.
Barbra Streisand, April 24.   Martha Graham, May 11.
Shirley MacLaine, April 24.   Don Rickles, May 8.
Ella Fitzgerald, April 25.   Charlotte Rae, April 22.
Carol Burnett, April 26.   Zubin Mehta, April 29.

THE GEMINI CHILD

is one born between May 21 and June 20.

The birthstone is the pearl.
The flower is the rose.
The color is violet.
    June was the fourth month of the old Roman calendar.
Its name source was the Latin word "junius."
    The symbol of the Sign of Gemini which rules June is
the Twins. The ruling planet of Gemini is Mercury.

Personality Characteristics:

If your child is born in Gemini he or she will be inclined
toward intellectual pursuits. He or she will live more in the
mental world of thoughts than in feelings, emotions, or the
material. Geminis will seldom finish one thing before com-
mencing another, causing them to appear unreliable and
indecisive. Actually it seems that their active minds and
thoughts race along too fast for their bodies to keep up. They
will be quick-witted, often very clever, expressing more in
words than in emotions.
    This child will be kind, willing, loving, and expressive in
disposition. He or she will exhibit curiosity and a desire to
learn about everything and everybody. Geminis can follow
two occupations at the same time. Their nature is sympathetic and sensitive as well as imaginative. They are very
idealistic, fond of study and research. The Gemini child will
enjoy adventure and travel. Although somewhat high-strung
and excitable, Geminis make friends easily. They love change
and must keep continually busy to be happy.
    The June child will stand and walk very erect with quick,
energetic, firm steps. Although he or she may not seem
overly strong, this child has much stamina and endurance
unless he or she overdoes.
    The Gemini child's restless, high-strung, impatient, indeci-

sive nature must be stabilized and channeled into conclusive accomplishments. He or she needs to understand the order and harmony of the universe and the relativity of all things. His or her indecision needs help to be overcome.

Talents and attributes:

Your Gemini child is inclined toward scientific, intellectual work as well as to education and government. Geminis will have many dual experiences, two courses of action, or two subjects of study often entering their lives, in which they will have to learn to make a choice. They will advance through educational progression. Geminis' associates and friends must be their intellectual equals or they will be unhappy. They have inventive abilities that may be of great help. Those born in Gemini make fine accountants, clerks, secretaries, editors, reporters, teachers, lawyers, translators, lecturers, and foreign diplomats. They generally succeed by following more than one occupation. They possess literary ability. Educational work is, however, one of their best outlets.

The Gemini child will usually find Aquarius, Libra, and to a lesser degree Aries and Leo people the most compatible.

Among great political leaders born in the Sign of Gemini are:

Queen Victoria of England, May 24.
John Fitzgerald Kennedy, 35th U.S. President, May 29.
Prince Philip of England, June 10.
Hubert H. Humphrey, U.S. Vice-President, May 27.
Henry Kissinger, U.S. Secretary of State, May 27.

Other internationally known persons born in the Sign of Gemini are:

Walt Whitman, poet, May 31.
Katherine Graham, Publisher, June 16.
Jeanette Rankin, Member, U.S. Congress, June 11.
Sally Ride, astronaut, May 26.
Jacques Cousteau, marine biologist, June 11.

Outstanding entertainment personalities:

John Wayne, May 26.
Brooke Shields, May 31.
Bob Hope, May 29.
Beverly Sills, May 25.
Paul McCartney, June 18.

Joan Rivers, June 8.
Barry Manilow, June 17.
Laurence Olivier, May 22.
Lionel Richie, June 20.
Lilli Palmer, May 24.

THE CANCER CHILD

is one born between June 21 and July 22.

The birthstone is the ruby.
The flower is the water lily.
The color is light green.

July was the fifth month of the old Roman calendar. Its name source was Julius, used in honor of Julius Caesar, who was born in this month.

The symbol of the Sign of Cancer is the Crab. The ruling planet of Cancer is the Moon.

Personality characteristics:

If your child is born in Cancer he or she has a sentimental and versatile nature and a constructive imagination. Cancer is sympathetic and talkative, loves home and family, and has a tenacious memory, especially for details and historical events. The Cancer child appreciates praise and is encouraged by kindness. This child will delight in beautiful scenery, romantic settings, and new adventures. Cancers are very conscientious but somewhat skeptical of new ideas until they understand them. However, they can adapt to different people and environments.

Cancer children appear retiring, but are really positive and tenacious and love to be noticed while appearing to be unassuming. They are not averse to fame, should recognition come.

Your Cancer child will be fond of older persons, ancient customs, and things connected with the past that have sentimental value. It seems that his or her fate is bound up with domestic ties and family interests, the home and home improvement. The Cancer individual often has a bright, alert, oval, or round face. He or she often worries over things others don't worry about and as a result may have slight indigestion or suffer from nervousness.

The Cancer child must learn to think and say, "I can," instead of "I can't." He or she must recognize and control moodiness, wavering and inconsistency. Your Moon child may fear ridicule and criticism and need help in meeting new people. Cancers need to be taught to avoid spending much time analyzing themselves and worrying over what people think of them. They can overstress the importance of people who do not agree with them. They should be encouraged to reach out for new horizons, leaving outmoded customs of the past behind.

Talents and attributes:

These imaginative, impressionable children make many changes in their lives until they find the position or occupation where they feel self-assured, well integrated, and appreciated. This person can succeed as a manager of a large corporation, a manufacturer, a public employee, or a utility worker, a job where there is much responsibility and a duty to perform. Persons in this sign make good nurses and managers in business, but their greatest attribute is their love of home. They can turn a cave into a paradise. Cancer people like the sea, employment with shipping lines, and sea travel.

The Cancer child will usually find Pisces and Scorpio, and to a lesser degree Taurus and Virgo people the most compatible.

Among great political leaders born in the Sign of Cancer are:

Simone Veil, President, European Parliament, July 13.
Julius Caesar, Roman emperor, July 12.
Calvin Coolidge, 30th U.S. President, July 4.
Haile Selassie, Emperor of Ethiopia, July 17.
Gerald Ford, 38th U.S. President, July 14.

Other internationally known persons born in the Sign of Cancer are:

Diana, Princess of Wales, July 1.
Helen Keller, blind educator, June 27.
John Paul Jones, U.S. Naval hero, July 6.
Rosalyn Yalow, Nobel scientist, July 19.
Roald Amundsen, explorer, July 16.

Outstanding entertainment personalities:

Ringo Starr, July 7.	Isaac Stern, July 21.
Cheryl Ladd, July 12.	Harrison Ford, July 13.
Van Cliburn, July 12.	Michele Lee, June 24.
Red Skelton, July 18.	Diana Rigg, July 20.
Vittorio de Sica, July 7.	Mariette Hartley, June 21.

THE LEO CHILD

· is one born between July 23 and August 22.

The birthstone is the sardonyx.
The flower is the gladiolus.
The color is light orange.
    August was the sixth month of the old Roman calendar
and was formerly called "Sextillis."
    Its name source was the Roman Emperor Augustus Caesar.
    The symbol of the Sign of Leo is the Lion. The ruling
planet of Leo is the Sun.

Personality characteristics:

If your child is born in Leo he or she is usually a happy
extrovert. He or she loves power. A child of the Sun is
sincere, honorable, and magnanimous, proud and impatient
with those who dare to question their intentions or motives.
As adults they are generally dignified and positive.
    The Leo child is philosophical, forceful, and demonstra-
tive. Because they are assured, they demonstrate faith, hope,
and fortitude. This child is apt to be overly energetic and lavish
in expenditure of energy and money when his or her sympathy or interest is aroused. Leos are usually popular, even-
tempered but quick to anger if their Leo pride is hurt. Ever
facing the Sun, Leo is sometimes superoptimistic. The Leo
person is powerful and commanding in determination and
ambitions. Although deeply emotional, he or she can triumph
over wrong desires. Leos trust those who believe in them,
until they are betrayed or deceived. Leos always aim for the
stars, and with their determination and self-confidence, Leo
children usually get there. They are rarely deceptive or
secretive.
    Leos can resist illness and recuperate from fatigue quickly.
They have a superabundance of vitality and wonderful
physiques.
    The Leo child is daring, unflinching, and unafraid and
must be taught to curb his or her exuberance. This child
tends to have too much false pride and may be boastful and
snobbish. Leos needs direction and control as children. Since
they always want to be at the head of things, they must be
made to realize that others like to be leaders, too.

Talents and attributes:

Leos' great organizing ability and commanding power usually bring success. They are charming and have the power to make people like them. Used beneficially this is a gift; used selfishly it is disastrous, to them as well as to their victims. These individuals make good managers, organizers, and military leaders. They are suited to a public career or professional life. They excel as artists, actors, and musicians, succeeding best where they have authority or where they hold a responsible, executive position.

The Leo child will usually find Sagittarius, Aries, and to a lesser degree Gemini and Libra people the most compatible.

Among great political leaders born in the Sign of Leo are:

Símon Bolívar, South American liberator, July 24.

Nancy Kassenbaum, U.S. Senator, July 29.

Napoleon I, Emperor of France, August 15.

Alexander the Great, Macedonian Greek world conqueror, July 23.

Tom Mboya, Kenya leader, August 15.

Other internationally known persons born in the Sign of Leo are:

Amelia Earhart, aviatrix, July 24.

Neil Armstrong, astronaut, August 5.

Maria Mitchell, astronomer, August 1.

CoCo Chanel, designer, August 19.

Bill Bradley, U.S. Senator and basketball player, July 28.

Outstanding entertainment personalities:

Shelley Winters, July 18.	Abby Dalton, August 15.
Lucille Ball, August 6.	Geoffrey Holder, August 1.
Peter O' Toole, August 2.	Lynda Carter, July 24.
Robert Culp, August 16.	Jason Robards, Jr., July 26.
Robert Redford, August 18.	David Steinberg, August 9.

THE VIRGO CHILD

is one born between August 23 and September 23.

The birthstone is the sapphire.

The flower is the aster.

The color is dark violet.

September was the seventh month of the old Roman calendar. Its name source was "septem" meaning "seven."

The symbol of the Sign of Virgo is the Virgin. The ruling planet of Virgo is Mercury.

Personality characteristics:

If your child is born in Virgo he or she is cautious, discreet, and not only contemplative but industrious. Virgos will enjoy the things money can buy and will gladly work for them. This child is self-assured, not easily content with the commonplace. He or she will learn quickly; this child may worry and have an overanxiety to succeed. Virgos will be sensitive to their surroundings and have a thirst for knowledge. They will be very careful of details, and can be very critical, leaving those they care for astounded. This Virgo child is methodical and spends little time speculating on the unknown.

Virgoans want facts; they are self-possessed and discreet. In business they work for greater improvements, sometimes unobserved and unappreciated. These individuals are greatly affected by marriage and expect purity and constancy in their mates.

The Virgo-born are persevering and ingenious and very intelligent, but rarely control their own lives or make changes unaided. There is a tendency to let the mentally less-developed give them orders. They earn money but spend it for pleasure and education instead of for material things. In emergencies, they may think of themselves before others.

The Virgo child can absorb and learn anything he or she is determined to learn. Virgos must correct selfishness and the continual criticism they usually practice. They must learn that their overanxiety dissipates their mental and physical energy.

Talents and attributes:

Virgo can succeed in life as an agent or intermediary for a large company, or can be a trusted executive assistant for a public or political figure. He or she excels in general commercial ventures, imports and exports, and matters connected with the good earth and its products. Virgo persons generally rise in life through their own merits, but can fail if they follow the wrong judgment of others. Writing, bookkeeping, recordkeeping, research, and the instruction of others lure this person.

The Virgo child will usually find Taurus, Capricorn, and to a lesser degree Cancer and Scorpio people the most compatible.

Among great political leaders born in the Sign of Virgo are:

William Howard Taft, 27th U.S. President, September 15.

Elizabeth I of England, September 7.

Lyndon B. Johnson, 36th U.S. President, August 27.

Geraldine Ferraro, U.S. Congresswoman and Vice-Presidential Candidate, August 26.

Daniel Inouye, U.S. Senator, September 7.

Other internationally known persons born in the Sign of Virgo are:

Leonard Bernstein, composer, August 25.

Jane Addams, social worker, September 6.

Maria Montessori, physician and educator, August 31.

Robert Schuller, religious leader and author, September 16.

Anna May (Grandma) Moses, painter, September 7.

Outstanding entertainment personalities:

Michael Jackson, August 29.

Bruce Springsteen, September 23

Bob Newhart, September 5.

Larry Hagman, September 21.

Rosemary Harris, September 19.

Bobby Short, September 15.

Lily Tomlin, September 1.

John Ritter, September 17.

Isabel Sanford, August 29.

Nell Carter, September 13.

THE LIBRA CHILD

is one born between September 24 and October 23.

The birthstone is the opal.

The flower is the cosmos.

The color is yellow.

October was the eighth month of the old Roman calendar. Its name source was "octo" meaning "eight."

The symbol of the Sign of Libra is the Balances. The ruling planet of Libra is Venus.

Personality characteristics:

If your child is born in Libra he or she loves justice and hates injustice. He or she is an extremely sensitive individual and likes to be shielded from the unhappy side of life. He or she has a tendency to cling to illusions, especially those about people one likes, usually to some detriment. Because Libra is happy, sincere, and honest, it is difficult for one to mistrust others. Your Libra child loves beauty, colors, music, and the arts. If not talented in the arts, he or she will deeply appreciate them. A great sense of sympathy toward people often deludes Libra into mistaking sympathy for love.

Libra children often have difficulty in learning from others or in learning through logic and reason. They seem to learn best from experience and intuition, which is amazingly developed.

These children are usually handsome or beautiful and well formed, as if their innate soul finds expression in the physical.

Be prepared to give your Libra child artistic surroundings and an education in the arts. Help him or her to face things as they are and to learn that the reality of things is often different from their appearance. Libra must learn the law of cause and effect, that all life has an interrelationship. This is the lesson of the Balances, as symbolized by the Sign of Libra. This child must learn self-control and that uncontrolled emotions or rampant impulses can never exalt one's soul or mind. Libra children will need help in making everyday decisions. They must not be allowed to avoid responsibility by justifying their procrastination.

Talents and attributes:

Libra's predominating talents are artistic. They may like work with beautiful fabrics, perfumes, clothing, jewelry designing, interior decorating, ceramics, stage designing, landscape architecture, drawing, painting, cartooning, flower gardening, music, singing and acting. They can be successful leaders by cultivating their talents along these lines. They love peace and harmony and are often outspoken exponents of these virtues.

The Libra child will usually find Aquarius, Gemini, and to a lesser degree Aries and Leo people the most compatible.

Among great political leaders born in the Sign of Libra are:
John Adams, 2nd U.S. President, October 19.
Dwight David Eisenhower, 34th U.S. President, October 14.
Mahatma Gandhi, leader in India, October 2.

Margaret Thatcher, British Prime Minister, October 13.
Eleanor Roosevelt, U.N. Ambassador, October 11.
Other internationally known persons born in the Sign of
Libra are:
Lee Iacocca, industrialist and author, October 15.
Melina Mercouri, Greek Cabinet Minister, October 18.
Giuseppe Verdi, opera composer, October 16.
Gertrude Ederle, English Channel Swimmer, October 23.
Jesse Jackson, civil rights leader, October 8.
Outstanding entertainment personalities:
Johnny Mathis, September 30.
John Lennon, October 9.
Angela Lansbury, October 16.
Johnny Carson, October 23.
Julie Andrews, October 1.
Jerome Robbins, October 11.
Mark Hamill, September 25.
Catherine Deneuve, October 22.
Barbara Walters, September 25.
Susan Sarandon, October 4.

THE SCORPIO CHILD

is one born between October 24 and November 22.

The birthstone is the topaz.
The flower is the chrysanthemum.
The color is red.
November was the ninth month of the old Roman calendar. Its name source was "novem" meaning "nine."
The symbol of the Sign of Scorpio which rules November is the Scorpion. The ruling planet of Scorpio is the fiery planet Mars.

Personality characteristics:

If your child is born in Scorpio he or she likes truth and dislikes falsehoods. A Scorpio child likes to visualize the completion and realization of his mental and physical efforts. He or she has an inner vision of the soul that can see beyond illusion. Scorpios tend to be secretive. Parents must earn their trust. This child has a tendency to go to extremes. There is also a tendency for Scorpios to be diverted from

their goals. Scorpios do not easily comply with the wishes and
dictates of others. If they do, it is often unwillingly. This
child is the most magnetic of all the children of the zodiac,
always attracting the admiration, attention, and often the
jealousy of the opposite sex.

Scorpio children are noted for their effervescent humor
and their attractiveness. Whether they are tall or short, dark
or light, they still attract people. They are quick and restless,
and tireless workers.

Scorpios, because of their great energy and force, should
be taught the difference between constructive and destruc-
tive power. They should be taught self-mastery and be given
careful direction so that their tremendous energy and drive is
channeled into creative activity. These children should also
be taught early in life that as they show understanding, so
will understanding and compassion be shown to them. The
study of psychology will help Scorpios to understand themselves and others. Another important lesson for the Scorpio
child to learn is to curb feelings of jealousy and envy. One of
the Scorpio weaknesses will be procrastination. The time to
do work is "now" and not tomorrow. Never listen to this
child's many excuses for putting things off. Another lesson to
be learned is the difference between impetuous physical at-
traction and deep, enduring affection. Scorpios' outbreaks,
moods and tempers should be traced to their motivating
causes and these corrected.

Talents and attributes:

The Scorpio child's talents are many and varied. He or she
is unusually talented in promotional activities, writing,
designing, modeling, and acting. Scorpios make good engi-
neers, electricians, contractors, surgeons, scientists, or chem-
ists. Scorpio will be excellent at research as well as a forceful
leader. Scorpios make loving spouses; they want to love and
be loved.

The Scorpio child will usually find Cancer, Pisces, and to a
lesser degree Virgo and Capricorn people the most compatible.

Among great political leaders born in the Sign of Scorpio
are:

Theodore Roosevelt, 26th U.S. President, October 27.
Indira Gandhi, Prime Minister of India, November 19.

Charles, Prince of Wales, November 14.
Sun Yat-sen, founder of modern China, November 12.
Charles de Gaulle, President of France, November 22.
Other internationally known persons born in the Sign of Scorpio are:
Pablo Picasso, painter, October 25.
Marie Curie, chemist, November 7.
Hanna Holburn Gray, university president, October 25.
Billy Graham, religious leader, November 7.
Isamu Noguchi, sculptor, November 17.
Outstanding entertainment personalities:
Katharine Hepburn, November 8.
Jane Pauley, October 30.
Sam Shepard, November 5.
Natalia Makarova, November 21.
Jane Alexander, October 28.
Marcello Mastroianni, November 18.
Lee Grant, October 31.
Burt Lancaster, November 2.
Bo Derek, November 20.
Charles Bronson, November 3.

THE SAGITTARIUS CHILD

is one born between November 23 and December 22.

The birthstone is the turquoise.
The flower is the narcissus.
The color, light shades of purple.
December was the tenth month of the old Roman calendar and is named from the Latin word "decem" meaning "ten."
The symbol of the sign of Sagittarius is the Archer. The ruling planet of Sagittarius is Jupiter.

Personality Characteristics:

If your child is born in Sagittarius he or she is intelligent, generous, and often possessive, especially of those who are loved. A child with this sun sign is hopeful and impressionable. He or she is quick and enterprising, demonstrative in affection, and loyal. This individual loves liberty and will vie with anyone to obtain it. Because of a firm belief in freedom of speech and expression, Sagittarians are opinionated and decidedly independent in their thinking and reasoning. If twenty-five people in a room agree on one point, the Sagittarius person would disagree vehemently. These children are often rebellious, with a tendency to be indifferent to law and order, especially if it affects their individual freedom. Their blunt characteristics often cause the people of this sign to lose friends. The Sagittarius child has a religious, philosophical, and psychological outlook on life. A Sagittarius child loves people and tries to understand them. This sign's sympathetic and methodical nature is well developed. Sagittarius is inquisitive and witty and has a penetrating mind.

Constitutionally this child is strong, but when his health is afflicted it usually comes from overactivity, excessive worry, and frustration over inability to solve problems. The Sagittarius child is a lover of beauty, above all the beauty of knowledge. These children take short cuts in almost everything they do. Often they got lost in petty details and forego the big things. This child is noble, sentimental, and impulsive, tactless and undiplomatic, but Sagittarius loves deeply and is usually artistic and refined.

The Sagittarius child needs help in learning discrimination in choosing friends, companions, and later, a mate. Sagittarians must learn to evaluate people. This child will have a desire to help humanity, especially the unfortunate, but with a lack of discrimination may end up sympathizing with those who seek only to take advantage. Sagittarians cannot judge people, for they have no guile. The Sagittarius child will love nature and the great outdoors. By understanding themselves, their talents, weaknesses, and rebellions, their lives can be so directed that they can accomplish anything they want to do.

Talents and attributes:

Sagittarians' talents expand best where they come in contact with others, such as in instructing classes in art, education, dancing, and the ministry. They may also enter into business deals, or be in any one of many professions, such as the law.

Among great political leaders born in the Sign of Sagittarius are:

Sir Winston Churchill, English statesman, November 30.

Mary, Queen of Scots, December 7.

Martin Van Buren, 8th U.S. President, December 5.

Zachary Taylor, 12th U.S. President, November 24.

Franklin Pierce, 14th U.S. President, November 25.

Other internationally known persons born in the Sign of Sagittarius are:

Chris Evert Lloyd, tennis player, December 21.

Margaret Mead, anthropologist, December 16.

Diego Rivera, muralist, December 8.

Gary Hart, U.S. Senator, November 28.

Shirley Chisholm, member U.S. Congresswoman, November 30.

Outstanding entertainment personalities:

Walt Disney, December 5.

Andy Williams, December 3.

Jane Fonda, December 21.

Sammy Davis, Jr., December 8.

Liv Ullman, December 16.

Woody Allen, December 1.

Dionne Warwick, December 12.

Frank Sinatra, December 12.

Steven Spielberg, December 18.

Lee Remick, December 14.

THE CAPRICORN CHILD

is one born between December 23 and January 20.

The birthstone is the garnet, which gives its wearer the virtue of constancy.

The flower is the carnation.

The color is deep blue.

January was the eleventh month of the old Roman calendar. Its name came from the ancient Roman diety Janus, the god of gates and doors, interpreted as the beginning of all things.

The symbol of the sign of Capricorn is the Goat. The ruling planet of Capricorn is Saturn.

Personality characteristics:

If your child is born in Capricorn he or she will have a quiet, somber meditative nature ruled by reason instead of impulse. Such children are thrifty, reserved, diplomatic, deep thinkers, and determined. They are painstaking, unusually slow and cautious in what they do. They give the appearance of self-confidence, yet they are not really too independent of others. They are often too cautious for their own rapid progression, often suspicious of ulterior motives in business dealings.

Capricornians are like the tortoise in the old fable, which kept plodding until it reached its desired goal. The Capricorn child is receptive to down-to-earth activities. Their tendency is to receive, but not give, to utilize others' work, abilities, and learning to their own advantage.

A Capricorn child must be taught the joy of sharing and giving. Capricorn children must learn to master trials and hardships and not blame others for their misfortunes. They must be helped to decide early in life that their achievements depend not only upon their faithful performance of duties but upon the exchange of ideas and trust in others. This child must be taught that to carry out mental and creative work the body must have good food, necessary rest, and exercise. These children may find themselves interested in mundane, earthly affairs, which is good if they do not forget that the soul needs beauty and spiritual things also. This child can be obstinate, jealous, and inclined to envy. Often life has to deal severely with Capricorn before this child realizes the lesson it is trying to teach. Children ruled by Capricorn limit themselves by their reluctance to make changes or to transcend their self-imposed limitations.

Talents and attributes:

Capricorns are industrious and ambitious. They often love wealth for the power and prestige it brings them. The Capricorn child is talented in mechanics, engineering, and politics. Literary and religious things interest them. They like positions and occupations that influence and impress others. They make good executives and love power in any field they enter, whether science, the arts, or the law. They are good managers of large businesses and are excellent in real estate. Capricornians often delay marriage until late in life, vacillating in their choice of a mate. Once married, however, they become faithful, devoted mates.

The Capricorn child will usually find Virgo and Taurus, and to a lesser degree Pisces and Scorpio people the most compatible.

Among great political leaders born in the Sign of Capricorn are:

Benjamin Franklin, American diplomat, January 17.
Woodrow Wilson, 28th U.S. President, December 28.
Maria Pintasilgo, Prime Minister of Portugal, January 18.
Anwar el-Sadat, Egyptian leader, December 25.
Mao Tse-tung, leader of Chinese revolution, December 26.

Other internationally known persons born in the Sign of Capricorn are:

Sir Isaac Newton, scientist, December 25.
Louis Pasteur, chemist, December 27.
Martin Luther King, Jr, civil rights leader, January 15.
Nancy Lopez, golfer, January 6.
Clara Barton, organizer of American Red Cross, December 25.

Outstanding entertainment personalities:

Elvis Presley, January 8.
Cary Grant, January 18.
Dolly Parton, January 19.
Federico Fellini, January 20.
James Earl Jones, January 17.
Frances Sternhagen, January 13.
Barbara Mandrell, December 25.
Danny Kaye, January 18.
Richard Widmark, December 26.
Marlene Dietrich, December 27.

THE AQUARIUS CHILD

is one born between January 21 and February 19.

The birthstone is the amethyst, which bequeaths its wearer the gift of sincerity.

The flower is the violet.

The color is light blue.

February was the twelfth month of the old Roman calendar and was named from Februa, the Roman festival of purification.

The symbol of the sign of Aquarius is the Water Bearer or the Sage. The ruling planet of Aquarius is Uranus.

Personality characteristics:

If your child is born under the Sign of Aquarius, he or she has a faithful and dependent nature and at times may be difficult to understand. He or she is patient, unobtrusive, faithful, kind, and inoffensive. The Aquarian child will not always defend itself against injustice. Aquarius is quiet when it would be better to speak up. Rather than argue with a person who is wrong, this child is apt to say, "Why should I argue or point out his errors? Let him find out his own mistakes." Many of this sign are interested in exploring the mysteries of nature. The Aquarian child is intuitive and honest, more mental than emotional. Love plays a part in Aquarius's life, but love does not dominate it. This child is too obsessed with learning, too curious about life and its mysteries to be possessed. The Aquarian child likes people and wants to be liked back. Aquarians are attracted to persons of intelligence and refinement. They may be tempted at times to let their idealism and dreams interfere or make them dissatisfied with reality.

The Aquarian child must be taught early in life that plans do not materialize overnight. Aquarians may want to start at the top instead of the bottom in anything they go into. The Aquarian child can learn whatever is desired if he or she uses persistence. Aquarius is capable of directing his or her interests to whatever is desired and succeeding in it. These children must learn the necessity of establishing a state of equilibrium between their higher consciousness and their lower selves. When this is accomplished Aquarius becomes a sage who can help others to higher understanding.

Talents and attributes:

Aquarius's talents are numerous. They can succeed in scientific research or as an executive or writer. They can sell anything to anyone. Consequently they are at their best when associated with large corporations, large promotional or pioneering activities. This child will be interested in international progress and reform. He or she may also become interested in archaeology, geology, physics, astronomy, or studies of the evolution of life.

Among great political leaders born in the Sign of Aquarius are:

Abraham Lincoln, 16th U.S. President, February 12.
Franklin D. Roosevelt, 31st U.S. President, January 30.
Isabel Peron, President of Argentina, February 6.
Ronald Reagan, 40th U.S. President, February 6.
Susan B. Anthony, suffrage leader, February 15.

Other internationally known persons born in the Sign of Aquarius are:

Charles A. Lindbergh, aviation pioneer, February 4.
Thomas A. Edison, inventor, February 11.
John McEnroe, tennis champion, February 16.
Elizabeth Blackwell, physician, February 3.
Ayn Rand, novelist, February 2.

Outstanding entertainment personalities:

Paul Newman, January 26.
Vanessa Redgrave, January 30.
Jack Lemmon, February 8.
Leontyne Price, February 10.
Carol Channing, January 31.
Telly Savalas, January 21.
Alan Bates, February 17.
Roberta Flack, February 10.
Blythe Danner, February 3.
Anna Pavlova, January 31.

THE PISCES CHILD

is one born between February 20 and March 20.

The birthstone is the bloodstone.
The flower is the daffodil.
The color is dark purple.

March was the first month of the Old Roman calendar. Its name source was Mars, the Roman god of war.

The symbol of the Sign of Pisces is the fishes. The ruling planet of Pisces is Neptune.

Personality characteristics:

If your child is born in Pisces he or she is affectionate, sympathetic, loyal, idealistic, kind, and forgiving. The Pisces child is the mystic, the seeker after hidden truths. Pisces is considered a dual sign, one fish battling odds and swimming upstream, and the other fish drifting along with the current.

Pisces children love peace, almost at any price. They cannot stand a discordant, inharmonious atmosphere. Loud noises, discordant voices, and arguments fill them with despair and make them very nervous. This child is sincere and truthful, and because of these qualities is not always able to see the "person behind the mask," so he or she may cultivate many wrong friends.

March children can enjoy a happy married life if they choose wisely. If they are not careful in choosing friends and a marriage partner, their lives can be full of sacrifice and service to those who are not appreciative of them.

The Piscean child often devotes his or her life to the cause of truth and justice. March children should cultivate the spiritual part of their natures. They must learn to search for facts. They should be taught to make decisions and come to conclusions. They should guard against jealousy and possessiveness and not let them interfere with happiness or with friendship with others. They must learn to trust their hunches and premonitions. Their lives should not be ruled by emotions and idealism.

It is important for Pisces children to develop confidence and self-assurance. If they do, they can attain their ultimate happiness. "For he who can master himself can master the world."

Talents and attributes:

This sign claims writers, poets, idealists, religious leaders, doctors, nurses, lawyers, all with the divine motivation of helping humanity as their objective. Pisceans like lovely clothes, beautiful things, poetry, and music. If they could realize the beautiful dreams in their minds and souls, they could bring about an earthly paradise.

The Pisces child will usually find Cancer and Scorpio, and to a lesser degree Capricorn and Taurus people the most compatible.

Among great political leaders born in the Sign of Pisces:
George Washington, 1st U.S. President, February 22.
José de San Martín, South American liberator, February 25.
Andrew Jackson, 7th U.S. President, March 15.
Edward Kennedy, U.S. Senator, February 22.

Grover Cleveland, 22nd U.S. President, March 18.
Other internationally known persons born in the Sign of Pisces are:

Ralph Nader, consumer advocate, February 27.
Albert Einstein, physicist, March 14.
Mary Lyon, educator, February 28.
Edna St. Vincent Millay, poet, February 22.
Caroline Hershel, astronomer, March 16.

Outstanding entertainment personalities:

Elizabeth Taylor, February 27.
Harry Belafonte, March 1.
Liza Minnelli, March 12.
Rex Harrison, March 5.
Sidney Poitier, February 20.
Renata Scotto, February 24.
Neil Sedaka, March 13.
Jerry Lewis, March 16.
Daniel J. Travanti, March 7.
Joanne Woodward, February 27.

Names for Girls

•

A

ABEBI—Nigerian: "We asked for her and she came." Abebe Bikila, Olympic marathon champion.

ABIGAIL—Hebrew: **Abigayil**. "My father is joy." Abigail Adams, wife of U.S. President John Adams, 1744–1818. English nicknames: **Abagael, Abbe, Abby, Abbey, Abbi, Abbie, Gail, Gale.** Foreign variations: **Abaigeal** (Irish).

ABRA—Hebrew: **Abraham.** "Mother of multitudes." Feminine form of **Abraham.** Abra was a favorite of Solomon in the Bible, and the heroine of the 16th-century European romance, *Amadis of Gaul.*

ACACIA—Greek: **Akakiá.** "The guileless"; a flower name. The feathery-blooming acacia symbolized immortality and resurrection. Also: **Casia, Cacia, Cacie, Kacie.**

ACANTHA—Greek: **Akantha.** "Sharp-pointed; thorned." Acanthus leaves were used as a decorative design in Greek architecture, honoring Acantha, legendary mother of Apollo.

ADA—Old English: **Eada.** "Prosperous, happy." St. Ada, 7th-century French abbess. English variations: **Adda, Aida.**

ADAH—Hebrew: **Adah.** "Tiara, crown or ornament. Adah Issacs Menken, famous 19th-century American actress.

ADALIA—Old German: **Adal** "Noble one," from the Greek seaport, Adalia. Also: **Adali, Adalie.**

ADAMINA—Latin: "of the red earth." A feminine form of **Adam.** English nicknames: **Ada, Addie, Mina.**

ADAR—Hebrew: "High eminent," or "fire." Adar is

29

the sixth month of the Jewish year.

ADARA—Greek: "beautiful," Arabic: "virgin."

ADDA—See **Ada**.

ADELA—See **Adelle**, **Adelaide**.

ADELAIDE—Old German: **Adal-heit** "Of noble rank." Old German: Adal-heida, "Noble-cheerful." St. Adelaide, of Burgundy, 10th century, called "Mother of kingdoms."
English nicknames: **Addie**, **Addy**, **Adela**, **Adel**, **Della**.
Foreign variations: **Adelheid** (German), **Adelaida** (Italian, Spanish).

ADELE—See **Adelle**.

ADELINE—See **Adelle**.

ADELLE—Old German: **Adal**. "Noble." Adela Rogers St. Johns, American writer; Adelle Davis, nutritionist. English nicknames: **Addie**, **Addy**, **Del**, **Della**. English variations: **Adela**, **Adaline**, **Adelina**, **Adelind**, **Adeline**, **Aline**, **Edeline**.
Foreign variations: **Adela**, **Adelina** (Spanish), **Adele**, **Adelina** (French), **Adelina** (Italian).

ADELPHA—Greek: **Adelph**. "Sisterly," beloved sister.

ADINA—Hebrew: **Adin**. "Voluptuous, beautiful."
English nickname: **Dina**. English variation: **Adine**, **Adena**.

ADITI—Hindi; "free and unbounded." In Hindi lore, Aditi is mother of the gods.

ADOLPHA—Old German: **Adal-wolf**. "Noble wolf." Feminine of **Adolf**.

ADONIA—Greek: **Adonis**. "Beautiful or godlike." Feminine of **Adonis** and the name of his festival.

ADORA—Latin: **Adoria**. "Gift, glory, renown." Also: **Adorée**.

ADORABELLE—Latin-French: **Adora-belle**. "Beautiful and adored."

ADORLEE—French: "Adored one."

ADRIA—Latin: **Adria**, **Hadria**. "Dark one." Greek: "girl from Adria, from the sea." Adrienne Barbeau, actress.
English variations: **Adriana**, **Adrea**.
Foreign variations: Adrienne (French), **Adriana** (Italian), **Adriane** (German).

ADRIANA—See **Adria**.

ADRIENNE—Popular varation of **Adria**.

AGATHA—Greek: **Agathe**. "Good, kind." St. Agatha, 3rd-century Sicilian martyr, Agatha Christie, noted English novelist. English nicknames: **Ag**, **Aggie**, **Aggy**. Foreign variations: **Agathe** (French, German), **Agata** (Italian), **Agueda** (Spanish), **Agata** (Irish).

AGAVE—Greek: **Agaue.** "Illustrious, noble." Agave was a daughter of Cadmus in Greek legends.

AGNELLA—Variation of **Agnes.**

AGNES—Greek: **Hagne.** "Pure one." St. Agnes, 4th-century Roman virgin martyr, Agnes De Mille, choreographer; Agnes Moorehead, actress.
English nicknames: **Aggie, Annis, Nessa, Nessi, Nessie, Nesta, Neysa, Nessy.**
Foreign variations: **Agnès** (French), **Agnese** (Italian), **Ines, Inez, Ynes, Ynez** (Spanish), **Aigneis** (Irish), **Agneta** (Swedish, Danish).

AIDA—See **Ada.**

AIDAN—Irish Gaelic: "little fire." In ancient Ireland fire symbolized purity and refinement. St. Aidan, 7th-century Irish bishop.
English variation: **Adan.**

AILEEN—Anglo-Irish: "light bearer." An Irish form of **Helen.**
English variations: **Aleen, Alene, Ailey, Aili, Eleen, Elene, Eileen, Ilene, Ileana, Ileane.**

AIMEE—See **Amy.** Aimee Semple MacPherson, American religious leader.

AISHA—Arabic: After Ayeska, favorite wife of the prophet Mohammed. Also, **Asia, Ashia, Asha.**

AISLINN—Irish Gaelic: "vision or dream."
English variation: **Isleen.**

ALAMEDA—North American Indian: "cottonwood grove." Spanish: "promenade."

ALANNA—Irish Gaelic: **Alain.** "Bright, fair, beautiful, harmonious." Hawaiian: "light and airy." A feminine form of **Alan, Allen.** Alanna Ladd, actress.
English variations: **Lana, Lanna, Alaine, Alayne, Allene, Allyn, Alina, Alana.**

ALARICE—Old German: **Alhric.** "Ruler of all." The feminine form of **Alaric.**
English variation: **Alarica.**

ALBERTA—Old English: **Adalbeorht,** "Noble, brilliant." St. Alberta, 3rd-century Christian martyr, Alberta Hunter, singer and songwriter.
English nicknames: **Allie, Berta, Bertie, Berti, Berte.**
English variations: **Albertina, Albertine, Elberta, Elbertine.**

ALBINIA—Latin: "white or blond." Feminine of **Alban** or **Albin.** A color name that has been used for centuries. Also, **Alba.**
English variations; **Albina, Alvina.**
Foreign variations: **Aubine** (French), **Albinia** (Italian).

ALCINA—Greek: **Alkinoe.** "Strong-minded." Feminine of **Alcinous.** A fairy with magical powers.

ALDA—Old German: "old, wise, rich." Feminine of **Otto**. St. Alda of Siena, Italy (1249–1309).

ALDORA—Old English: **Aeldra**. "Of superior rank, noble gift."

ALERIA—Middle Latin: **Alario**. "Eaglelike."

ALESIA—Greek: "helper."

ALETA—Greek: "wanderer."

ALETHEA—Greek: **Aletheia**. "Truthful one." See **Alice**. English variations: **Aleta, Aletta**. Foreign variation: **Aletea** (Spanish, Italian).

ALEXANDRA—Greek: **Alexandros**. "Helper and defender of mankind." Princess Alexandra of Kent (England), cousin of Queen Elizabeth II; Alexandra, wife of England's King Edward VII; Alexandra Danilova, ballerina. English nicknames: **Alex, Alexa, Alexine, Alexis, Alla, Lexie, Lexi, Lexine, Sandi, Sandie, Sandy, Sandra, Zandra**. Foreign variations: **Alexandrine** (French), **Alessandra** (Italian), **Alejandra** (Spanish).

ALEXIS—See **Alexandra**. Alexis Smith, actress. Popular form of **Alexandra**.

ALFONSINE—Old German: **Adal-funs**. "Noble and ready." Feminine of **Alfonso**. English variations: **Alphonsine, Alonza**.

ALFREDA—Old English: **Aelf-raed**. "Elf-counselor, good counselor." With wisdom and diplomacy this woman counselled others. English nicknames: **Alfi, Alfie, Freda**. English variations: **Elfreda, Elfrieda, Elfrida, Elva**.

ALICE—Greek: **Alethia**. "Truthful one." Alice is also a version of **Adelaide**. Princess Alice of England; Alice Marble, tennis champion; Alicia Markova, ballerina; Alice Walker, writer. English nicknames: **Allie, Ellie, Elsie, Elsa**. English variations: **Alicea, Alicia, Alissa, Alithia, Allys, Alyce, Alys**. Foreign variations: **Alicia** (Italian, Spanish, Swedish), **Ailis** (Irish).

ALIDA—Late Latin: **Ala-ida**. "Little winged one"; or Spanish: "noble." Alida was also a city in ancient Asia Minor. Alida Valli, Italian actress. English nicknames: **Dela, Lela, Leeta**. English variations: **Aleda, Aleta, Elida, Elita, Alita, Leda, Lita, Adela, Oleda, Oleta**. Foreign variations: **Aletta** (Italian), **Aleta, Adelita, Adelina** (Spanish), **Alette** (French).

ALIMA—Arabic: "learned in dancing and music."

ALINA, ALINE—Celtic:

"fair, harmonious"; or Russian, Polish: "bright." Aline MacMahon, actress.
English variations: **Alena, Alene, Alina.**

ALISA—Modern Hebrew name: "a joy." Also: **Alyssa, Alissa.**

ALISON—Irish Gaelic: **Allsun.** "Little truthful one." A Gaelic form of **Alice** and **Louise.** Ali McGraw, Ally Sheedy, actresses.
English nicknames: **Alie, Allie, Ali, Ally, Lissie, Lissy.**
English variations: **Allison, Allyson, Alyson.**
Foreign variation: **Allsun** (Irish Gaelic).

ALIZA—Hebrew: "joyous."

ALLA—See **Alexandra.** Alla Nazimova, famous actress (1879–1945).

ALLEGRA—Italian: "cheerful, gay." Allegra Kent, ballerina.

ALLENE—See **Alanna.**

ALLIE—See **Alison, Alice, Alberta.** Also: **Aly, Ally.**

ALLISON—See **Alison.**

ALMA—Spanish, Italian: "soul or spirit"; or Latin: "nourishing, supportive, spiritually helpful." Alma Gluck, famous opera singer (1884–1938).

ALMIRA—Arabic: "fulfillment of the word," or "truth without question."

English variation: **Elmira.**

ALOHA—Hawaiian: "love, kindness, greetings, or farewell." Aloha is the greeting and farewell from that fair state, Hawaii.

ALONZA—See **Alfonsine.**

ALOYSIA—See **Louise.**

ALPHA—Greek: "first one." Alpha is the first letter of the Greek alphabet.
English variation: **Alfa.**

ALTA—Latin: **Altus.** "High or lofty."

ALTHEA—Greek: **Althaia.** "Wholesome, healer." Althea Gibson, tennis champion.
English nickname: **Thea.**
English variations: **Elthea, Altheda, Altha, Eltha.**

ALULA—Late Latin: **Alula.** "Winged one"; or Arabic: **Al-ula.** "The first." Alula is a star in Ursa Major.

ALURA—Old English. **Alhraed.** "Divine counselor." Feminine of Old English **Alurea.** Also: **Allura.**

ALVA—Latin: **Alba.** "Blond one." Alva Belmont, American philanthropist. See **Albinia.**

ALVINA—Old English: **Aethel-wine.** "Noble friend." Alternate origin, Old English: **Aelf-wine.** "Elf-friend." Feminine of Alvin. Also: **Elvina, Elvena, Elvine.**

ALYCE—see **Alice.** Also: **Alys.**

ALYSSA—Greek: "sane one, rational." Named for the fragrant sweet alyssum flower.

ALZENA—Arabic-Persian: **Alzan.** "The woman." Also: **Alzina, Alzena.**

AMABEL—Latin: **Amabilis.** "Loveable one, amiable." English nicknames: **Ama, Belle, Mab.** English variation: **Amabelle.**

AMADEA—Middle Latin: **Amadeus.** "Loved of God." Feminine of **Amadeus.** English variation: **Amadee.**

AMANDA—Latin: "worthy of love, lovable, loved, and esteemed." Amanda Sewell, American painter (1859–1926). English nicknames: **Manda, Mandy.** English variation: **Mandaline.** Foreign variations: **Amandine** (French), **Amata** (Spanish).

AMARIS—Hebrew: **Amaryah.** "God has promised." Feminine of Hebrew **Amariah.**

AMARYLLIS—Greek: "a sparkling stream"; used to personify an ideal country girl, and thus "shepherdess" and "sweetheart."

AMBER—Old French: **Ambre.** "The amber jewel." Arabic: "jewel." Gaelic: "fierce." Usage famed from the novel and motion picture *Forever Amber* by Kathleen Winsor.

AMBROSINE—Greek: Am-

brotos. "Divine, immortal one." Feminine of **Ambrose.**

AMELIA—Gothic: **Amala.** "Industrious one." Also traced to Latin: **Aemilia.** "Flattering, winning one." See **Emily.** Amelia Earhart, famous aviatrix (1898–1937); Amelia Bloomer, 19th century feminist. English nicknames: **Amy, Em, Emmie, Emmy.** English variations: **Amalea, Amalia, Amilia, Emilia, Ameline, Emelina, Emeline, Amelita, Emelita, Emmeline, Emelie, Amalie.** Foreign variations: **Amélie** (French), **Amalia** (German, Spanish, Dutch) **Amelia** (Italian, Portuguese).

AMELINDA—Latin-Spanish: **Ami-linda.** "Beloved and pretty."

AMETHYST—Greek: **Amethystos.** "Wine-color, a jewel." The amethyst was accredited with the power of the preventing intoxication in ancient Greece. A name sometimes given to girls born in February.

AMI—See **Amy.**

AMINTA—Latin: **Amyntas.** "Protector." Amynta was a shepherdess in Greek myths. Also: **Amynta.** English nicknames: **Minta, Minty.**

AMITY—Old French: **Amiste.** "Friendship."

AMY—French: **Aimée,** Latin: **Amare.** "Beloved, a friend." Amy Lowell, American poet, Pulitzer Prize winner (1874–1925); St. Amata, niece of St. Clare of Assissi, died 1250; Amy Grant, singer.
English nickname: **Ame.**
English variations: **Aimee, Amie.**
Foreign variations: **Aimée** (French, **Amata** (Italian, Swedish, Spanish).

ANASTASIA—Greek: **Anastasios.** "Of the Resurrection." Famous from the Russian Grand Duchess Anastasia, believed by some to have escaped death in 1918 when the Czar's family were assassinated.
English nicknames: **Stacie, Stacia, Stacey, Stacy, Tasia.**
English variation: **Anstice.**
Foreign variation: **Anastasie** (French).

ANATOLA—Greek: **Anatolios.** "From the East; from Anatolia."

ANDREA—Latin: "womanly." Greek: "A man's woman; fearless." Feminine form of **Andreas** or **Andrew.**
English variations: **Andria, Andreana, Andriana, Andri.**
Foreign variations: **Aindrea.** (Irish), **Andrée** (French).

ANDRIA—Latin: "maiden of Andros, a Greek island."
See **Andrea.**

ANEMONE—Greek: "windflower." a breath, legendary Greek nymph pursued by the wind was changed into the beautiful anemone flower.

ANGELA—Greek: "angel or messenger." St. Angela of Foligno, Italy (1248–1309), great religious mystic; Angela Lansbury, Angie Dickinson, actresses.
English nicknames: **Angie, Angy.**
English variations: **Angelina, Angeline, Angel, Angelita.**
Foreign variations: **Aingeal** (Irish), **Angèle** (French).

ANGELICA—Latin: **Angelicus.** "Angelic one." Also: **Anjelica.** Angelica Catalini, 19th-century Italian singer; Anjelica Huston, actress.
Foreign variations: **Angelika** (German), **Angélique** (French).

ANGELINE—See **Angela.**

ANITA—See **ANN.** Anita Loos, novelist.

ANN, ANNE—Hebrew. **Hannah.** "Graceful one." Mother of the prophet Samuel. St. Anne was the mother of the Virgin Mary. Anne Boleyn and Anne of Cleves, wives of England's King Henry VIII, Queen Anne of England, 1664–1714; Anna Pavlova, ballet dancer; Annie Oakley, western heroine; Anne Bancroft, actress.
English nicknames: **Annie, Anny, Nan, Nancy, Nita.**
English variations: **Anne, Anna, Ana, Anette, Anita,**

Nina, Ninon, Hannah,
Annora, Annah, Annice,
Nanna, Annina.
Foreign variations: **Ana,
Anita, Nita** (Spanish),
Annette, Nanette (French),
Anna (German, Italian,
Dutch, Swedish, Danish).

ANNABELLE—Hebrew-Latin:
Hannah-bella. "Graceful-beau-
tiful."
English nicknames: **Annie,
Belle.**
English variation: **Annabella.**
Foreign variation: **Annabla**
(Irish).

ANNETTE—See **Ann.**

ANNIS—Greek: "whole, complete." Also: **Annys.**

ANNUNCIATA—Latin:
Annuntiatio. "Bearer of
news." A name honoring
the Annunciation. Used for a
daughter born in March,
the month of the Annunciation.
Foreign variations: **Annunziata**
(Italian), **Anunciación**
(Spanish.

ANONNA—Latin: "yearly
crops." Annona was the
Roman goddess of crops.

ANORA—English: **Ann-nora.**
Combination of **Anne** and
Nora.

ANSELMA—Old Norse:
Anshelm. "Divinely pro-
tected." A feminine form of
Anselm.
English nicknames: **Selma,
Zelma.**

ANTHEA—Greek: **Antheia.**

"Flower." Antheia was a name
for Aphrodite as the Greek
goddess of flowers.

ANTOINETTE—See **Antonia.**

ANTONIA—Latin: "inesti-
mable; priceless." The price-
less jewel of kindness is
encased within our hearts. A
feminine form of **Anthony.**
Famous from Queen Marie
Antoinette of France, Willa
Cather's novel *My Antonia,*
Antonia Fraser, British
author.
English nicknames: **Tonie,
Toni, Tony, Tonia, Netta,
Nettie, Netty, Toinette.**
Foreign variations: **Antoinette**
(French), **Antonietta** (Italian),
Antonie (German), **Antonetta**
(Swedish, Slavic).

APOLLINE—Greek: **Apollon.**
"Sun or sunlight." St.
Apolline of Alexandria,
martyred. A.D. 249.

APRIL—Latin: **Aprilis.**
"Opening; born in April."
April was the beginning of
spring in the old Roman and
Greek calendars. Also:
Aprille, Averil, Averyl, Avril.

ARA—Greek: "an altar."
Ara was the Greek goddess of
vengeance and destruction.

ARABELLA—Latin: "beau-
tiful altar"; or Old German:
"eagle heroine."
English nicknames: **Bella, Belle.**
Foreign variations: **Arabella**
(Italian, Dutch), **Arabelle**
(French, German), **Arabela**
(Spanish).

ARDATH—Hebrew: **Aridatha.** "A flowering field."

ARDEEN—Latin: "ardent."

ARDELLE—Latin: **Ardere.** "Warm, enthusiastic." English variations: **Arda, Ardelia, Ardis, Ardine, Ardene, Ardeen, Ardella.**

ARETHA—Greek: "excellence, virtue, valor." Aretha Franklin, singer. English variations: **Aretta, Areta.** Foreign variation: **Arette** (French).

ARGENTA—Latin: **Argentum.** "Silvery one."

ARIA—Italian: "a melody." English variations: **Arietta, Ariette.**

ARIANA—Latin: **Ariadna.** "Very holy or very pleasing one." Ariadne, daughter of a king of ancient Crete, extricated the hero Theseus from the labyrinth.

ARIELLA—Hebrew: **Ariel.** "Lioness of God." Feminine of **Ariel.** Since Shakespeare, this name has come to symbolize the airy or ethereal.

ARLEEN—See **Arlene.**

ARLENE—Irish Gaelic: **Airleas.** "A pledge." Feminine of **Arlen.** Arlene Francis and Arlene Dahl, actresses. English nicknames: **Arlie, Lene, Lena.** English variations: **Arleen,** Arlena, Arleta, Arlette, Arline, Arlyne.

ARMIDA—Latin: "little armed one." A name used by Tasso for a famous beauty in his 16th-century work, *Jerusalem Delivered.*

ARMILLA—Latin: "bracelet-wearing battle-maid." Also Icelandic, Teutonic.

ARMINA—Old German: **Harimann.** "Warrior-maid." English variations: **Armine, Arminie, Erminie.**

ARNALDA—Old German: **Arn-wald.** "Eagle-ruler" or "eagle-strong." Feminine form of **Arnold.**

ARNINA—Hebrew, of uncertain meaning, probably "inspired singer." Also **Arona,** both feminine forms of **Aaron.**

ARVA—Latin: **Arvus.** "Pastureland or seashore."

ASELMA—Gaelic: "the fair."

ASHLEY—Anglo-Saxon: "from the ash-tree meadow or lea." Popular modern U.S. name.

ASTA—Greek: **Aster.** "Star, starlike." English variation: **Astra.**

ASTRID—Old Norse. **Astryd.** "Divine strength, strong in love." The name of many Scandinavian queens and princesses. Also: **Astryr, Astrud.**

ATALANTA—Greek: **Atalante.**
"mighty bearer." Feminine of
Atlas, the hero who carried
the world on his shoulders.
Atalanta was a huntress in
Greek myths.
English variation: **Atlanta.**

ATALAYA—Spanish: "guardian."

ATARA—Hebrew: "a crown."
Also: **Atera, Ateret.**

ATHALIA—Hebrew: **Athale-
yah.** "God is exalted."
English variation: **Atalia.**

ATHENA—Greek: **Athene.**
"Wisdom." Athena, Greek
goddess, one of who taught
that knowledge and experience result in wisdom.
English nicknames: **Athie,
Attie.**

ATLANTA—See **Atalanta.**

AUDREY—Old English:
Aethelthryth. "Noble strength."
St. Audrey, died A.D. 679,
famous English abbess;
Audrey Hepburn, actress.
English variations: **Audrie,
Audry.**

AUGUSTA—Latin: "majes-
tic one." Kaiserin Augusta,
wife of Willhelm II, the
German Emperor during
World War I.
Foreign variations: **Auguste**
(German, French, Dutch,
Danish).

AURA—Latin: "gentle
breeze."
English variations: **Aurea,
Auria.**

AURELIA—Latin: "golden."
Roman goddess of the
dawn. Gold was the symbol of
refinement and purity. St.
Aurelia, 11th-century French
princess; Aurelia Reinhart,
noted American educator.
English variations: **Oralia,
Orelia.**
Foreign variation: **Aurélie**
(French).

AURORA—Latin: "daybreak."
Foreign variation: **Aurore**
(French).

AUSTINE—Latin: **Augustinus.**
"Majestic little one."
Feminine form of **Augustine**
and **Austin.**

AVA—Latin: **Avis.** "Birdlike."
Ava Gardner, actress.

AVELINE—see **Evelyn.**

AVENA—Latin: "oats or
oatfield."

AVERA—Hebrew: **Aberah.**
"Transgressor."

AVERIL—Old English:
"born in the month of April;
or Old English: **Efer-hild.**
"Boar warrior-maid."
English variations: **Averyl,
Avril.**

AVICE—Old French:
"warlike."

AVIS—See **Ava.**

AVIVA—Hebrew: "springtime youthfully fresh." Also:
Avivah, Viva, Auvit.

AYN—See **Ann.** Ayn Rand,
novelist.

AZALEA—Latin: "dry earth." A flower name, for the azalea which thrives even in dry earth.

AZELIA—Hebrew: **Aziel.** "Helped by God."

AZURA—Old French from Persian: **Azur.** "Blue sky."

B

BAB—Arabic: **Bab.** "From the gateway." see **Barbara.**

BABE—See **Barbara.**

BABETTE—Hawaiian: **Barbara.** Greek: "little Barbara, stranger, foreigner." Sometimes a diminutive of **Elizabeth,** "God has promised."

BALBINA—Latin-Italian: **Balbina.** "Little stammerer."

BAMBI—Italian: **Bambino.** "Child."

BAPTISTA—Latin: "baptizer." Foreign variations: **Batista** (Italian), **Baptiste** (French), **Bautista** (Spanish).

BARBARA—Latin: "stranger, foreigner." Beautiful, but a stranger to the land. St. Barbara, early Christian martyr; Barbara Hutton, American heiress; Barbara Stanwyck, actress; Barbra Streisand, singer.
English nicknames: **Bab, Babb, Babs, Barbie, Barby,**
English variations: **Babette, Barbette, Babita, Barbra.**
Foreign variations: **Barbe** (French), **Bárbara** (Spanish), **Varvara, Varina** (Slavic).

BASILIA—Greek: **Basileus.**

"Queenly, regal." A feminine form of **Basil.**

BATHILDA—Old German: **Badu-hildi.** "Commanding battle-maiden."
Foreign variation: **Bathilde** (French).

BATHSHEBA—Hebrew: "daughter of the oath; seventh daughter." Bathsheba was the wife of the Biblical King David.

BATISTA—See **Baptista.**

BEATA—Latin: **Beata.** "Blessed, happy one."

BEATRICE—Latin: **Beatrix.** "She who makes others happy." Beatrice was the famous heroine of Dante's 13th-century *Divine Comedy.* Beatrice Lillie, entertainer. English nicknames: **Bea, Bee, Trixie, Trixy.**
Foreign variations: **Béatrice** (French), **Beatrix** (German, Spanish), **Beitris** (Scottish).

BEDA—Old English: **Beadu.** "Warrior maiden."

BELA—Czech: "white." Also **Bel, Belia, Bell.**

BELINDA—Old Spanish: **Bellalinda.** "Beautiful, pretty."

Belinda Montgomery, actress.
English nicknames: **Belle, Binnie, Linda.**

BELLANCA—Italian: "blond one."
Foreign variation: **Blanca** (Spanish).

BELLE—French: "beautiful one." see also **Belinda, Isabelle.**
English variations: **Bell, Bella, Belva, Belvia.**

BELVA—See **Belle.** Belva Plain, novelist.

BENEDICTA—Latin: "blessed one." Feminine of **Benedict.**
English nicknames: **Bennie, Benita, Binnie, Dixie.**
Foreign variations: **Benoite** (French), **Benedikta** (German), **Benedetta** (Italian), **Benita** (Spanish).

BENIGNA—Latin: "kind, gentle, gracious."

BENITA—See **Benedicta.** Spanish: "little Benedicta," blessed one. Benita Hume, English actress.

BERDINE—Old German-French: "glorious one."

BERENGARIA—Old English: **Beran-gari.** "Bear-spear maid." Berengaria was the queen of England's famous King Richard the Lion-Hearted, 1157–1199.

BERNADETTE—French: "brave as a bear." Feminine of **Bernard.** St. Bernadette of Lourdes, 1844–1879.

Bernadette Peters, actress.
English Nicknames: **Bernie, Berny.**
English variations: **Bernadine, Bernadene, Bernita.**
Foreign variation: **Bernardina** (Italian, Spanish).

BERNIA—Old Anglo-Latin: **Beornia.** "Battle maid."

BERNICE—Greek: **Berenike.** "Harbinger of victory."
English nicknames: **Bernie, Berny, Bunny, Nixie.**
English variations: **Berenice, Veronica.**
Foreign variations: **Berenice, Veronique** (French), **Veronike** (German).

BERTHA—Old German: **Perahta.** "Shining, glorious one." Bertha was the old German fertility goddess.
English nicknames: **Berta, Bertie, Berty.**
Foreign variations: **Berthe** (French), **Berta, Berthe** (German), **Berta** (Italian, Spanish).

BERTILDE—Old English: **Beorht-hilde** "Shining battle maid."

BERTRADE—Old English: **Beortht-raed.** "Shining counselor."

BERYL—Greek: **Beryllos.** "The sea-green jewel." The beryl was an emblem of good fortune.

BETHANY—Aramaic: "house of poverty." Place name, near Jerusalem.

BETHEL—Hebrew: "house of God."
English variation: **Beth.**

BETHIA—English, from Hebrew: "house of God."
English nickname: **Beth.**

BETSY—See **Elizabeth.**

BETTE—A variant on **Betty.** Bette Davis, actress; Bette Midler, singer.

BETTY—See **Elizabeth.**

BEULAH—Hebrew: "the married one." Beulah Bondi, noted American actress.
English variation: **Beula.**

BEVERLY—Old English: **Beo-for-leah.** "Dweller at the beaver-meadow." Beverly Garland, American actress; Beverly Sills, singer.

BEVIN—Irish Gaelic: **Bebhinn.** "Melodious lady." Bebhinn or Bevin was the daughter of Brian Boru, most famous of all Irish kings, 11th century.

BIANCA—Italian: "white." Bianca Jagger, actress.

BIBI—Arabic: "lady." Bibi Anderson, Swedish actress. Also: **Bebe.**

BILLIE—Old English: **Willa.** "Resolution; willpower." See also **Wilhelmina.** Billie Burke, American actress; Billie Jean King, tennis player.
English variation: **Billy.**

BINGA—Old German: **Binge.** "From the kettle-shaped hollow."

BIRDIE—English: "little birdlike one."

BIRGIT—See **Bridget.**

BLAIR—Teutonic, Celtic: "From the plains."

BLANCA—See **Bellanca, Blanche.**

BLANCHE—Old French: **Blanch.** "White, fair one." Blanche of Castile, Queen of France, 1187–1252; Blanche Thebom, noted opera singer.
Foreign variations: **Bianca** (Italian), **Blanka** (German), **Blanca** (Spanish), **Blinnie, Bluinse** (Irish).

BLASIA—Latin: **Blasius.** "Stammerer." Alternate origin, Old German: **Blas.** "Firebrand." **Blasia** is the feminine form of **Blasius** or **Blaze.**

BLESSING—Old English: **Bletsung.** "Consecrated one."

BLISS—Old English: **Bliths.** "Gladness, joy."

BLITHE—See **Blythe.**

BLOSSOM—Old English: **Blostm.** "Fresh, lovely." Blossom Seeley, American vaudeville actress, singer.

BLYTHE—Old English: **Blithe.** "Joyful, cheerful one."
English variation: **Blithe.**

BO—Chinese: "precious." Also a nickname for **Bonita.** Bo Derek, actress.

BONITA—Spanish: "pretty, also good." Bonita Granville, American actress.
English nicknames: **Bo, Bonie, Nita.**

BONNIE—Middle English: **Bonie.** "Good one." See also **Bonita.**
English variations: **Bonny, Bunni, Bunnie, Bunny.**

BRANDY—Dutch, after the sweet, strong liquor. Also: **Brandi, Brandie.** Popular modern U.S. name.

BRENDA—Irish Gaelic: **Breandan.** "Little raven"; or Old English: **Brand.** "Firebrand." American actress Brenda Vaccaro.

BRENNA—Irish Gaelic: **Brann.** "Raven, with raven tresses."
Feminine form of **Brennan.**

BRIANNA—Irish Gaelic: "strong one." A feminine form of **Brian.** Also: **Briana, Breanne, Brianne, Brina, Bryana, Bryanna, Bryna.**
English nicknames: **Briny, Briney, Bri.**

BRIDGET—Irish. Gaelic: **Brighid.** "Protective, strong. St. Brigid of Kildare, patroness of Ireland; St. Brigitta of Sweden; actress Brigitte Bardot.
English nicknames: **Biddie Biddy, Bridie, Brita, Brydie.**
Foreign variations: **Brigitte, Birgitta, Bergette**

(French, German), **Brigida** (Italian, Spanish). Also: **Birget** (Norwegian); **Brigid, Berget, Brietta.**

BRITA—See **Bridget.**

BRITTANY—Latin: "from England." Also: **Britta, Brit, Brett, Brittni.**

BRONWEN—Old Welsh: **Brangwen.** "White bosomed." In ancient Welsh lore Bronwen was the daughter of Llyr, the sea god, and sister of Bran, King of Ireland.

BROOKE—Old English: "from the brook." Also from a surname; a feminine form of **Brook.** Actresses Brooke Shields, Brooke Adams.

BRUCIE—Old French: **Bruis.** "From the thicket, a forest sprite," Feminine of **Bruce.**

BRUNELLA—Old French: "brown-haired one."

BRUNETTA—Italian: "brunette."

BRUNHILDA—Old German: **Bruni-hilde.** "Armored warrior maiden." Brunhilda was a queen in the old Germanic Siegfried legend.

BUENA—Spanish: "the good one."

BUFFY—See **Elizabeth.**

BUNNY—See **Bernice, Bonnie.**

C

CADENCE—Late Latin: "rhythmic."
English variation: **Cadena.**
Foreign variations: **Cadenza** (Italian), **Cadence** (French).

CADY—Modern U.S., from a last name, after Elizabeth Cady Stanton, 19th-century feminist.

CAITLIN—An Irish form of **Catherine.** Also: **Catlin, Caitlan, Catlee.**

CALANDRA—Greek: **Kalandros.** "Lark."
English nicknames: **Cal, Callie, Cally.**
Foreign variations: **Calandre** (French), **Calandria** (Spanish).

CALANTHA—Greek: **Kalanthe.**
"Beautiful blossom."
English nicknames: **Cal, Callie, Cally, Calli.**
Foreign variation: **Calanthe** (French).

CALEDONIA—Latin: "from Scotland." Caledonia is an ancient name for Scotland.

CALIDA—Spanish: "warm, ardent."

CALISTA—Greek: **Kallisto.** "Most beautiful one."

CALLA—Greek: **Kalos.** "Beautiful."

CALLULA—Latin: "little beautiful one."

CALYPSO—Greek: **Kalypso.** "Concealer." Calypso was a sea nymph who kept Odysseus captive seven years in the Homeric Odyssey.

CAMEO—Italian: **Cammeo.** "A sculptured jewel."

CAMILLE—Latin: **Camilla.** "Young ceremonial attendant." Camilla was a Volscian queen in Virgil's Aeneid; Camille was the heroine of a novel by Dumas.
English nicknames: **Cam, Cammie, Cammy, Millie, Milly.**
Foreign variations: **Camille** (French), **Camilla** (Italian), **Camila** (Spanish).

CANACE—Greek: **Kanake.** "Daughter of the wind." In Greek myths Canace was the daughter of Aeolus, god of the winds.

CANDACE—Greek: **Kandake.** "Glittering, glowing white."
English nicknames: **Candee, Candie, Candy, Dace, Dacey.**
English variation: **Candice.**
Candice Bergen, actress.

CANDIDA—Latin: **Candide.** "Bright-white." See **Candace.** St. Candida of Naples, died A.D. 78, was said to have welcomed St. Peter to Italy; Candida is the heroine of the play by that name by Bernard Shaw.
Foreign variation: **Candide** (French).

CAPRICE—Italian: **Capriccio.** "Fanciful."

CARA—Italian: "dear, beloved one"; or Irish Gaelic: **Caraid.** "Friend"; or Vietnamese: "precious jewel." English variations: **Carina, Carine, Kara.**

CARESSE—French: "endearing one."

CARI—Turkish: "flowing like water." Also: **Carrie, Kairee.** Nickname for **Carol, Caroline.**

CARISSA—Latin: "dear or artful one."

CARITA—Latin: "beloved, dear one."

CARLA—See **Caroline, Charlotte.**

CARLINE—See **Caroline, Charlotte.** Also: **Carleen.**

CARLING—Gaelic. "Little champion." Carling Bassett, tennis player.

CARLITA—see **Caroline, Charlotte.**

CARLOTTA—Italian form of **Caroline, Carla.** See **Charlotte.**

CARLY—Teutonic: "little womanly one." Pet name for **Caroline;** a feminine form of **Charles.** Also: **Carla, Karla, Carlita.** Carly Simon, singer.

CARMA—Sanskrit: **Karma.** "Fate or destiny."

CARMEL—Hebrew: **Kar-** mel. "Garden," or "God's vineyard." Mount Carmel in Palestine is famed in the Bible. English nicknames: **Carma, Carmie, Carmy, Lita.** Foreign variations: **Carmela** (Italian, Spanish), **Carmelita** (Spanish), **Carmelina, Melina** (Italian).

CARMEN—Latin: **Carmea.** "A song." Carmen is the heroine of Bizet's opera by that name. From Santa Maria del Carmen in honor of St. Mary. Additional French and Spanish meaning: "crimson." English nicknames: **Carma, Carmia.** English variations: **Carmina, Carmine, Carmita, Charmaine.** Foreign variation: **Carmencita** (Spanish).

CARNATION—French: "flesh color."

CAROL—Latin: **Carola.** "Strong and womanly." The feminine of **Charles** and **Carl.** Alternate origin, Old French: **Carole.** "A song of joy." See **Caroline.** Carol Heiss, American skater, actresses Carol Burnett and Carol Channing. English nicknames: **Carrie, Caro.** English variations: **Carel, Caryl.**

CAROLINE—Latin-French: "little, womenly one." Queen Caroline, wife of England's King George II;

Carrie Nation, American reformer; Princess Caroline of Monaco.
English nicknames: **Carrie, Caro, Carol, Lina, Line.**
English variations: **Carline, Charleen, Charlene, Charline, Sharleen, Sharlene, Sharline.**
Foreign variations: **Carolina** (Italian, Spanish), **Karoline, Karla** (German), **Karolina** (Polish).

CASEY—Irish Gaelic: **Cathasach.** "Valorous, brave, watchful." Traditionally male, but now popular U.S. female usage. Also: **Kasey, Kacie, Kaci, Caci.**

CASSANDRA—Greek: **Kassandra.** "Helper of men," or "disbelieved by men." Cassandra in Greek legend was a Trojan princess whose prophetic warnings went unheeded; also a character in Shakespeare's play, *Troilus and Crossida.*
English nicknames: **Cassie, Sandy.**
Foreign variations. **Cassandre** (French), **Cassandra** (Spanish).

CASSIDY—Irish: **Casidhe.** "Ingenious, clever one, curly-haired one." Commonly a masculine name; popular in modern U.S. for girls.
Nickname: **Cassie.**

CATHERINE—Greek: **Katharos.** "Pure one." St. Catherine of Alexandria, 4th century, escaped martyrdom on a spiked wheel known later as a "Catherine wheel." Other famous Catherines: Catherine the Great, Empress of Russia, died 1796; Catherine of Aragon, first wife of England's King Henry VIII; St. Catherine of Siena, 14th century; Katharine Cornell, Katharine Hepburn, Catherine Deneuve, actresses.
English nicknames: **Cat, Cathie, Cathy, Kate, Kathy, Kati, Katie, Katy, Kit, Kitty, Kay, Kaye.**
English variations: **Catharine, Katharine, Katherine, Cathleen, Kathleen, Kathlene, Kathline.**
Foreign variations: **Katerine, Katrina, Katti, Ketti** (German), **Catalina** (Spanish), **Catarina, Caterina** (Italian), **Katinka, Kassia** (Slavic), **Caitlin, Caitria** (Irish), **Catriona** (Scottish), **Ekaterina** (Russian).

CATHLEEN—See Catherine.

CEARA—Irish Gaelic: "Spear."

CECILIA—Latin: **Caecilia.** "dim-sighted one," originally, but since St. Cecelia is the patron saint of music, also, "musical one." Cecilia Holland, author; Cicely Tyson, actress, Cecile Dionne of the famous quintuplets. Also: **Cicely, Cicily, Cecyl, Cecyle, Cecely.**
English nicknames: **Cele, Celia, Celie, Ciel, Cissie, Sissie.**

Foreign variations: **Cacilia, Cacilie** (German), **Cecile, Celie** (French), **Celia** (Swedish), **Cecilia** (Spanish, Italian), **Sisile, Sile** (Irish), **Sileas** (Scottish).

CELANDINE—Greek: **Cheladon.** "The swallow."

CELENE—See **Selene.**

CELESTE—Latin: **Caelestis.** "Heavenly." Celeste Holm, actress.
English nicknames: **Cele, Celia.**
English variations: **Celesta, Celestina, Celestine.**

CELESTINE—See **Celeste.**

CELIA—See **Cecilia, Celeste.**

CELOSIA—Greek: **Keleos.** "Flaming, burning."

CERELIA—Latin: **Cerelia.** "Of the spring."

CERYL—See **Cheryl.**

CHANDRA—Sanskrit: **Candra.** "Moon; moonlike." Chandra Cheeseborough, Olympic runner.

CHARISSA—Greek: **Charis.** "Loving." see **Charity.**

CHARITY—Latin: **Caritas.** "Benevolent, charitable." Introduced as a given name to America by the Pilgrim Fathers.
English nicknames: **Charissa, Charita, Charry, Cherry.**

CHARLA—See **Carla.**

CHARLEEN—See **Caroline, Charlotte.**

CHARLENE—see **Caroline, Charlotte.**

CHARLOTTE—French: **Charlotte.** "Little womanly one." A feminine form of **Charles.** Charlotte, queen of England's George III; Charlotte Corday, heroine of French Revolution; Charlotte Brontë, English author; Carlotta, 19th-century Mexican empress; Lola Montez, actress. English nicknames: **Carla, Charyl, Cheryl, Sheryl, Sheree, Sherrill, Sherry, Karla, Lotta, Lottie, Lotty, Lola, Loleta, Lolita.**
English variations: **Carlotta, Carlene, Carline, Charleen, Charlene, Charline, Karline, Sharleen, Sharlene.**
Foreign variations: **Carlota** (Spanish), **Carlotta** (Italian), **Charlotta** (Swedish), **Karlotte** (German).

CHARMAINE—Latin: **Carmen.** "Singer" or Greek: "joy, delight."
See **Carmen.** Made popular by the song of the 1920s, written by Rapee and Pollack, and as heroine of the play and film, *What Price Glory.*
English variations: **Charmain, Charmian, Charmion.**

CHARYL—see **Charlotte.**

CHELSEA—Old English: "a port of ships." Also: **Chelsey.**

CHERIE—French: "dear, cherished, beloved one." Cher, popular singer.

English variations: **Cher,
Cheri, Chery, Cheree,
Cherry.**

CHERRY—Old North
French: **Cherise.** "Cherry-
like." See **Charity.**

CHERYL—Popular U.S.
variant of **Carol** or **Charlotte;**
sometimes from **Cherie.**
Also: **Sherrell, Charyl.**

CHIQUITA—Spanish: "little one."

CHLOE—Greek: "young
verdant." grass; The shepherdess heroine of Longus'
romance *Daphnis and Chloe.*
Chloe was the Greek deity
of green grain. Also: **Cloe.**

CHRISTABELLE—Latin-
French: **Christe-belle.** "Beau-
tiful Christian."
English variation: **Cristabel.**

CHRISTINE—French: "Chris-
tian." Christina, 17th-century
Swedish queen; Christina
Rossetti, 19th-century English
poet; Chris Evert Lloyd,
tennis player; Christie Brink-
ley, model and author; Tina
Turner, singer.
English nicknames: **Chris,
Chrissie, Chrissy, Christie,
Christy, Tina, Tine, Tiny.**
English variations: **Christina,
Christiana, Christiane, Cris-
tina.**
Foreign variations: **Cristina**
(Italian, Spanish), **Kirsten,
Kirstin, Kristin** (Scandina-
vian), **Christiane, Kristel**
(German), **Cristiona, Cristin**
(Irish), **Cairistiona** (Scottish).

CHRYSEIS—Latin: "daughter of the golden one." In the
Greek *Iliad* she was a
beautiful maiden captured by
the Greeks and given to the
hero Agamemnon.

CICELY—See **Cecilia.**

CINDERELLA—French:
Cendrillon. "Little one of the
ashes." From the fairy tale of
the poor girl miraculously found
by and married to a prince.
English nicknames: **Cindie,
Cindy, Ella.**

CINDY—See **Lucinda,
Cynthia, Cinderella.**

CLAIRE—See **Clara.**

CLARA—Latin: "brilliant,
bright, illustrious." St. Clara
of Assisi, born A.D. 1193,
follower and aide of St.
Francis, known in Italy as
Santa Chiara; Clara Barton,
founder of the Red Cross,
died 1912; Klara Schulmann,
19th-century German com-
poser; Clare Booth Luce,
American writer, diplomat;
Claire Bloom, actress.
English nicknames: **Clarey,
Clari, Clarie, Clary.**
English variations: **Claire,
Clare, Clarette, Clarinda,
Clarine, Clarita.**
Foreign variations: **Claire**
(French), **Chiara** (Italian),
Klara (German), **Clara,
Clareta, Clarita** (Spanish),
Sorcha (Scottish).

CLARABELLE—French:
Clarabelle. "Brilliant, beautiful."

CLARAMAE—English: **Claramay.** Modern compound of Clara and May. Claramae Turner, opera singer.

CLARESTA—English: "most brilliant one."

CLARETTE—See **Clara.**

CLARICE—French: **Clarice.** "Little brilliant one." English variations: **Clarissa, Clarisse, Clarrisse, Clerissa.**

CLARIMOND—Latin-German: "brilliant protector."

CLARINDA—Spanish: "brilliant, beautiful."

CLARISSA—Latin: **Clarissima.** "Most brilliant one." See **Clarice.**

CLAUDETTE—see **Claudia.**

CLAUDIA—Latin: "the lame one." Feminine form of **Claude** or **Claudius,** a famous Roman family and imperial name, and, as the emperor treated captives well, "magnanimous." Claudia Weill, film director; Claudette Colbert, Claudia Cardinale, actresses.
English nickname: **Claudie.**
English variations: **Claudette, Claudina, Claudine.**
Foreign variations: **Claude, Claudette, Claudine** (French), **Gladys, Gwladys** (Welsh), **Claudia** (German, Italian, Spanish).

CLEMATIS—Greek: **Klematis.** "Vine or brushwood." From the sweet-smelling clematis flower.

CLEMENCY—See **Clementia.**

CLEMENTIA—Latin: "mild, calm, merciful." Popularized by the song, "Oh, My Darling Clemetine."
English nicknames: **Clem, Clemmie, Clemmy.**
Foreign variations: **Clemence** (French), **Klementine** (German).

CLEMENTINE—see **Clementia.**

CLEO—Greek: "glory, fame." See **Cleopatra.** Cleo Laine, singer.

CLEOPATRA—Greek: "father's glory or fame." A father's pride and joy. Cleopatra, 69–30 B.C.. Queen of Egypt; heroine of Shakespeare's play, *Antony and Cleopatra.*

CLEVA—Middle English: **Cleve.** "Dweller at the cliff." Feminine of **Cleve** and **Clive.**

CLIANTHA—Greek: **Kleianthe.** "Glory-flower." This child has the splendor and beauty of a flower from heaven.
English variation: **Cleantha.**
Foreign variation: **Cleanthe** (French).

CLIO—Greek: **Kleio.** "The proclaimer." A woman who made known her opinion. Clio was the ancient Greek Muse of History.

CLORINDA—Latin: fictional name formed by Tasso, 16th century, for a character in *Jerusalem Delivered*. Possible meanings: "renowned," or "verdant, beautiful."

CLOTILDA—German: **Chlodhilde**. "Famous battle-maid." A girl who fought beside the man she loved. St. Clotilda, 6th century, was the wife of Clovis I, King of France.
Foreign variations: **Clothilde** (French), **Klothilde** (German), **Clotilda** (Italian, Spanish).

CLOVER—Old English: **Claefer**. "Clover blossom."

CLYMENE—Greek: **Klymene**. "Renowned, famed one." Clymene in Greek myths was the daughter of Oceanus and the mother of Atlas and Prometheus.

CLYTIE—Greek: **Klytai**. "Splendid or beautiful one." Clytie, a nymph, daughter of Oceanus in Greek legends, was changed into a heliotrope flower because she loved the sun and could then always turn her face toward it.

CODY—Old English: "a cushion." Also: **Codi, Codie**.

COLETTE—Greek-French: "victorious army." A French nickname form of **Nicolette**, from **Nicholas**. Colette, French novelist; Nicolette Larson, singer.

Foreign variation: **Collette** (French).

COLLEEN—Irish Gaelic: **Cailin**. "Girl, maiden." Colleen Dewhurst, actress. Also: **Coleen**.

COLUMBA—Latin: "the dove." An ancient symbol of peace in all nations St. Columba, born in Ireland, became the greatest religious benefactor of Scotland, 6th century. His name is used by both men and women.
English nicknames: **Collie, Colly**.
English variations: **Coline, Columbia, Columbine**.
Foreign variations: **Colombe, Coulombe** (French).

COMFORT—French: **Confort**. "Strengthening aid and comfort." A Puritan name first popularized in the 18th century.

CONCEPTION—Latin: **Conceptio**. "Beginning." Used in Spain and Latin America in honor of Santa Maria de la Concepción.
Foreign variations: **Concepcíon, Concha, Conchita** (Spanish).

CONCHA—See **Conception**.

CONCHITA—See Conception.

CONCORDIA—Latin: "harmony." At peace with man and nature. Concordia was a Roman goddess representing peace after war.

CONRADINE—Old Ger-

man: **Kuon-rad.** "Bold, wise counselor." The feminine of **Conrad.**
English nicknames: **Connie, Conny.**

CONSOLATA—Italian: "consolation." Used in honor of St. Mary.

CONSTANCE—Latin: **Constantia.** "Firmness, constancy." St. Constance, 2nd-century Roman martyr; Constance Towers, actress.
English nicknames: **Connie, Conny.**
English variations: **Constancy, Constanta, Constantina.**
Foreign variations: **Constanza** (Italian, Spanish), **Konstanze** (German).

CONSUELA—Spanish: "consolation." A wonderful friend when needed. Consuelo Vanderbilt, American heiress.
Foreign variations: **Consuelo** (Italian, Spanish).

CORA—Greek: **Kore.** "The maiden." In Greek mythology Kore was the daughter of the goddess Demeter. Corinne Calvet, actress; Coretta Scott King, civil rights activist.
English nicknames: **Corrie, Cory.**
English variations: **Kora, Corella, Corette, Corrina, Correne, Corene, Coretta, Corra.**
Foreign variation: **Corina** (Spanish).

CORABELLE—Greek-French: **Kore-Belle.** "Beautiful maiden."

CORAL—Latin: **Corallum.** "Coral from the sea," or Old French: **Coral.** "Cordial, sincere." Coral Brown, English actress.
English variation: **Coraline.**
Foreign variation: **Coralie** (French).

CORDELIA—Middle Welsh: **Creiddylad.** "Jewel of the sea; Latin: "warm-hearted." In Welsh legends Cordelia was the daughter of King Lear, ruler of the sea. In Shakespeare's *King Lear* she was the only daughter who remained loyal.
English nicknames: **Cordie, Delia, Della.**
Foreign variations: **Cordélie** (French), **Kordula** (German).

CORINNE—See **Cora.**

CORISSA—Latin-Greek: "most maidenly."
English variation: **Corisa.**

CORLISS—Old English: **Carleas.** "Cheerful, goodhearted."

CORNELIA—Latin: "yellowish or horn-colored"; or Latin, "queenly, womanly, enduring." The feminine of **Cornelius.** The corneal tree was sacred to Apollo in Greek myths. St. Cornelia, an early North African Christian martyr; Cornelia Otis Skinner, noted actress and writer.
English Nicknames: **Cornie, Nela, Nella, Nelia, Nelli, Nellie.**
English variations: **Cornela, Cornella, Cornelle.**

Foreign variation: **Cornélie** (French).

CORONA—Spanish: "crown, crowned one."

CORY, COREY—See **Cora**.

COSETTE—French: "victorious army." A French feminine nickname from **Nicholas**.
Foreign variation: **Cosetta** (Italian).

COSIMA—Greek: **Kosmos**. "Order, harmony; the world." Feminine form of **Cosmo**. Cosima Wagner, wife of composer Richard Wagner.

COURTNEY—Old French: **Courtenay**. "Dweller at the court or farmstead." Also masculine; modern U.S. usage usually feminine.

CRESCENT—Old French: **Creissant**. "To increase or create."
Foreign variation: **Crescentia** (Italian).

CRISPINA—Latin: "curly-haired." Feminine form of **Crispin**.

CRYSTAL—Latin: **Crystallum**. "Clear as crystal." Chrystal Herne, American actress; Krystal Carrington, character on TV's "Dynasty."

English variations: **Chrystal, Krystal**.

CYNARA—Greek: **Kinara**. "Thistle or artichoke." Famed from the writings of Horace, ancient Roman poet, and from Ernest Dowson's poem.

CYNTHIA—Greek: **Kynthia**. "The moon." Among the ancient Greeks, Cynthia was an epithet for Artemis or Diana, the moon goddess, who was born on Mount Cynthos on the island of Delos. Cynthia Gregory, ballerina; Cyndi Lauper, rock singer.
English nicknames: **Cynth, Cynthie, Cindy, Cindie, Cinny, Cyn, Cyndi**.

CYPRIS—Greek: **Kipris**. "From the island of Cyprus."

CYRENA—Greek: **Kyrene**. "From Cyrene." Cyrene was a goddess of Cyrenaica, an ancient North African country. In Greek myths Cyrene was a water nymph loved by Apollo.

CYRILLA—Latin: "lordly one." Feminine form of **Cyril**. Foreign variation: **Cirila** (Spanish).

CYTHEREA—Greek: **Kythereia**. "From the island of Cytherea." Cytherea was an epithet for Aphrodite or Venus.

D

DACIA—Greek: **Dakoi**. "From Dacia." Dacia was an ancient Eastern European country.

DAFFODIL—Old French: **Afrodille**. "The daffodil flower." Touched by Pluto and turned to gold from white, according to the Greek myth.

DAGMAR—Old German: **Dagomar**. "Day glorious"; or Old German: Dank-mar. "Famous thinker, glory of the Danes. Also "joy of the land."

DAHLIA—Old Norse: **Dal-r**. "From the valley." Latin form of the surname of A. Dahl, Swedish botanist, for whom the flower was named.

DAISY—Old English: **Daeges-eage**. "Eye-of-the-day." A miniature symbol of the sun. In France this flower is called Marguerite. *Daisy Miller*, novel by Henry James.

DALE—Old English: **Dael**. "From the valley." Alternate origin, Greek: **Damalis**. "Heifer, gentle one." Dale Evans Rogers, noted actress, entertainer. English variations: **Daile, Dayle.**

DAMARIS—Greek: "wife." Also: **Damara.**

DAMITA—Spanish: "little noble lady."

DANA—Celtic: "from Denmark"; or for Dana, mother of the gods in Scandinavian mythology. Dana Hill, actress.

DANICA—Old Slavic: **Danika**. "Star, morning star."

DANIELA, DANIELLE—Hebrew: **Dani'el**. "God is my judge." Feminine form of **Daniel**. Danielle Brisebois, actress.
English variations: **Danella, Danelle.**
Foreign variations: **Danielle** (French), **Daniela** (Spanish).

DANYA—Modern U.S. form, a feminine form of **Daniel**.

DAPHNE—Greek: "laurel or bay tree; laurel maiden; victorious." Also: **Daphna**. The fragrant laurel branches were used to crown victors. Daphne, daughter of the river god, was changed into a laurel tree in Greek mythology. Daphne du Maurier, English novelist.

DARA—Hebrew: "House of compassion or wisdom."

DARCIE—Old French: **D'Arcy**. "From the fortress." Feminine version of **D'Arcy**. Also Irish Gaelic: **Dorchaidhe**. "Dark man."

DARIA—Greek: **Dareios**. "Wealthy, queenly." Feminine form of **Darius**, from the famous Persian ruler.

DARLENE—Old Anglo-French: **Darel-ene**. "Little dear one, little darling." Also: **Darleen, Darline.**

DARRELLE—Old Anglo-French: **Darel**. "Little dear one."

English variations: **Darryl,
Daryl.**

DAVIDA—Hebrew: **David.**
"Beloved one." Feminine form of **David.**
English variations. **Davina,
Davita.**

DAWATHA—Swahili: "last
one."

DAWN—Old English:
Dagian. "The dawn of day."
Dawn Addams, actress.

DEANNA—See **Diana.**

DEBORAH—Hebrew: "the
bee." Deborah was a famous
Biblical prophetess who
helped free Israel from the
Canaanites. Debbie Reynolds, Deborah Kerr, actresses.
English nicknames: **Deb,
Debbie, Debby, Debs.**
English variations: **Debora,
Debra, Devorah, Debera.**

DECIMA—Latin: "the
tenth daughter."

DEE—Welsh: **Du.** "Black;
dark one." A short form of
Dierdre; Delia, Diana. Also:
Didi, Dee Dee, Dede.

DEIRDRE—Irish Gaelic:
Deardriu. "Complete wanderer"; or Irish Gaelic:
"Sorrow and compassion."
Dierdre was the tragic
heroine of an old Irish legend.
She fell in love and fled to
England with Naoise, later,
when they returned, her
lover was killed and she died
on his grave.

DELCINE—See **Dulcine.**

DELFINE—Greek:
larkspur or delphinic
flower." Named for its
flower-center, which resembles a dolphin-fish or
delphinos. Also, Greek:
"calm, serene, loving
sister."
English variations: **Delfina,
Delphina, Delphine.**

DELIA—Greek: **Delos;
Delia.** "Visible." Delia was a
name for Artemis, the
Greek moon goddess who was
born on the Isle of Delos.

DELICIA—Latin: **Deliciae.**
"Delightful one."

DELIGHT—Old French:
Delit. "Delight or pleasure."

DELILAH—Hebrew: **Delilah.**
"Languishing or gentle."
Delilah was the betrayer of
Samson in the Bible.
English variations: **Delila,
Dalila.**

DELLA—See **Adelle, Adeline,
Adelaide.** Della Reese, singer.

DELMA—Spanish: **Delmar;** French: **Delmare.** "Of
the sea."

DELORA—See **Dolores.**

DELORES—See **Dolores.**

DELPHINE—See **Delfine.**

DELTA—Greek: "fourth
letter of the Greek alphabet."
A name for a fourth
daughter.

DEMETRIA—Greek: **Demetrios.** "Belonging to
Demeter, Greek fertility

. Demetria,
　stian martyr, died

　—Old English: **Denu.**
　n the valley." Feminine
　n of **Dean.**
　nglish variations: **Deana,
Deane, Dina.**

DENISE—French: "adherent of Dionysus, Greek god of wine." The feminine form of **Dennis.** Denise Levertor, poet.
English variations: **Denice,
Denyse, Denyce.**

DESIREE—French: **Desirée.** "Desired; longed-for."

DESMA—Greek: **Desmos.** "A bond of pledge."

DESMONA—Greek: **Dysdai-monia.** "Ill-starred one." A shortening of Desdemona, famous character in Shakespeare's *Othello.*

DEVA—Sanskrit: "divine." A name for the moon goddess.

DEVONA—Old English: **Defena.** "From Devonshire." Devonshire was named for the ancient Celtic tribe called Defena, believed to mean "deep valley people." Also: **Devonna.**

DEXTRA—Latin: **Dexter.** "Skillful, dexterous."

DIAMANTA—French: **Diamant.** "Diamondlike."

DIANA, DIANE—Latin: **Diana.** "Goddess; divine one." Diana was the Roman moon goddess and deity of the hunt. Notable namesakes include Diana, Princess of Wales; Diahann Carroll, singer; Diane Keaton, actress. English nicknames: **Di, Dian, Dee.**
English variations: **Deana, Deanna, Dianna, Dyana, Dyane, Diahann.**

DIANTHA—Greek: **Diosanthus.** "Flower of Zeus, divine flower."
English variations: **Dianthe, Dianthia.**

DIDO—Greek: Obscure meaning, possibly, "teacher, enlightener." Dido, an ancient princess of Tyre, was the reputed founder of the famous North African city of Carthage.

DINAH—Hebrew: "judged." Dinah was a daughter of Jacob and Leah in the Bible. Actresses Dinah Shore, Dina Merrill, Dinah Manoff. English variation: **Dina.**

DISA—Old Norse: **Diss.** "Active sprite"; or Greek: **Dis.** "Twice or double." Dis was an ancient Nordic fairy guardian.

DIXIE—French: **Dix.** "Ten or tenth." Dixie Land, the Southern states, was so named without substantiation, from ten-dollar bills called "Dixies." Dixie Lee Ray, Governor of Washington.

DOANNA—American compound of Dorothy and Anna.

DOCILA—Latin: **Docilis.** "Gentle, teachable."

DOLLY—see **Dorothy.** Dolly Parton, singer.

DOLORES—Spanish: "sorrows." Usage from Santa Maria de los Dolores, referring to the seven sorrowful occasions in the life of St. Mary. Dolores Hart, Dolores del Rio, actresses. English and Spanish nicknames: **Lola, Lolita.** English variations: **Delores, Deloris, Delora, Dolorita.**

DOMINA—Latin: "lady."

DOMINICA—Latin: "belonging to the Lord." Feminine of **Dominic.** Foreign variations: **Dominique** (French), **Domenica** (Italian), **Dominga** (Spanish).

DONALDA—Scottish Gaelic: **Domhnull.** "World ruler." Feminine of **Donald.** English variation: **Donis.**

DONATA—Latin: **Donatio.** "Donation; gift."

DONIA—See **Donalda.**

DONNA—Italian: "lady." Donna Reed, actress; Donna De Varona, Olympic swimmer. Foreign variation: **Doña** (Spanish).

DORA—Greek: **Doron.** "Gift." See **Dorothy, Theodora.** English nicknames: **Dori, Dorrie.** English variations: **Doralin,** Doralynne, Dorelia, Dorena, Dorette, Doreen.

DORCAS—Greek: **Dorkas.** "A gazelle." In the Bible, Dorcas was raised from the dead by St. Peter.

DORÉ—French: "golden one." Also: **Dorée.**

DOREEN, DORENE—Irish Gaelic: **Doire-ann.** "The sullen one." Also, Greek: "bountiful"; French: "golden." English variations: **Dorine, Dorina.**

DORINDA—Greek-Spanish: **Doron linda.** "Beautiful gift."

DORIS—Greek: "from the ocean, bountiful." Also, Hawaiian: "from the sea." In Greek myths Doris was the daughter of Oceanus, god of the sea. Doris Day, actress; Doris Lessing, author. English variations: **Doria, Dorice, Dorise, Dorris.**

DOROTHY—Greek: **Dorothea.** "Gift of God." See **Theodora.** St. Dorothea, early Christian martyr; writers Dorothy Thompson, Dorothy Parker, Dorothy Kilgallen, Dorothy Sayers; Dorothea Dix, humanitarian. English nicknames: **Dot, Dottie, Dotty, Dol, Dollie, Dolly.** English variations: **Dorothea, Dorotea, Dorthea, Dorthy.** Foreign variations: **Dorothea** (German), **Dorothée** (French), **Dorotea** (Italian, Spanish).

DRUSILLA—Latin: "descendant of Drusus, the strong one."
English nicknames: **Dru, Drusa, Drucie, Drusie.**

DUANA—Irish, Gaelic: **Dubhain.** "Little dark one"; or Irish Gaelic: **Duan.** "Song."
English variations: **Duna, Dwana.**

DUENA—Spanish: **Dueña.** "Chaperon."

DULCIANA—See **Dulcie.**

DULCIBELLE—See **Dulcie.**

DULCIE—Latin: **Dulcis.** "Sweet one."
English variations: **Delcine, Dulce, Dulcea, Dulcine, Dulcinea, Dulcibelle, Dulciana.**

DURENE—Latin: **Durus.** "Enduring one."

DYAN—See **Diana.** Dyan Cannon, actress.

E

EARLENE—Old English: **Eorl.** "Noble woman." The feminine form of **Earl.** Alternate, Irish Gaelic: **Airleas.** "A pledge."
English nicknames: **Earlie, Earley.**
English variations: **Earline, Erlene, Erline.**

EARTHA—Old English: **Ertha.** "Child of the earth, earthly, earthy, worldly, realistic." Eartha Kitt, vocalist, actress.
English variations: **Erda, Ertha, Herta, Hertha.**

EASTER—Old English: **Eastre.** "Born at Easter time." Eostre was the ancient Anglo-Saxon goddess of spring.

EBBA—Old English: "flowing back of the tide." See **Eve.**

EBONY—Modern U.S.: "blackness"; the word used as a name.

ECHO—Greek: **Echo.** "Reflected sound." In Greek myths Echo, a nymph, pined away for the love of Narcissus, until nothing was left but her voice.

EDA—Old English: **Eada.** "Prosperity, blessedness"; or Old Norse: **Edda.** "Poetry." Eda Le Shan, author. See **Edith.**

EDANA—Irish Gaelic: **Aiden, Eideann.** "Little fiery one." St. Edana of Ireland, 6th century.

EDE—See **Eda.** Also Greek: "generation." Alternate, Old English: **Eadda.** "Prosperous."

EDELINE—See **Adeline.**

EDEN—Hebrew: 'eden. "Delight, pleasure."

EDINA—Scottish: "From the city of Edinburgh"; or Old English: **Ead-wine.** "Prosperous friend." See **Edwina.** Poetical name for the capital city of Scotland.

EDITH—Old English: **Eadgyth.** "Rich gift." Edith Wharton, American novelist; Dame Edith Evans, English actress; Edith Hamilton, American mythology writer; Edith Piaf, French chanteuse; Edie Adams, singer, actress; Eydi Gorme, singer.
English nicknames: **Eda, Ede, Edie, Eyde, Eydie.**
English variations: **Editha, Edithe, Ediva, Edyth, Edythe.**
Foreign variation: **Edita** (Italian).

EDLYN—Old English: **Eathelin.** "Noble little one"; or Old Anglo-French: **Ead-elin.** "Prosperous little one."

EDMONDA—Old English: **Eadmund.** "Prosperous protector." Feminine of **Edmund.**
English variation: **Edmunda.**

EDNA—Hebrew: 'ednah. "Rejuvenation." Edna, wife of Enoch in the Biblical Apocrypha; Edna St. Vincent Millay, American poet; Edna Ferber, American novelist.
English nicknames: **Ed, Eddie.**

EDREA—Old English: **Ear-ric.** "Prosperous, powerful." Feminine of **Edric.** English variation: **Edra.**

EDWARDINE—Old English: **Ead-weard.** "Prosperous guardian. Feminine of **Edward.**

EDWINA—Old English: **Ead-wine.** "Prosperous friend." Feminine of **Edward.** English variation: **Edina.**

EGBERTA—Old English: **Ecgbeorht.** "Bright, shining sword." Feminine of **Egbert.**
English variation: **Egbertina, Egbertine.**

EGLANTINE—Old French: **Aiglentine.** "Sweetbrier rose; woodbine." Eglentyne was a prioress in Chaucer's 14th-century writings.

EILEEN—Irish Gaelic: **Eibhlin.** "Light." The Irish form of **Helen.** Eileen Farrell, operatic singer; Eileen Heckart, actress.

EIR—Old Norse: "peace, clemency." Eir was the Norse goddess of healing.

EKATERINA—see **Catherine.** Ekaterina Szabo, Romanian gymnast.

ELA—See **Elaine, Ella.**

ELAINE—See **Helen.** The old French form of **Helen,** popularized by Tennyson's "Elaine, the Lily Maid of Astolat." Elaine May, author/director.

Elata   58

English variations: **Elane, Elayne.**

ELATA—Latin: **Elatus.** "Lofty, elevated."

ELBERTA—See **Alberta.** Clara Elberta Rumph, after whom the Elberta peach was named.

ELDORA—Spanish: **El dorado.** "Gilded one"; Teutonic: "gift of wisdom."

ELDRIDA—Old English: **Ealdraed.** "Old, wise counselor." Feminine form of **Eldred.**

ELEANOR—Old French: **Elienor.** "Light." An old form of **Helen.** Eleanor of Aquitaine, English queen, died 1204; Nell Gwyn, famous 17th-century English actress; Eleonora Duse, Italian actress; Eleanor Roosevelt, wife of President Franklin D. Roosevelt; Eleanor Powell, actress. English nicknames: **El, Ella, Ellie, Nelda, Nell, Nellie, Nelly, Nora.** English variations: **Eleanore, Elinor, Elinore, Eleonore, Eleonora, Elnore, Elaine, Leonore, Lenore.** Foreign variations: **Elenora** (Italian), **Eléonore** (French), **Leanor** (Spanish), **Elenore** (German, Danish).

ELECTRA—Greek: **Elektra.** "Brilliant one." Electra was the daughter of the hero Agamemnon in Greek history.

ELENA—See **Helen.** Elena Verdugo, actress.

ELFRIDA—Old English: **Aelfraed.** "Good counselor, wise and peaceful." See **Alfreda.** Elfreda, second wife of England's 10-century King Edgar. English variations: **Elfreda, Elfrieda.**

ELGA—Gothic: **Alhs**; Slavic: **Olga.** "Holy, consecrated."

ELINOR—See **Eleanore.**

ELISE—See **Elizabeth.**

ELISSA, ELYSSA—See **Elizabeth.**

ELIZABETH—Hebrew: **Elisheba.** "Consecrated to God; oath of God." St. Elizabeth, mother of John the Baptist; Elizabeth I and II, English queens; Elizabeth Barrett Browning, English poet; actresses Elizabeth Taylor, Elizabeth Ashley. English nicknames: **Bess, Bessie, Bessy, Beth, Betsey, Betsy, Bett, Betta, Bette, Bettina, Betty, Buffy, Elsa, Else, Elsie, Libby, Lisa, Lise, Liza, Lizzie, Lizzy.** English variations: **Elisabeth, Elisa, Elise, Elissa, Eliza, Elyse, Elyssa, Lisbeth, Lizabeth.** Foreign variations: **Elisabeth, Elise, Lisette, Lizette, Babette** (French), **Elisabetta, Elisa** (Italian), **Elisabeth, Elsa, Else** (German, Dutch, Danish), **Isabel, Belita,**

Elisa, Ysabel (Spanish),
Elisabet (Swedish), **Eilis**
(Irish), **Ealasaid Elspeth**
(Scottish).

ELLA—Old English: **Aelf.**
"Elf; beautiful fairy maiden."
See **Eleanore, Ellen.** Ella
Fitzgerald, jazz vocalist.
English nicknames: **Ellie,
Elly.**

ELLAMAY—Compound of
Ella and **May.**

ELLEN—See **Helen.** Ellen
Terry, famous English actress
(1848–1928).

ELLICE—Greek: **Elias.**
"Jehovah is God." A feminine
form of **Ellis** and **Elias.**

ELMA—Greek: **Elmo.**
"Amiable." Also; Turkish:
"apple." Feminine of
Elmo.

ELMIRA—Old English:
Aethel-Maere. "Noble famous
one." Feminine of **Elmer.**
See **Almira.**

ELNA—See **Helen.**

ELNORA—See **Eleanore.**

ELOISE—See **Louise.**

ELRICA—Old German:
Alh-ric. "Ruler of all."

ELSA—Old German: "no-
ble one." See **Elizabeth.** Elsa,
bride of Lohengrin in
German legends; Elsa Max-
well, writer, lecturer; Elsa
Lanchester, actress.

ELSIE—Old German: **Elsa.**
"Noble one." See **Elizabeth.**

ELVA—Old English: **Aelf-a.**
"Elfin, good."
English variations: **Elvia,
Elvie, Elfie.**
Foreign variation: **Ailbhe**
(Irish).

ELVINA—Old English:
Aelfwine. "Elfin friend."
Feminine form of **Elvin.**

ELVIRA—Latin: **Albinia.**
"White, blond"; Spanish:
"Elfin." Donna Elvira, in
Mozart's famous opera *Don
Giovanni*.
English variation: **Elvera.**
Foreign variations: **Elvire**
(French), **Elvira** (Italian).

ELYSE—See **Elizabeth,
Elysia.**

ELYSIA—Latin: "sweetly
blissful." Elysium in Roman
myths was the dwelling place
of happy souls.
English variations: **Elise,
Elyse, Ilise, Ilysa, Ilyse.**

EMERALD—Old French:
Esmeraude. "The bright
green gem."
English nicknames: **Em,
Emmie.**
English variation: **Emerant.**
Foreign variations: **Emeraude**
(French), **Esmeralda** (Spanish).

EMILY—Gothic: **Amala.**
"Industrious one"; or Latin:
Aemilia. "Flattering, win-
ning one." See **Amelia.** Emily
Brontë, English novelist;
Emily Dickinson, American
poet; Emily Post, etiquette
arbiter;

English nicknames: **Em, Emmie, Emmy.**
English variations: **Emelda, Emilie, Emlyn, Emlynne, Emera.**
Foreign variations: **Emilie** (French), **Emilie** (German), **Emilia** (Italian, Spanish, Dutch), **Eimile** (Irish), **Aimil** (Scottish), **Emmali,** (Iranian).

EMINA—Latin: **Eminens.** "Lofty, prominent one."

EMMA—Old German: **Imma.** "Universal one"; or German: **Amme.** "Nurse." Emma Willard, 19th-century American educator; Lady Emma Hamilton, 18th-century English beauty; Emmylou Harris, singer.
English nicknames: **Em, Emmie, Emmi, Emmy.**
English variations: **Emelina, Emeline, Emelyne, Emmaline.**
Foreign variations: **Emma** (Italian, German), **Ema** (Spanish).

EMMALINE—See **Emma.**

EMOGENE—See **Imogene.**

ENA—Irish Gaelic: **Aine.** "Little ardent or fiery one." Princess Victoria Ena, born 1887, later Queen of Spain.

ENGELBERTA—Old German: **Engel-berthta.** "Bright angel." A little one haloed by golden hair.

ENID—Old Welsh: **Enit.** "Woodlark, purity." Celtic: "pure in soul"; English:

"fair." In the old English Arthurian legends Enid was the wife of Geraint. Enid Bagnold, English writer.

ENNEA—Greek: "nine; ninth child."

ENRICA—Italian: "ruler of an estate or home." The Italian feminine form of **Henry.**

EOLANDE—See **Yolande.**

ERANTHE—Greek: **Earanthemos.** "Spring flower.

ERDA—See **Eartha, Herta, Hertha.**

ERICA—Old Norse: **Eyrekr.** "Ever powerful; ever-ruler." Feminine of **Eric.** Greek: "the heather flower." Erica Jong, author.
Foreign variation: **Erika** (Swedish).

ERIN—Irish Gaelic: **Erinn.** "From Ireland." Erin Gray, actress.

ERLINE—See **Earlene.**

ERLINDA—Hebrew: "lively."

ERMA—Old German: **Heriman.** "Army maid;" or Latin: **Herminia.** "Noble one." English variations: **Ermina, Erminia, Erminie, Hermia, Hermine, Herminie, Hermione.**

ERNA—Old English: **Earn.** "Eagle." See **Ernestine.** English variation: **Ernaline.**

ERNESTINE—Old English: **Earnest.** "Earnest one." Feminine of **Ernest.** English nickname: **Erna.**

ERTHA—See **Eartha.**

ERWINA—Old English: **Earwine.** "Sea friend." Feminine of **Erwin.**

ESME—See **Esmeralda.**

ESMERALDA—Spanish: "emerald"; Latin: "adorned one." A character in Victor Hugo's *The Hunchback of Notre Dame.* English nickname: **Esme.**

ESTA—Italian: **Est.** "From the East."

ESTELLE—French: **Estoile.** "A star." Estelle Winwood, Stella Stevens, actresses. English nicknames: **Essie, Stella, Stelle.** English variation: **Estella.** Foreign variations: **Estelle** (French), **Estrella, Estrellita** (Spanish).

ESTHER—Hebrew: **Ester;** Persian: **Esthur.** "A star." The Biblical Esther was queen of Persia; Esther Forbes, American Pulitzer Prize winner, history, 1943; Esther Williams, swimmer and actress. English nicknames: **Essa, Essie, Ettie, Etty, Hetty.** English variations: **Ester, Hester, Hesther.** Foreign variations: **Ester** (Italian, Spanish), **Hester,** (Dutch), **Eister** (Irish).

ETHEL—Old English: **Aethel.** "Noble one." Ethel Barrymore, Ethel Merman, actresses. English variations: **Ethelda,** Ethelinda, Etheline, Ethelyn, Ethyl.

ETHELINDA—Old German: **Athal-lindi.** "Noble serpent." The serpent was a symbol of wisdom and life without end. See **Ethel.**

ETHELJEAN—Modern compound of **Ethel** and **Jean.**

ETTA—Old German: **Etta.** "Little one." See **Henrietta.**

EUCLEA—Greek: **Eukleia.** "Glory."

EUDICE—Modern Israeli form of Hebrew Judith, "praise."

EUDOCIA—Greek: **Eudoxos.** "Of good repute." English nicknames: **Docie, Doxie, Doxy.** English variations: **Eudosia, Eudoxia.**

EUDORA—Greek: **Eudora.** "Generous." Eudora Welty, author. English nickname: **Dora.** Foreign variation: **Eudore** (French).

EUGENIA—Greek: **Eugenios.** "Well-born; noble." Feminine form of **Eugene.** Eugénie, Empress of France, 1826–1920; St. Eugenia, 3rd-century Roman martyr. English nicknames: **Genie, Gene.** Foreign variations: **Eugénie** (French), **Eugenia** (Italian, German, Spanish).

EULALIA—Greek: **Eulalos.** "Fair speech; well-spoken

one." St. Eulalia, 4th-century martyr, patron of Barcelona.
English nicknames: **Eula, Lallie.**
Foreign variations: **Eulalie** (French), **Eulalia** (Italian, Spanish).

EUNICE—Greek: **Eunike.** "Happy, victorious one." Eunice was the mother of Timothy in the Bible; Eunice Shriver, humanitarian.

EUPHEMIA—Greek: **Eu-phemia.** "Auspicious speech; good repute." St. Euphemia, 4th-century virgin martyr, is greatly venerated.
English nicknames: **Effie, Effy.**
Foreign variations: **Euphémie** (French), **Euphemia** (German), **Eufemia** (Italian, Spanish), **Eadaoine** (Irish).

EUSTACIA—Latin: **Eusta-thius.** "Stable, tranquil"; or Latin: **Eustachus.** "Fruit-ful." Feminine form of **Eustace.**
English nicknames: **Stacie, Stacey, Stacy, Stace.**

EVA—See **Eve.**

EVADNE—Greek: "sweet singer."

EVALEEN—See **Eve.**

EVANGELINE—Greek: **Euangelos.** "Bringer of good news." Famous from Longfellow's poem, *Evangeline*.
English nicknames: **Eve, Eva, Vangie, Vangy.**

EVE—Hebrew: **Chavva.** "Life-giving." The Biblical mother of mankind, wife of the first man, Adam. Actresses Eva Le Gallienne, Eve Arden, Eva Gabor, Eva Marie Saint.
English variations: **Eva, Eba, Ebba, Evelina, Eveline, Evelyn, Evlyn.**
Foreign variations: **Eve** (French), **Eva** (German, Italian, Spanish, Danish, Portuguese), **Aoiffe, Evaleen** (Irish).

EVELYN—See **Eve.** Also Irish Gaelic: **Eibhilin.** "Light." A form of **Helen.**

EYVETTE—Modern U.S. variant of **Yvette,** from the French: "hero with yew-bow."

F

FABIA—Latin: **Fabiana.** "Bean grower." Feminine of **Fabian.**

FAITH—Middle English: **Fayth.** "Ever true, always faithful."
English nickname: **Fay.**

FALLON—Modern U.S.

name. From Fallon, a character in TV's "Dy-nasty." Originally a surname.

FANCHON—French: **Fran-çoise.** "Free." An old French derivative of **Frances.**

FANNY—See **Frances.**

FARICA—see **Frederica**.

FARRAH—Modern U.S.; from a surname. Farrah Fawcett, actress.

FAUSTINE—Latin: **Fausta**. "Lucky, auspicious." Feminine form of **Faust**.
English variations: **Faustina, Fausta**.
Foreign variations: **Faustina** (Italian), **Faustine** (French).

FAVOR—Old French: "Help, approval; good will conferred."

FAWN—Old French: **Faon** "Young deer; reddish-brown colored."

FAY—Old French: **Fae**. "A fairy or elf"; or Irish Gaelic: **Feich**. "Raven." See **Faith**. Faye Dunaway, Faye Grant, actresses.

FAYANNE—Compound of **Fay** and **Anne**.

FAYETTE—Old French: "little fairy." "O, thou art fairer than the evening air, clad in the beauty of a thousand stars."—Marlowe.

FAYME—Old French: **Fame**. "Lofty reputation; renown."

FEALTY—Old French: **Feelté**. "Fidelity, allegiance." "To God, thy country and thy friend be true."—Vaughan.

FEDORA—See **Theodora**.

FELDA—Old German: **Felda**. "From the field."

FELICE—Latin: **Felicia**. "Happy one." Feminine form of **Felix**. Felice is a character in *Piers Plowman*, 14th-century English allegorical poem. Felicia Farr, actress.
English variations: **Felicia, Felicity, Felis**.
Foreign variations: **Félice, Félise** (French), **Felicia** (Italian), **Felicidad** or **Feliciana** (Spanish).

FENELLA—Irish Gaelic: **Fionnghuala**. "White-shouldered one." Fenella was an elflike character in Scott's *Peveril of the Peak*.
English variation: **Finella**.

FEODORA—See **Theodora**.

FERN—Old English: **Fearn**. "A fern; fernlike."

FERNANDA—Gothic: **Fairhonanth**. "World-daring; life-adventuring." A feminine form of **Ferdinand**.
English variations: **Ferdinanda, Fernandina**.

FIDELLA—Latin: **Fidelis**. "Faithful one." Beethoven opera, *Fidelio;* Imogene called herself "Fidele" in Shakespeare's *Cymbeline*.

FIFI—See **Josephine**.

FILIPA—See **Philippa**.

FIONA—Irish Gaelic: **Fionn**. "Fair one." Greek: "violet." Fiona MacLeod was a character in Sharp's writings.

FLANNA—Irish Gaelic: **Flann**. "Red-haired."

FLAVIA—Latin: feminine of Flavius. "Yellow-haired one."

FLETA—Old English: Fleotig. "Swift, fleet one."

FLEUR—French: "a flower." English variation: **Fleurette**.

FLEURETTE—see **Fleur**.

FLORA—Latin: "flower." Flora was the Roman goddess of flowers. Flora MacDonald, Scottish 18th-century heroine; Flora Robson, English actress.
English nicknames: **Florrie, Florry**.
English variations: **Flore, Floria**.
Foreign variations: **Flore** (French), **Fiora** (Italian), **Flor** (Spanish).

FLORENCE—Latin: Florentia. "Blooming, flourishing, prosperous." Florence Nightingale, founder of nursing system (1820–1910); Florence Reed, actress.
English nicknames: **Flo, Florrie, Flossie**.
English variations: **Florance, Florinda, Floris, Florine**.
Foreign variations: **Fiorenza** (Italian), **Florencia** (Spanish) **Florentia** (German).

FLOWER—Old French: Fleur. "A blossom."

FONDA—Middle English: Fonned. "Affectionate, tender"; Latin: **Fundus**. "Foundation."

FORTUNE—Latin: Fortuna. "Fate; destiny."

Foreign variation: **Fortuna** (Italian, Spanish).

FRANCES—Latin: **Franciscus**. "Free one," or "from France." Frances Willard, 19th-century educator; Frances Perkins, former U.S. Secretary of Labor; Fran Lebowitz, author; Francesca Annis, English actress; Fanny Brice, actress and comedienne.
English nicknames: **Fan, Fannie, Fanny, Fran, Frannie, Franny, Francie, Francy, Frankie**.
English variations: **Francine, Francyne**.
Foreign variations: **Françoise** (French), **Francesca, Cecca** (Italian), **Franziska** (German), **Francisca** (Spanish), **Franciska** (Polish).

FRANCINE—See **Frances**.

FREDA—See **Frieda**.

FREDELLA—Modern compound of **Frieda** and **Ella**. Also, **Fredelle**.

FREDERICA—Old German: **Fridu-ric**. "Peaceful ruler." Frederika, Queen of Greece.
English nicknames: **Freddie, Freddy**.
English variations: **Frederika, Frerika, Farica**.
Foreign variations: **Frédérique** (French), **Federica** (Italian, Spanish), **Friederike** (German).

FREYA—Old Norse: Freyja. "Noble lady." Freya was the Norse goddess of love and beauty.

FRIEDA—Old German:
Frida. "Peaceful one." See
Winifred.
English variations: **Freda,**
Frida.

FRITZI—Old German:
Frida-ric. "Peaceful ruler." A

German feminine form of
Fritz from **Frederick.**

FRONDE—Latin: **Frondis.**
"A leafy branch."

FULVIA—Latin: "tawny or
yellow-colored."

G

GABRIELLE—Hebrew: **Gab-
hriel.** "Heroine of
God, God gives me strength."
The feminine form of **Gabriel.**
Gabriela Mistral, Nobel
Prize winner, literature;
Gabriela Sabatini, tennis
player.
English nicknames: **Gabie,**
Gaby.
English variations: **Gabriela,**
Gabriella.

GAEA—Greek: **Gaia.** "The
earth." Gaia was the Greek
deity of the earth, the
mother of Uranus.
English variation: **Gala.**

GAIL—Old English: **Gal.**
"Gay, lively one." see **Abigail.**
Gail Parent, author; Gail
Storm, actress.
English variations: **Gale,**
Gayle, Gayel.

GALATEA—Greek: **Galateia.**
"Milky white." In the Greek
legend, Pygmalion fash-
ioned an ivory statue he called
Galatea, which Aphrodite
caused to come to life.

GALE—Old Norse: **Gala.**

"To sing; singer." See **Gail,**
Abigail.

GALIENA—Old German:
Galiana. "Lofty one."

GARDA—see **Gerda.**

GARDENIA—New Latin:
"the fragrant white gardenia
flower." The gardenia was
named for Alexander Garden,
18th-century American botanist.

GARI—Teutonic: "spear
maiden." Feminine of **Gary.**

GARLAND—Old French:
Garlande. "A wreath or crown
of flowers."

GARNET—Middle English:
Gernet. "The garnet gem."
English variation: **Garnette.**

GAVRILA—Hebrew: "her
oine." The feminine of
Gabriel.

GAY—Old French: **Gai.**
"Bright and lively."

GAYLE—see **Gail.**

GAZELLA—New Latin:
"gazelle or antelope." Also:
Gazelle.

GELASIA—Greek: **Gelastikos.** "Inclined to laughter."

GEMMA—Italian: "a gem or precious stone." Gemma Craven, Gemma Jones, English actresses.

GENE—See **Eugenia.** Gene Tierney, actress.

GENEVA—Old French: **Genèvre.** "Juniper tree."

GENEVIEVE—Old German: **Geno-wefa.** "White wave." See **Guinevere.** St. Genevièvre, A.D. 420–519, patron of Paris; Genevieve Bujold, actress.

GEORGETTE—see **Georgia.**

GEORGIA—Latin: "farmer." Feminine of **George.** Georgia Neese Clarke, Treasurer of the U.S.; Georgia O'Keeffe, artist; Georgette de la Plante, French modiste after whom "Georgette crepe" was named.
English nicknames: **Georgia, Gregory.**
English variations: **Georgene, Georgette, Georgina, Georgine.**
Foreign variations: **Georgine, Georgienne, Georgette** (French), **Giorgia** (Italian), **Georgina** (German, Dutch).

GEORGIANA—See **Georgia.**

GERALDINE—Old German: **Ger-walt.** "Spear-mighty." Feminine of **Gerald.** Geraldine Ferraro, politician; Geraldine Page, actress.

English variation: **Geraldina.**
English nicknames: **Gerrie, Gerry, Jeri, Jerri, Jerry.**
Foreign variations: **Géraldine** (French), **Giralda** (Italian), **Gerhardine** (German).

GERANIUM—Greek: **Geranion.** "Crane." From usage, refers to the geranium flower.

GERDA—Old Norse: **Garth-f.** "Enclosure; protection." Gerda was the wife of the god Freyr in Norse myths; also a child in Andersen's fairy tale, *The Snow Queen.* English variation: **Garda.**

GERMAIN—French: **Germaine;** or Latin: **Germanus.** "A German." Germaine Greer, author and feminist.

GERTRUDE—Old German: **Ger-trut.** "Spear-loved." Gertrude was one of the German mythical Valkyries. Notables include St. Gertrude the Great, 13th-century German mystic; Gertrude Stein, writer; Gertrude Lawrence, actress.
English nicknames: **Gert, Gertie, Getty, Trudie, Trudy.**
Foreign variations: **Gertrud** (German), **Gertrude** (French), **Gertrudis** (Spanish), **Geltruda** (Italian).

GIACINTA—Sée **Hyacinth.**

GIANINA—Italian: "God is gracious." Feminine form of **Giovanni, John.** Also: **Giannina.**

GILBERTA—Old German:

Gisil-berhta. "Brilliant pledge or hostage."
English nicknames: **Gillie, Gilly.**
English variations: **Gilberte, Gilbertina, Gilbertine.**

GILDA—Old English: **Gyldan.** "Covered with gold." Gilda was daughter of Rigoletto in the Verdi opera; Gilda Radner, actress.

GILLIAN—Latin: **Juliana.** "Youthful, downy-haired one." One of the most popular names in the Middle Ages. English nicknames: **Gill, Gillie, Gilly, Jill.**

GINA—Variant of **Eugenia**; also Japanese: "silvery." See **Regina.** Gina Lollobrigida, Italian actress.

GINEVRA—see **Guinevere.**

GINGER—Latin: **Gingiber.** "Ginger spice or ginger flower." See **Virginia.** Ginger Rogers, actress, dancer.

GISELLE—Old German. **Gisela.** "Pledge or hostage." Gisela, daughter of a French king, married in A.D. 880. Rollo or Rolf, 1st Duke of Normandy, ancestor of William the Conqueror; Gisele MacKenzie, actress, singer.
English variations: **Gisela, Gisella, Giselle.**
Foreign variations: **Gisèle** (French), **Gisela** (Italian, Spanish).

Gitana—Spanish: "a gypsy."

GLADYS—Old Welsh: **Gwladys**; Latin: **Claudia.** "Lame one"; or Latin: **Gladiolus.** "Small sword or gladiolus flower."
English nickname: **Glad.**
English variation: **Gleda.**

GLEDA—Old English: **Gled.** "Glowing; glad one." Icelandic: "make happy, gladden." See **Gladys.**

GLENDA—Old Welsh: **Glyn**; Irish Gaelic: **Ghleanna.** "Dweller in a valley or glen." Feminine form of **Glenn.** Glenda Jackson, Glynis Johns, actresses.
English variations: **Glenna, Glynis, Glynnie.**

GLORIA—Latin: "glory, glorious one." Actresses Gloria Swanson, Gloria Grahame; Gloria Steinem, feminist.
English variations: **Glori, Gloriana, Gloriane, Glory.**

GLORIANA—See **Gloria.**

GLYNIS—See **Glenna.**

GODIVA—Old English: **Godgifu.** "Gift of God." Lady Godiva of Coventry, wife of Leofric, Earl of Mercia, was heroine of the legend and poem by Tennyson.

GOLDA—Old English: "Golden one, golden-haired." English variations: **Goldie, Goldy.** Golda Meir, Prime Minister of Israel, Goldie Hawn, actress.

GRACE—Latin: **Gratia.** "Graceful, attractive one." Grace Coolidge, wife of U.S. President Calvin Coolidge; Princess Grace Kelly Grimaldi of Monaco; Grace Jones, singer.
Foreign variations: **Grazia** (Italian), **Engracia** (Spanish), **Giorsal** (Scottish).

GREER—See **Gregoria.**

GREGORIA—Latin: **Gregorius.** "Watchful one." A feminine form of **Gregory.** Greer Garson, actress.
English variation: **Greer.**

GRETA, GRETCHEN, GRETE, GRETEL—See **Margaret.**

GRISELDA—Old German: **Grisja-hilde.** "Gray battle-maiden." A character in Boccaccio's *Decameron.*
English nicknames: **Selda, Zelda.**
English variations: **Chriselda, Grishilda, Grizelda.**
Foreign variations: **Grishilde, Griseldis** (German, Dutch), **Griselda** (French, Italian).

GUENNA—See **Gwendolyn, Guinevere.**

GUIDA—Italian: **Guida.** "A guide." A woman ordained to guide or teach others.
Alternate, Old German: **Wido.** "Warrior maid."

GUILLA—See **Wilhelmina**

GUINEVERE—Old Welsh: **Gwenhwyvar.** "White wave, white phantom." The wife of King Arthur in English legends. See **Gwendolyn, Genevieve.**
English variations: **Gaynor, Gaenna, Gwenore, Jennifer, Genevieve, Vanora.**
Foreign variations: **Ginevra** (Italian).

GUNHILDA—Old Norse: **Gunn-hildr.** "Warrior battle-maid." A daughter of the Norsemen who fought beside the man she loved.
Gunhilda, daughter of a Polish duke, was the queen of Danish King Sweyn Forkbeard and mother of King Canute of Denmark and England, 11th century.

GUSTAVA—Swedish: **Gustaf.** "Staff of the Goths."
English nicknames: **Gussie, Gussy.**

GWENDA—See **Gwendolyn.**

GWENDOLYN—Old Welsh: "White-haired one; lady of the new vision." Gwendolyn was the wife of Merlin the magician in old Welsh legends. See **Guinevere.**
English nicknames: **Gwen, Gwennie, Gwenda, Guenna, Gwyn, Gwenyth, Wendy.**
English variations: **Gwendaline, Gwendolen, Gwendoline.**

GWYNETH—Old Welsh: **Gwynedd.** "White, blessed one."

GWYNNE—Old Welsh: **Gwyn.** "White or fair one."

GYPSY—Old English:

Gypcyan. "A gypsy, a wanderer." Gypsy Rose Lee, actress.

GYTHA—Old English: "A gift"; or Old Norse: Guthr.

"Warlike." The Danish Countess Gytha was the wife of 11th-century Godwin, Earl of Wessex, England. English variation: Githa.

H

HADRIA—See Adria.

HAGAR—Hebrew: Haghar. "Forsaken." Hagar in the Bible was an Egyptian slave of Sarah, the wife of Abraham. "Abraham sent Hagar with her son into the wilderness." —Gen 21:14.

HAIDEE—Greek: Aidoios. "Modest; honored." Haidee was a Greek girl in Byron's *Don Juan*.

HALCYONE—Greek: Halkyon. "Sea-conceived; kingfisher bird." In Greek myths Halcyone, daughter of Acolus, in grief for her drowned husband, threw herself into the sea and was changed into a kingfisher.

HALDANA—Old Norse: Half-Dan. "Half Danish." Feminine of Halden.

HALFRIDA—Old German: Hali-frid. "Peaceful heroine"; or Old English: Heall-frith. "Peaceful hall or home."

HALIMEDA—Greek: Halimdes. "Thinking of the sea." English nicknames: Hallie, Meda.

HANNAH—Hebrew: Khannah. "Graceful one." See Ann. Hannah in the Bible was the mother of the prophet Samuel. Hannah Arendt, philosopher, Hana Mandlikova, tennis player. English nicknames: Hannie, Hanny, Annie, Nan, Hanna, Nanny. English variations: Anna, Anne, Hana.

HARALDA—Old Norse: Harvald. "Army ruler." Feminine of Harold. English nicknames: Hallie, Hally.

HARMONY—Latin: Harmonia. "Concord, harmony." English variations: Harmonia, Harmonie.

HARRIET—Old French: Hanriette. "Estate or home ruler." See Henrietta. Harriet Beecher Stowe, American writer (1812–1896); Harriet Tubman, conductor on the Underground Railroad during America's Civil War.

HATTIE—See Henrietta.

HAYLEY—Modern U.S.:

"clever, ingenious one."
Hayley Mills, actress. Also,
Haley.

HAZEL—Old English:
Haesel. "Hazelnut tree."
Among the ancient people
of Europe the hazel branch
was an insignia of rulership.
Foreign variation: **Aveline**
(French).

HEATHER—Middle En-
glish: **Hadder.** "The heather
flower or shrub." Heather
McCrae, actress.

HEBE—Greek: **Hebe.**
"Youth." Hebe, daughter of
Zeus in Greek myths, was
the goddess of youth.

HEDDA—Old German:
Hadu. "Strife." From the Ibsen
play, *Hedda Gabler*, and
from Hedda Hopper, noted
columnist, actress. See
Hedwig.
English variations: **Heddi,
Heddy, Hedy.**

HEDWIG—Old German:
Haduwig. "Strife, fight."
English variations: **Heda,
Hedwiga.**
Foreign variations: **Hedwig,
Hedda** (German), **Hedvige**
(French), **Hedy** (Slavic).

HEDY—Greek: **Hedy.**
"Sweet, pleasant." See
Hedda, Hedwig. Hedy
Lamarr, actress.

HEIDI—Originally a nickname for **Adelaide:** "noble
one." Made famous by the
novel *Heidi* by Johanna Spyri.

HELEN—Greek: **Helene.**
"Light; a torch." St. Helena,
mother of the Emperor
Constantine; Helen Keller,
deaf, dumb, blind lecturer
and writer; Helen Hayes,
noted American actress.
English nicknames: **Nell,
Nellie, Nelly, Lena, Lina.**
English variations: **Helena,
Helene, Eleanore, Elenore,
Elinore, Elaine, Elane, Ella,
Ellie, Elna, Ellen, Ellene,
Ellyn, Elyn, Ellette, Nellette,
Nelliana, Ileana, Elene,
Leonora, Leonore, Lenore,
Leora, Lora, Lana, Nora,
Norah.**
Foreign variations: **Helena,
Helene** (German), **Hélène**
(French), **Elena** (Italian,
Spanish).

HELENA—See **Helen.**

HELENE—See **Helen.**

HELGA—Old German:
Halag. "Pious, religious,
holy." See **Olga.**

HELICE—Greek: **Helike.**
"Spiral." Helike was a Greek
nymph in mythology.

HELMA—Old German:
Helm. "Helmet or protection." Also a shortened
form of **Wilhelmina.**
English variation: **Hilma.**

HELOISE—See **Louise.**
Heloise was a 12th-century
French abbess and scholar,
renowed for her romance with
Abelard.

HENRIETTA—French:

Henriette. "Estate or home ruler." A feminine form of **Henry.** Henriette Maria, wife of England's King Charles I; Henrietta (Hetty) Green, American financier.
English nicknames: **Hettie, Hetty, Hattie, Hatty, Ettie, Etta, Netta, Nettie, Netty, Yetta.**
English variations: **Harriet, Harriette, Harriott, Henriette.**
Foreign variations: **Henriette** (French, German), **Hendrika** (Dutch), **Henrika** (Swedish), **Enrichetta** (Italian), **Enriqueta** (Spanish), **Eiric** (Scottish).

HENRIKA—See **Henrietta.**

HERA—Greek: "ruling lady; queen." Hera was the Greek queen of heaven, the wife of Zeus.

HERMIA—See **Hermione, Erma.**

HERMINA—See **Hermoine, Erma.**

HERMINE—See **Hermoinc, Erma.**

HERMIONE—Greek: "of the world or earth." See **Erma.** In Greek myths Hermione was the daughter of Menelaus and Helen of Troy. She was a queen in Shakespeare's *A Winter's Tale.* Namesakes include Hermione Baddeley, Hermione Gingold, English actresses.

English variations: **Hermia, Hermine, Herminia.**

HERMOSA—Spanish: "beautiful."

HERTHA—Old English: **Ertha.** "Earth." Hertha was the old Teutonic goddess of peace and fertility.
English variations: **Herta, Eartha, Ertha, Erda.**

HESPER—Greek: **Hesperos.** "Evening or evening star." "The evening star, love's harbinger."—Milton. Hesperia was the Greek name for Italy. See **Esther.**
English variations: **Hespera, Hesperia.**

HESTER—Greek: **Aster** "Star." See **Esther.** Hester Prynne, heroine of Hawthorne's *The Scarlet Letter.*
English variation: **Hesther.**

HIBERNIA—Latin: "Ireland."

HIBISCUS—Latin: "the marsh-mallow plant and flower."

HILARY—Latin: **Hilaria:** "Cheerful one." The name Hillaria is in the English "Hundred Roll's" dated 1273. Also: **Hillary.**

HILDA—Old German: **Hilde.** "Battle maid." Hilda was one of the Valkyrie in Norse myths, a beautiful maiden who escorted souls to Valhalla. St. Hild, an abbess, A.D. 614–680.
English variations: **Hild, Hilde, Hilda, Hildie, Hildy.**

HILDEGARDE—Old German: **Hildi-gard.** "Battle wand, battle maiden, battle stronghold." Hildegard, chanteuse and actress; St. Hildegarde, German 11th-century abbess.

HILDEMAR—Old German: **Hildi-mar.** "Battle-celebrated or glorious."

HILDRETH—Old German: **Hildi-reth.** "Battle counselor." A feminine adviser on battle strategy.

HILMA—see **Helma.**

HOLDA—Old German: "concealed" or "beloved." Frau Holda in German myths led the spirits in a swift, celestial flight. Foreign variations: **Holde, Holle, Hulda** (German).

HOLLY—Old English: **Holea.** "Holly tree"; or Old English: **Halig.** "Holy." Named for the decorative Christmas holly; or for a child born at Christmas.

HONEY—Old English: **Hunig.** "Sweet one." See **Honbria.**

HONOR—Latin: **Honoria**: "Honor." Honor Moore, writer; Honor Blackman, actress.

HONORIA—Latin: "Honor; honorable one." English nicknames: **Honey, Nora, Norah, Norry.**

HOPE—Old English: "hope, expectation, desire." A name first popularized by the Puritans. Hope Lange, actress.

HORATIA—Latin: **Horatius.** "Keeper of the hours." Feminine form of **Horace.** English variation: **Horacia.**

HORTENSE—Latin: **Hortensia.** "Of the garden, a gardener." Hortense Calisher, novelist. English variation: **Hortensia.** Foreign variations: **Hortensia** (German, Dutch, Danish), **Ortensia** (Italian).

HOSHI—Japanese: "star."

HUBERTA—Old German: **Hugi-beraht.** "Brilliant mind." Feminine of **Hubert.**

HUETTE—Old English: **Hugiet.** Feminine of **Hugh.** English variations: **Hughette, Hugette, Huetta.**

HULDA—Old German: **Hulda.** "Gracious or beloved." Hebrew: **Huldah.** "Weasel." Huldah was an ancient Biblical prophetess. English nicknames: **Huldie, Huldy.**

HYACINTH—Greek: **Hyakinthos.** "Hyacinth flower or purple hyacinth color." English nicknames: **Cinthie, Cynthie, Jackie, Jacky.** English variations: **Hyacintha, Hyacinthia, Jacintha, Jacinthe.** Foreign variations: **Hyacinthe**

(French), **Hyacinthie** (German), **Giacinta** (Italian), **Jacinta** (Spanish).

HYPATIA—Greek: **Hypate.** "Highest." Hypatia was a beautiful, wise 5th-century martyred philosopher and mathematician.

I

IANTHA—Greek: **Ianthinos.** "Violet-colored flower." English variations: **Ianthina, Janthina.**

IDA—Old German: "industrious"; or Old English: **Eada.** "Prosperous, happy." Mount Ida in Crete was famous in Greek myths, the place where Jupiter was concealed as a baby. Namesakes include Ida Tarbell, writer; Ida Lupino, actress. English variations: **Idalia, Idalina, Idaline.**

IDUNA—Old Norse: "Lover"; or Old German: **Ida.** "Industrious." In Norse myths Iduna was the keeper of the golden apples of youth. English variation: **Idonia.**

IERNE—Late Latin: "Ireland."

IGNATIA—Latin: "fiery, ardent one." A girl whose temper flared between her mirth and tears. Feminine form of **Ignatius.**

ILA—Old French: **Isle.** "From the island"; or Old English: **Idle.** "Battle."

ILEANA—Greek: **Iliona.** "From the city of Ilion or Troy." Ileana is a name used by Greek royalty.

ILKA—Slavic: **Milka.** "Flattering or industrious." Ilka Chase, actress-writer.

ILONA—Hungarian: "beautiful one." Greek: "a light." See **Helen.** Ilona Massey, actress. Also: **Ilone.**

ILSA—Teutonic: "noble maiden." English variations: **Ilse, Elsa, Else.**

IMOGENE—Latin: **Imaginis** "An image or likeness." Imogene Coca, comedienne. Also: **Imogen.**

IMPERIA—Latin: **Imperialis.** "Imperial one."

INA—Latin: **Ina.** A Latin feminine name-suffix added to masculine names. See **Catherine.** Namesakes: Ina Claire, Ina Balin, actresses.

INEZ—Spanish form of **Agnes.** See **Agnes.**

INGRID—Old Norse: **Ingrida.** "Hero's daughter; beautiful." Ing was an ancient Norse name for a deity, hero, or son. Ingrid Bergman, actress. Scandinavian variations: **Inga,**

**Inge, Inger, Ingunna,
Ingaberg.**

INIGA—Latin: **Ignatia.**
"Fiery, ardent one." A
transposed spelling of
Ignatia, from the Spanish
"Inigo."

IOLA—Greek: **Iole.** "Dawn
cloud; violet color." In Greek
myths Iole was a princess
captured by Hercules.
English variation: **Iole.**

IOLANTHE—Greek: "vio-
let flower." Popularized by a
light opera by Gilbert and
Sullivan. See **Yolanda.**

IONA—Greek: "violet."
Celtic: the name of an island
where many ancient Celtic
kings are buried. Also: **Ione,
Ionia.**

IRENE—Greek: **Eirene.**
"Peace." Irene was the Greek
goddess of peace. Irene
Joliot-Curie, chemist; Irene
Dunne, actress.
English nicknames: **Rene,
Rena.**
English variations: **Irena,
Irina, Eirena, Erena.**

IRIS—Greek: "the rainbow;
the iris flower." Iris was the
messenger of the Greek
gods, also representing the
rainbow. Iris Murdoch,
British novelist.

IRMA—Latin: **Herminia.**
"High-ranking person"; or Old
German: **Era-man.** "Hon-
orable, noble person. See
Erma.

IRVETTE—Old English:

Earwine. "Sea friend."
Feminine form of **Irving.**

ISA—Old German: **Isan.**
"Iron-willed one." See **Isabel.**

ISABEL—Old Spanish:
Ysabel. "Consecrated to
God." The Spanish form of
Elizabeth. Isabel (Isabella)
Queen of Spain, patroness
of Columbus; Isabella Bird,
19th-century explorer.
English nicknames: **Issie,
Issy, Bella, Belle, Ib, Isa.**
English variations: **Isabella,
Isabelle.**
Foreign variations: **Isabeau**
(French), **Isabella** (Italian),
Isabel (Spanish), **Isabelle**
(German), **Iseabal** (Scottish).

ISADORA—Greek: "gift of
Isis." Feminine form of
Isidore. Isadora Duncan,
dancer and teacher.

ISIS—Egyptian: **Ast.** "Supreme goddess or spirit." Isis
was the ancient Egyptian
goddess of motherhood,
fertility, and the moon.

ISLEEN—see **Aislinn.**

ISOLDE—Old Welsh:
Eyslk. "The fair one." In the
old English King Arthur
legends Isolde or Iseult was
the wife of Tristan; Isolde is
also in German myths and
celebrated from Wagner's
opera *Tristan and Isolda.*
Also: **Isolda.**

ITA—Old Irish Gaelic: **Itu.**
"Thirst." St. Ita or Ytha of
Ireland, 6th century.

IVA—Old French: Ive. "Yewtree." See Jane. English variation: Ivanna.

IVY—Old English: Ifig. "Ivy vine." The Ivy was sacred to Dionysus and Bacchus in Greek and Roman myths. Ivy Baker Priest, former Treasurer of the U.S. Also: Ivory.

J

JACINTA—Spanish, Greek: "hyacinth, purple." Also: Jacinth, Jacinna, Jacynth.

JACOBA—Late Latin: Jacoba. "The supplanter." A feminine form of Jacob, James. English variations: Jacobina, Jacobine.

JACQUELINE—Old French: "the supplanter." A feminine form of Jacob, James, Jacques. Jacqueline Kennedy Onassis, editor; Jaclyn Smith, actress; Jacqueline Cochran, aviatrix. English nicknames: Jackie, Jacky. English variations: Jacquelyn, Jacquetta, Jackelyn, Jaclyn.

JADE—Spanish: Ijada. "Jade stone."

JAEL—Hebrew: "wild mountain goat." Also, a Biblical heroine. Used in Israel for both girls and boys.

JAMIE—Modern U.S., feminine form of James. English variations: Jamee, Jami, Jayme, Jaymee, Jaime, Jaimie.

JAMILA—Arabic: "beautiful."

JAN—See Jane.

JANE—Hebrew: Y-hohhanan. "God is gracious." A feminine form of John. Jane Austen, English novelist, Jane Addams, social worker; actresses Jane Russell, Jane Powell, Jane Wyman, Jane Fonda, Jayne Mansfield. English nicknames: Janie, Janey, Janny, Jeanie, Jeaney, Jennie, Jenny, Netta, Zaneta. English variations: Jan, Janae, Janet, Janette, Janice, Janis, Janina, Janna, Jayne, Jean, Jeanne, Jennette, Joan, Joanne, Joana, Joanna. Foreign variations: Jeanne, Jeannette (French), Johanna (German), Gianina, Giovanna (Italian), Juana, Juanita (Spanish), Sinead, Shena, Sheena (Irish), Sine, Seonaid (Scottish).

JANELLE—A compound of Jane and Ellen. Janelle Taylor, novelist.

JANET—see Jane.

JANICE—see Jane.

JANINA—See Jane.

JANTHINA—See Ianthe.

JASMINE—Persian: **Yasaman.** "The jasmine flower." Jessamyn West, writer.
English variations: **Jasmina, Jasmin, Jessamine, Jessamyn.**
Foreign variations: **Yasmine, Yasiman** (India).

JAYNE—Sanskrit: **Jina.** "Victorious one." See **Jane.**

JEAN—French: **Jeanne.** "God is gracious." See **Jane.** St. Jeanne D'Arc (Joan of Arc), 15th-century French martyr; Jean Simmons, actress.

JEANNETTE—See **Jane.**

JEMIMA—Hebrew: **Yemimah.** "A dove." An ancient symbol of purity and peace. In the Bible, Jemima was a daughter of Job.
English nicknames: **Jemie, Jemmie, Mimi.**

JENILEE—Modern combination of **Jenny** and **Lee.** Also: **Jenalee.** Jennilee Harrison, actress.

JENNIFER—See **Guinevere.** "White-cheeked, white wave, white phantom." Popular modern U.S. name.
English nicknames: **Jenny, Jennie, Jenni, Jen.**
English variations: **Gennifer, Genna, Genni, Gennie.**

JENNY—See **Jane, Jennifer.**

JEREMIA—Hebrew: **Yirmeyah.** "Exalted of the Lord." Feminine form of **Jeremiah.**
English nicknames: **Jeri, Jerrie, Jerry.**

JERI—See **Geraldine, Jeremia.**

JERRI, JERRY—See **Geraldine, Jeremia.**

JERUSHA—Hebrew: **Yerushah.** "Possessed or married."

JESSAMINE—See **Jasmine.**

JESSICA—Hebrew: **Yishay.** "Wealthy one." Jessica was Shylock's daughter in Shakespeare's *The Merchant of Venice.* Jessica Tandy, Jessica Lange, actresses.
English variations: **Jessie, Jessalynn, Jyssica, Jesseca.**

JESSIE—See **Jessica.**

JEWEL—Old French: **Juel.** "A precious thing or gem."

JILL—See **Julia, Gillian.** Jill St. John, actress.
English nicknames: **Jilly, Jilli, Jillie.**

JINX—Latin: **Inyx.** "Spell." Jinx Falkenburg, actress.
English variation: **Jynx.**

JOAKIMA—Hebrew: **Jehoaiakim.** "The Lord will set up or judge." Feminine of **Joachim.**

JOAN—See **Jane.** Actresses Joan Crawford, Joan Fontaine; Joan Benoit, Olympic marathon champion.

JOANNA—see **Jane.**

JOBINA—Hebrew: **Iyyobh.** "Afflicted, persecuted." "The gem cannot be polished without friction, nor man perfected without trials." —Chinese Proverb.

English variation: **Jobyna.**

JOCASTA—Italian: "Light-hearted."

JOCELYN—Old English: **Goscelin.** "The just one." Latin: "playful, merry." A feminine variation of **Justin.** English variations: **Jocelyne, Jocellne, Joscclyne, Josceline, Justine.**

JOCOSA—Latin: **Jocosus.** "Humorous, joking."

JODY—See **Judith.** Also: **Jodie.** Jodie Foster, actress.

JOELLE—Hebrew: "the Lord is willing." Feminine of **Joel.** Also: **Joella, Joela.**

JOHANNA—See **Jane.**

JOLETTA—See **Julia.**

JOLINE—Hebrew: "she will increase." Modern form of **Josephine.** Feminine of **Joseph.** Also: **Joleen, Jolene.**

JORDANA—Hebrew: **Yarden.** "The descending." Feminine form of **Jordan.**

JOSEPHA—See **Josephine.**

JOSEPHINE—Hebrew: **Yoseph.** "she will add; increaser." Feminine of **Joseph.** Josephine, Empress of France, 1763–1814; Josephine Hull, American actress. English nicknames: **Jo, Josie.** English variations: **Josepha, Josephina, Joette, Josette.** Foreign variations: **Josephe, Josephine, Fifi, Fifine** (French), **Josepha** (German),

Giuseppina (Italian), **Josefa, Josefina, Pepita** (Spanish), **Seosaimhthin** (Irish).

JOVITA—Latin: **Jovialis.** "Joyful."

JOY—Latin: **Joia.** "Joyful one." Also: **Joie.** English variations: **Joice, Joyce, Joyous.**

JOYCE—French: **Joyeuse.** "Joyful." See **Joy.**

JUANITA—See **Jane.**

JUDITH—Hebrew: **Yehudith.** "Praised." Judith's story is in the Apocrypha, an appendix to the Bible. Judith Anderson, actress. English nicknames: **Judie, Judy, Jody.** Foreign variations: **Guiditta** (Italian), **Siobhan** (Irish), **Siubhan** (Scottish).

JUDY—See **Judith.**

JULI—See **Julia.**

JULIA—Latin: "youthful one." Feminine form of **Julius.** Julia Ward Howe, poet, (1819–1910); Juliana, Queen of the Netherlands; actresses Julie Andrews, Julie Harris. English nicknames: **Julie, Jill, Juli, Gillie.** English variations: **Juliet, Julietta, Juliette, Juliana, Julina, Juline, Joletta.** Foreign variations: **Giulia, Giulietta** (Italian), **Julie, Juliette** (French), **Julia, Julieta** (Spanish), **Julie**

(German), **Sile** (Irish), **Sileas** (Scottish).

JULIET—See **Julia**.

JUNE—Latin: **Junius**. "Born in June." Actresses June Havoc, June Allyson.
English variations: **Junia, Juniata, Junette, Junine**.

JUNELLA—Compound of **June** and **Ella**.

JUNO—Latin: "heavenly one." Juno was the queen of the goddesses in Roman myth.

JUSTINE—Latin: **Justus**. "The just one." A feminine form of **Justus**.
English variations: **Justina, Justa, Joscelyn**.
Foreign variations: **Giustina** (Italian), **Justina** (Spanish).

K

KALA—Hindi: "black, time."

KALILA—Arabic: "sweetheart, loved one." Also: **Kalilla, Kaylee**.

KAMA—Sanskrit: "love." The Hindu love god Kama, a handsome youth, rode a parrot and carried a bow of sugar cane with a bowstring of bees, each arrow tipped with a flower.

KAMEKO—Japanese: "child of the tortoise," which symbolizes longevity.

KARA—See **Cara**.

KAREN—Popular form of **Catherine**. Greek: "pure." Also: **Karin, Korin**. Karen Horney, psychologist, writer; Karen Black, actress.

KARLA—Modern variant of **Carol, Caroline**: "strong, womanly." Also: **Kari**.

KASMIRA—Old Slavic:

Kazatimiru. "Commands peace."

KATE—Popular diminutive of **Katherine**: "the pure one." English nicknames: **Kati, Katie, Katy, Katina**.

KATHERINE—See **Catherine**.

KATHLEEN—See **Catherine**.

KAYE—See **Catherine**.

KEELY—Irish Gaelic: **Cadhla**. "Beautiful one." Keely Smith, singer.

KEISHA—Popular modern U.S. name of unclear origin. See **Lakeisha**.

KELDA—Old Norse: "a spring." English nickname: **Kelly**.

KELILAH—Hebrew: "laurel, crown, victory." Also: **Kelula, Kyla, Kyle**.

KELLY—Irish Gaelic:

Ceallach. "Warrior-maid."
Used for both girls and
boys.

KENDA—Modern U.S.:
"child of pure water."

KENYA—Modern U.S.: the
name of the country used as a
first name.

KENYATTA—Modern U.S.:
the surname of the African
leader, Jomo Kenyatta,
used as a first name. Also:
Kenyetta.

KERRY—Irish Gaelic:
Ciarda. "Dark one."

KETTI—See **Catherine.**
Ketti Frings, writer, dramatist.

KETURA—Hebrew: **Qeturah.**
"Incense." Named for the
incense that perfumed the
air during religious services.

KIM—Old English: **Cyne.**
"Chief, ruler." Also a
shortened form of **Kimberley.**
Actresses Kim Stanley, Kim
Novak, Kim Hunter.

KIMBERLEY—Old En-
glish: **Cyne-burh-leah.** "From
the royal-fortress meadow."

KINETA—Greek: **Kinetikos.**
"Active one."

KIRSTIN—Originally a Scandinavian form of Christine;
modern U.S. usage. See
Christine, Kristen.

KIZZY—Modern U.S. Alex
Haley claims an African origin
for this name in *Roots,* but
evidence suggests it is a form
of Keziah, a Biblical name
from the Hebrew, "Cassia,"
for the cassia tree. Also:
Kizzie.

KORA—See **Cora.**

KOREN—Greek: **Kore.**
"The maiden."

KRISTEN—Originally a
Scandinavian form of Chris-
tine; now a popular U.S.
name. See **Christine.** Also:
**Kirsten, Kirstin, Kristina,
Krista, Kristel, Krysten,
Kristyn, Kristy, Krystyna.**

KYNA—Irish Gaelic: **Conn.**
"Intelligence, wisdom"; or
Irish Gaelic: **Con.** "High,
exalted." Feminine of **Conan.**

L

LAKEISHA—Modern U.S.
name gaining in popularity.
A combination of La- and a pet
name which can also be
used independently. Also:
**Lashawn, Latanya, Latonya,
Latasha, Latisha, Latoya,
Latrice.**

LALA—Slavic: "the tulip
flower."

LALAGE—Greek: "free of
Speech." Also: **Lalia.**

LALITA—Sanskrit: "pleasing, artless."

LANA—See **Helen, Alanna.**
Lana Turner, actress.

LANETTE—Old Anglo-French: **Lane-et.** "From the little lane."

LANI—Hawaiian: "sky."

LANNA—see **Helen, Alanna.**

LARA—Latin: "shining, famous one"; or **Etruscan**: "lordly." Russian form of **Lanssa**, from Greek; "Cheerful." In Roman myths Lara was a daughter of the river god Almo.

LARAINE—Latin: **Larus.** "Seabird; gull." See **Lorraine.** English variations: **Larine, Larina.**

LA REINA—Spanish: "the queen."
English variations: **Lareina, Larena.**
Foreign variation: **La reine** (French).

LARISSA—Greek: "cheerful one." A Greek princess, namesake of cities and monuments.

LARK—Middle English: **Larke.** "Singing lark or skylark."

LA ROUX—French: **Roux.** "Redhead."

LASSIE—Middle English: **Lasse.** "Little girl." A Scottish derivation.

LATONIA—Latin: **Latona.** "Sacred to Latona." Latona was the mother of Apollo and Diana in Roman myths.

LATOYA—See **Lakeisha.**
Latoya Jackson, singer.

LAURA—Latin: **Laures.** "A crown of laurel leaves." A wreath of laurel leaves was the ancient emblem of victory. Feminine of **Lawrence.** Loretta Young, Laurette Taylor, actresses; Lorna Doone, fictional heroine. English nicknames: **Laurie, Lori, Lorrie.**
English variations: **Laurel, Lauvelle, Lauren, Laureen, Laurena, Laurene, Lauretta, Laurette, Lora, Loren, Lorena, Lorene, Loretta, Lorette, Lorine, Lorita, Lorna.**
Foreign variations: **Lorenza** (Italian), **Laure, Laurette** (French), **Laura** (Spanish, German).

LAUREN—See **Laura.**
Also **Laurel, Laurelle.** Lauren Bacall, actress; Lauren Hutton, model.

LAVEDA—Latin: **Lavare.** "Purified one."
English variations: **Lavetta, Lavette.**

LA VERNE—Old French: **La vergne.** "From the alder-tree grove." or Latin: **Vernis.** "Springlike." Also: **Laverine.**

LAVINIA—Latin: **Lavare.** "Purified"; or Latin: **Lavinia.** "Lady from Latium."
English variation: **Lavina.**

LEA—See **Lee, Leah.**

LEAH—Hebrew: "weary

one." Leah was Jacob's wife in
the Bible.
English variations: **Lea, Lee,
Leigh, Lia, Liah.**

LEALA—Old French: **Leial.**
"Faithful, loyal one."
English variations: **Lealia,
Lealie.**

LEANA—See **Liana.**

LEANDRA—Latin: "like a
lioness." Also **Leodora,
Leoine, Leoline, Leona,
Leoarrie, Leonelle.**

LEANNE—Compound of
the names **Lee** and **Anne.**
See **Liana.**

LEATRICE—Compound of
Leah and **Beatrice.**

LEDA—See **Letitia.** In
Greek myths Leda was the
mother of Helen of Troy.

LEE—Old English: **Leah.**
"From the pasture meadow";
or Irish Gaelic: **Laoidheach.**
"Poetic." Lee Remick, actress.

LEILA—Arabic: **Layla.**
"Dark as night." Leila was the
heroine of an ancient
Persian legend, "Leila and
Majnum."
English variations: **Leilia,
Lela, Lila.**

LEILANI—Hawaiian: **Lei-
Lani.** "Heavenly flower."

LELA—See **Leila.**

LEMUELA—Hebrew: **Lemu'el**
"Consecreated to God."
Feminine of **Lemuel.**

LENA—Latin: "she who

allures." See **Madeline,
Helen.** Lena Horne, singer, actress; Lina Wertmuller,
film director.
English variation: **Lina.**

LENIS—Latin: "smooth
soft, mild."
English variations: **Lena,
Lene, Leneta, Lenita,
Lenos.**

LENORE—See **Eleanore,
Helen.**

LEODA—Old German:
Leute. "Woman of the
people."
English variation: **Leota.**

LEOLA—Latin: "lion";
Teutonic: "dear." A feminine
form of **Leo.**

LEOMA—Old English:
"light, brightness."

LEONA—French: **Léonie.**
"Lion."
English variations: **Leonie,
Leoine, Leonelle.**

LEONARDA—Old Frankish:
Leon-hard. "Lion-brave."
Foreign variations: Leonarde
(Italian), **Leonarda** (Ger-
man, Spanish).

LEONORE—See **Elea-
nore, Helen.** Leonora,
heroine of Beethoven's
opera *Fidelio.*

LEONTINE—Latin: **Leo.**
"Lionlike." Leontyne Price,
opera singer.
English variation: **Leontyne.**

LEOPOLDINE—Old Ger-
man: **Leut-pald.** "Bold for the
people."

English variations: **Leopolda,**
Leopoldina.

LEOTA—See **Leoda.**

LEOTIE—North American
Indian: "prairie flower."

LESLIE—Scottish Gaelic:
Liosliath. "Dweller at the gray
fortress."
English variation : **Lesley.**

LETA—See **Letitia.**

LETHA—Greek: **Lethe.**
"Forgetfulness." In Greek
myths, the river of oblivion
whose waters caused forgetful-
ness.
English variations: **Lethia,**
Leitha, Leithia, Leda,
Leta.

LETITIA—Latin: **Laetitia.**
"Gladness." Letitia Baldridge,
author.
English nicknames: **Leta,**
Leda, Letty, Tish.
English variations: **Leticia,**
Letice.
Foreign variations: **Letizia**
(Italian), **Léetice** (French),
Leticia (Spanish).

LETTY—See **Letitia.**

LEVANA—Late Latin: "the
rising sun." A sister of the
dawn. The Roman goddess
Levana was the patron of
childbirth, lifting newborn
children from the earth.

LEVIA—Hebrew: "to join."

LEVINA—Middle English:
Levene. "A flash, lightning."

LEWANNA—Hebrew: **Le-**
bhanah. "The beaming, white
one; the moon."

LEXINE—See **Alexandra.**

LEYA—Spanish **Ley.** "Loy-
alty or law."

LIANA—French: **Liane.** "A
climbing vine."
English variations: **Liane,**
Lianna, Lianne, Leana.

LIBERTY—Middle English:
"Free." Also: **Libby.**

LIBBY—See **Elizabeth.**
Libby Holman, actress,
chanteuse.

LILA—Hindi: "capricious-
ness of fate"; Persian: "lilac";
Polish, short for Leopoldine,
"defender of the people."
Also: **Lilia.** Lila Kedrova,
actress.

LILAC—Persian: **Nilak.**
"Bluish color; a lilac flower."

LILIAN—see **Lillian.**

LILITH—East Semitic:
Lilitu. "Belonging to the
night." Lilith, the first wife
of Adam in ancient Eastern
mythology.

LILLIAN—Latin: **Lilium.**
"A lily flower." Lillian Russell,
actress, singer (1861–1922):
Lily Pons, opera singer;
Lillian Gish, actress.
English nicknames: **Lil, Lili,**
Lilli, Lilly, Lily.
English variations: **Lilian,**
Liliana, Liliane, Lilyan,
Lilias.
Foreign variations: **Lili**

(German), **Lis** (French), **Lilies** (Scottish).

LILY—See **Lillian**.

LILYBET—Cornish form of **Elizabeth**, "God's promise."

LINA—See **Lena, Caroline, Adeline**.

LINDA—Spanish: "pretty one, beautiful." Actresses Linda Evans, Lynda Day George.
English variations: **Lynda, Lindy**.

LINDSAY—Old English: "from the linden tree island." Lindsay Wagner, actress.
Also: **Lindsey**.

LINETTE—Old French: **Linette**. "The linnet bird, " based on Latin: **Linum**. "Flax." The linnet feeds on flax seeds. In the King Arthur legends Lynette was the beloved of Gareth.
English variations: **Linnet, Linetta, Lynette**.

LINNEA—Old Norse: **Lind**, "Limetree."
English variation: **Lynnea**.

LISA—Popular modern variation of **Elizabeth**. Lisa Del Giocondo, subject of Da Vinci's "Mona Lisa." Also: **Leesa**.

LISBETH—See **Elizabeth**.

LISSA—Old English: "honey."

LITA—See **Carmel**.

LIVANA—Hebrew: "white" or "the moon." Also: **Lsuana**.

LIVIA—See **Olivia**.

LIZA—See **Elizabeth**. Liza Minnelli, actress-singer.

LIZABETH—See **Elizabeth**. Lizabeth Scott, actress.

LODEMA—Old English: Ladmann. "Pilot or guide."

LOIS—See **Louise**.

LOLA—See **Dolores, Charlotte**. Lola Montez, renowned 20th-century actress.

LOLITA—See **Dolores**.

LONA—Middle English: **Al-one**. "Solitary, lone one." A lady waiting for her knight in armor.

LORA—See **Laura, Helen**.

LORELEI—German: **Lurlei**. "Siren of the River Rhine."

LORENA—See **Laura**.

LORETTA—See **Laura**.

LORI—See **Laura**.

LORNA—See **Laura**.

LORRAINE—Old German: **Lothar-ingen**. "Place of Lothar." Lothar, an ancient warrior name, meant "famous army." Lotharingen was known by the French as the Duchy of Lorraine.
English variation: **Loraine**.

LOTTA—See **Charlotte**. Also: **Lotte**.

LOTUS—Greek: **Lotos**. "The lotus flower." The sacred Nile River lily of ancient Egypt.

LOUELLA—See **Luella.**

LOUISE—Old German: **Hlutwig.** "Famous warrior-maid." Louisa M. Alcott, Louise Bogan, authors.
English nicknames: **Lu, Lou, Lulie, Lulu.**
English variations: **Louisa, Eloisa, Eloise, Aloisa, Aloisia, Aloysia, Alison, Allison, Ludwiga, Lois, Loise, Louisette, Loyce.**
Foreign variations: **Louise, Héloïse, Lisette** (French), **Luise, Ludovika** (German), **Luisa** (Italian, Spanish), **Liusadh** (Scottish), **Labhaoise** (Irish).

LOVE—Old English: **Lufu.** "Tender affection."

LOYCE—See **Louise.** Loyce Whiteman, singer.

LUANA—Old German-Hebrew: **Lud-khannah.** "Graceful battle maid."
Popularized by the heroine of the stage play, *Bird of Paradise.*
English nicknames: **Lou, Lu.**
English variations: **Luane, Louanna, Luwana.**

LUCERNE—Latin: "circle of light." Also: **Lucerna.**

LUCIANNA—Italian compound from **Lucy** and **Anne.** Lucianna Paluzzi, Italian actress.

LUCILLE—See **Lucy.** Lucille Ball, film and television actress; St. Lucilla, 3rd-century Roman martyr.

LUCINDA—See **Lucy.** A 17th-century poetic spelling of **Lucy.**
English nickname: **Cindy.**

LUCITA—Spanish: "Mary of the light."

LUCRETIA—Latin: "riches; reward." Lucretia, a virtuous Roman wife, was immortalized in Shakespeare's poem. *The Rape of Lucrece.*
Lucrezia Borgia, Italian Duchess of Ferrara (1480–1519); Lucretia Mott, 19th-century American reformer;
Foreign variations: **Lucrèce** (French), **Lucrezia** (Italian), **Lucrecia** (Spanish).

LUCY—Latin. **Lucia.** "Light; bringer of light." St. Lucy of Syracuse, famous 3rd-century virgin martyr; Lucy Stone, 19th-century pioneer in advancement of women.
English nicknames: **Lou, Lu, Luce.**
English variations: **Luciana, Lucida, Lucinda, Lucile, Lucille, Lucette.**
Foreign variations: **Lucie, Lucienne** (French), **Lucie** (German), **Lucia** (Italian), **Lucia, Luz** (Spanish), **Liusadh** (Scottish), **Luighseach** (Irish).

LUDMILLA—Old Slavic: **Ljudumilu.** "Beloved by the people." Ludmilla Tcherina, ballerina.
Foreign variation: **Ludmila** (German).

LUELLA—Old English: **Hlud-self.** "Famous elf." Louella O. Parsons, noted columnist; English variations: **Louella, Loella, Luelle, Ludella.**

LUNETTA—Italian: "little moon." Derived from Luna, the name of the Roman moon goddess.

LUPE—Spanish-Mexican: Santa Maria de Guadalupe. A shortening through usage of the last syllables of the saint's name. Alternate, Latin: **Lupus.** "Wolf." Lupe Velez, actress.

LURLINE—German: **Lurlei.** "Siren." Circe, the temptress of Ulysses, was another siren. See **Lorelei.** Lurline Matson, wife of the founder of the shipping lines, after whom several liners were named. English variations: **Lura, Lurleen, Lurlene, Lurette.**

LUVENA—Middle-English-Latin:

Luve-ena. "Little beloved one."

LUZ—Spanish: "Mary of the light."

LYDIA—Greek: **Lydia.** "A woman of Lydia." Lydia, an ancient country of Asia Minor, was famed for its kings, Midas and Croesus, who became symbols of wealth. Foreign variations: **Lydie** (French), **Lidia** (Italian, Spanish), **Lidija** (Russian).

LYNN—Old English: **Hlynn.** "A waterfall or pool below a fall." Lynn Fontanne, actress. Also: **Lyn, Linn, Lynette.**

LYRIS—Greek: **Lyristes.** "Player on a lyre or harp." English variation: **Lyra.**

LYSANDRA—Greek: **Lysander.** "Liberator of men." The feminine of **Lysander,** an ancient Greek hero-name.

M

MAB—Irish Gaelic: **Meadhbh.** "Mirth, joy." Mab, Queen of the Fairies in Irish myths, was used in that role by Shakespeare in *Romeo and Juliet.* English variations: **Mave, Meave, Mavis.** Foreign variations: **Mab, Meave** (Irish), **Mavis** (French).

MABEL—Latin; **Amabilis.** "Lovable one." English variations: **Mabelle, Mable, Maybelle.** Foreign variations: **Mabelle** (French), **Maible** (Irish), **Moibeal** (Scottish).

MADELINE—Greek: **Magdalene.** "From Magdala." Magdala, meaning "ele-

vated, magnificent," on the
Sea of Galilee in Palestine,
was the birthplace of St. Mary
Magdalene, whose sins
were forgiven by Jesus Christ.
Namesakes include Made-
line, daughter of King Francis
I of France, who became
queen of James V of Scotland;
Madeline Kahn, actress.
English nicknames: **Mada,
Maddie, Maddy, Mala,
Lena, Lina, Maud.**
English variations: **Madeleine,
Madalena, Madelon, Madlen,
Madlin, Madel, Madella,
Madelle, Magdala, Magdalen,
Magdalene, Malena, Malina,
Marleen, Marlene, Marline.**
Foreign variations: **Madelaine,
Madeleine, Madelon** (French),
Magdalena, Madalena (Span-
ish), **Magdalene, Marlene,
Madlen, Magda, Mady**
(German), **Maddalena**
(Italian), **Maighdlin** (Irish).

MADELLE—See **Madeline.**

MADGE—See **Margaret.**

MADONNA—Latin: "my
lady." Madonna, rock star.

MADORA—See **Media.**

MADRA—Spanish: **Madre.**
"Mother."

MAE—See **May.**

MAGDA—See **Madeline,
Maida.**

MAGDALENE—See **Made-
line.**

MAGGY—See **Margaret.**

MAGNILDA—Old Ger-

man; **Magan-hildi.** "Powerful
battle-maiden"; or Latin-
German: **Magn-hildi.** "Great
battle-maiden."

MAGNOLIA—New Latin:
"magnolia flower and tree."
The magnolia was named
for Pierre Magnol, 17th-
century French botanist.
English nicknames: **Mag,
Maggie, Nola, Nolie.**

MAHALA—Hebrew: **Mahalah.**
"Tenderness." Mahalia Jack-
son, noted singer.
English variations: **Mahalah,
Mahalia.**

MAIA—Greek: "nurse or
mother." The month of May
was named for her, mother
of Mercury.

MAIDA—Old English:
Maegth. "A maiden."
English nicknames: **Maidie,
Mady.**
English variations: **Maidel,
Mayda, Mayde, Maydena.**
Foreign variations: **Magd,
Mady, Magda** (German).

MAISIE—See **Margaret.**

MAJESTA—Latin: **Majesta.**
"Majestic one." Majesta or
Maia, consort of Vulcan,
was the Roman goddess of the
month of May.

MALA—See **Madeline.**
Mala Powers, actress.

MALINA—See **Madeline,
Malinda.**

MALINDA—Greek: **Meilichos.**
"Mild, gentle one."

English nicknames: **Mailie,
Mally, Lindy.**
English variations: **Malinde,
Melinda, Malena, Malina,
Melina.**

MALLORY—Old German:
Madel-hari. "Council army;
army counselor"; or Old
French: **Mail-hair-er**
"Unfortunate; strong." Often
used as a masculine name.
Modern U.S. feminine.

MALVA—Greek: **Malako.**
"Soft, slender"; or Latin:
Malva. Mallow flower."
English variations: **Melva,
Melba.**

MALVINA—Irish Gaelic:
Maolmin. "Polished chief;
Latin: "sweet friend, sweet
wine." Feminine of **Malvin**
and **Melvin.** In ancient Irish
myths that were called the
Fenian Cycle, Malvina was
a heroine.
English nicknames: **Malva,
Malvie, Melva, Melvie,
Mal, Mel.**
English variations: **Melvina,
Melvine.**

MANDA—Spanish: "battle
maiden." Also: **Armanda,
Mandy.**

MANDISA—Xhosa (South
African): "sweet."

MANDY—Popular U.S.
form of **Amanda:** "worthy of
love." Also **Mandi, Mandie.**

MANSI—Hopi Indian:
"plucked flower."

MANUELA—Spanish: "God's
with us." A Spanish feminine
form of **Emmanuel.**

MARA—Hebrew: **Marah.**
"Bitter." A form of Mary.
English variations: **Maralina,
Maraline, Mari, Damara.**

MARALINE—See **Mara.**

MARCELLA—Latin: "be-
longing to Mars; martial one",
Teutonic: "intelligent con-
testant." A feminine form of
Marcus. Marcella, a Roman
widow, was a 4th-century
disciple of St. Jerome;
Marcella Sembrich, operatic
soprano.
English nicknames: **Marcie,
Marcy.**
English variations: **Marcelle,
Marcellina, Marcelline,
Marcile, Marcille.**
Foreign variations: **Marcelle**
(French), **Marcela** (Spanish).

MARCIA—Latin: "belong-
ing to Mars; martial one." A
feminine form of **Marcius**
and **Marcus.** St. Marcia was
an early Christian martyr.
Marsha Mason, actress.
English nicknames: **Marcie,
Marcy.**
English variations: **Marcelia,
Marcile, Marcille, Marchita,
Marquita, Marsha.**
Foreign variations: **Marcie**
(French), **Marcia** (Italian).

MARCILE—See **Marcella,
Marcia.**

MARE—Irish: **Maire.** See
Mary. Mare Winningham,
actress.

MARELDA—Old German:
Marhildi. "Famous battle-
maiden."
English variation: **Marilda.**

MARELLA—See **Mary.**

MARETTA—See **Mary.**

MARGARET—Latin: **Mar-
garita.** "A pearl." Honoring
Margaret, patron saint of
Scotland. Notables: Princess
Margaret of England; Margaret
Mitchell, author of *Gone with
the Wind*: Margaret Mead,
anthropologist.
English nicknames: **Marga,
Marge, Margie, Margo,
Madge, Mag, Maggie, Maggi,
Maisie, Meg, Meta, Greta,
Peg, Peggie, Peggy, Rita.**
English variations: **Margareta,
Margarita, Margery, Margory,
Marget, Margette, Margalo,
Margita, Marguerite, Mar-
jorie, Marjory, Miriam.**
Foreign variations: **Margherita**
(Italian), **Margarita, Rita**
(Spanish), **Marguerite, Margot**
(French), **Margarethe,
Margarete, Grete, Gretal,
Grethel, Gretchen** (German),
Margarete, Margreth (Dan-
ish), **Margaretha** (Dutch),
Mairghread (Irish, Scottish).

MARGOT—See **Margaret.**

MARI—See **Mary.** Mari
Gorman, actress.

MARIA, MARIE—See
Mary. Namesakes: Maria
Theresa, Empress of Austria
(1717–1780); Marie Curie,
co-discoverer of radium;
Maria Tallchief, ballerina.
Also: **Mariah.**

MARIAH—See **Marie.**
Also: **Maraya.**

MARIAN—Hebrew-English:
Mary-Anne. "Bitter-graceful."
or Old French: **Mari-on.**
"Little Mary." See **Mary,
Anne.** St. Mariana, Spanish,
"Lily of Madrid," 1565–1624;
Marian Anderson, singer.
English variations: **Marion,
Mariana, Marianna, Mari-
anne, Maryanne.**
Foreign variations: **Marianna**
(Italian), **Marianne** (French),
Mariana (Spanish), **Marianne**
(German).

MARIEL—Modern U.S.
name, a combination of **Mary**
and **Ellen.** Mariel Hemingway,
actress.

MARIETTA—See **Mary.**

MARIGOLD—English: **Marygold**
"The golden marigold flower."
A girl with hair like yellow
gold.

MARILYN—See **Mary.**
Marilyn Miller, Marilyn
Monroe, actresses.
English variations: **Marilin,
Marylin.**

MARINA—Latin: "of the
sea." St. Marina of Alexan-
dria, early Christian martyr;
Princess Marina of Greece
was married to Prince
George of England, 1934.
Marisa Berenson, actress.
English variations: **Marni,
Marna, Maris, Mari, Marinna,
Marisa, Marissa, Meris.**

MARJORIE—Old French:
Margerie. "A pearl." An early
form of **Marguerite**, the
French spelling of **Margaret**.
Marjorie Kinnan Rawlings,
writer, actress Marjorie Main.
English nicknames: **Marge,
Margie, Margy, Margo,
Marje, Marjie, Marjy.**
English variations: **Marjory,
Margery, Margory.**
Foreign variations: **Meadhbh**
(Irish), **Marcail** (Scottish).

MARLA—See *Mary.*

MARLENE—See **Madeline.**
Marlene Dietrich, actress.
English variations: **Marleen,
Marleene, Marlena, Mar-
line.**

MARMARA—Greek: **Mar-
mareous.** "Flashing, glittering,
radiating." Also: **Marmee.**

MARSHA—See **Marcia.**

MARTA—Variant of Aramaic
Martha, "lady of the house,
mistress. "Marta Heflin,
singer.

MARTHA—Aramaic: **Mar-
tha.** "Lady or mistress." A
woman of discretion, the
queen of her home. Martha
was the sister of Mary and
Lazarus in the Bible. The
most famous American with
this name was Martha
Washington; others include
Martha Raye, actress.
English nicknames; **Mart,
Marth, Martie, Marty,
Mattie, Matty, Pat, Patty.**
English variations: **Marthena,
Martita, Martella.**

Foreign variations: **Marthe**
(French, German), **Marta**
(Italian, Spanish, Swedish),
Moireach (Scottish).

MARTINA—Latin: "mar-
tial, warlike one." A name
from planet Mars, which
the ancients called the god of
war. Martina Navratilova,
tennis champion; Martine
Van Hamel, dancer and
choreographer.
English nicknames: **Marta,
Martie, Marty, Tina.**
Foreign variation: **Martine**
(French).

MARVEL—Old French:
Merveille. "A miracle; a
wonderful thing."
English variations: **Marva,
Marvela, Marvella, Mar-
velle.**

MARY—Hebrew: **Marah:
Miryam.** "Bitter or bitter-
ness." Call me not Naomi
(the pleasant), call me Mara
(the bitter) for the Almighty
hath dealt very bitterly with
me."—Ruth, 1.20. Marah
was the Hebrew word for the
bitter resin myrrh, used in
Biblical times as incense and
perfume. One of the world's
most popular names, Mary
stands for the mother of
Jesus Christ and is also the
name of many saints and
European queens. Namesakes
include Mamie Eisen-
hower; writers Mary Roberts
Rinehart, Mary Gordon;
actresses Mary Pickford, Mary

Martin, Maria Schell, Mamie Van Doren.
English nicknames: **Mame, Mamie, Mayme, May, Mari, Moll, Mollie, Molly, Polly.**
English variations: **Mara, Mare, Maria, Marie, Maretta, Marette, Marella, Mariette, Marietta, Marilla, Marilyn, Marla, Marya, Miriam, Muriel.**
Foreign variations: **Marie, Manette Manon, Maryse** (French), **Maria, Marita, Mariquita** (Spanish), **Maire, Maura, Maureen, Mearr, Moira, Moire, Moya, Muire** (Irish), **Marya** (Slavic), **Mairi, Moire, Muire** (Scottish).

MARYANN—A compound of **Mary** and **Ann**. See **Marian.**

MARYLOU—A compound of **Mary** and **Louise.**

MARYRUTH—A compound of **Mary** and **Ruth.**

MARYSE—See **Mary.**

MATHILDA—Old German: **Mat-hilde.** "Mighty battle-maiden." Matilda was the queen of William the Conqueror, Norman-French ruler who subjugated England in 1066.
English nicknames: **Mat, Matti, Mattie, Matty, Tilda, Tildy, Tillie, Tilly.**
English variations: **Matilda, Maud, Maude.**
Foreign variations: **Mathilde** (German, French), **Matelda** (Italian), **Matilde** (Spanish), **Maitilde** (Irish).

MATTEA—Hebrew: **Mattithyah.** "Gift of God." A feminine form of **Matthew.**
English variations: **Matthea, Matthia, Mathea, Mathia.**

MAUDE—See **Mathilda.** Maude Adams, actress.

MAUREEN—Irish Gaelic: **Mairin.** "Little Mary." See **Mary.** Alternate, Old French: **Maurin.** "Of dark complexion." A feminine form of **Maurice.** Maurine Neuberger, U.S. Senator; Maureen O'Hara, actress.
English variations: **Mora, Moira, Moreen, Moria, Maurine.**
Foreign variations: **Morena** (Spanish), **Maurizia** (Italian).

MAUVE—Latin: **Malva.** "Violet or lilac-colored." A name for a violet-eyed little girl.
English variation: **Malva.**

MAVIS—French: **Mauvis.** "Song thrush." See **Mab.**

MAXINE—Latin: **Maxima.** "Greatest." In legend and in history, greatness of character is recorded. Maxene Andrews, singer.
English nicknames: **Maxie, Maxi, Maxy.**

MAY—Latin: **Maia.** "Great one." Used for daughters born in May. Maia was the Roman goddess of spring, wife

of Vulcan. See **Mary**. May
Robson, Mae West, actresses.
English variations: **Mae,
Maia, Maya, Maye.**

MAYBELLE—Latin-French:
Maia-belle. "Great and
beautiful one." See **Mabel.**

MAYDA—See **Maida.**

MAYLEA—Hawaiian: "wild-
flower."

MAYME—See **Mary.**

MEARA—Irish Gaelic:
"mirth."

MEDIA—Greek: **Medeon.**
"Ruling"; or Latin: **Media.**
"Middle child." Medea was
an ancient Greek enchantress.
English variations: **Medea,
Madora, Medora.**

MEDORA—See **Media.**

MEGAN—Greek: **Megas.**
"Great mighty one"; or Irish
Gaelic: **Meghan.** "Margaret."
Also Welsh. See **Margaret.**
Popular U.S. name. Also:
Meagan, Meaghan.

MEHITABEL—Hebrew:
Meheytabel. "Benefited by
God." Popularized by the
Archie and Mehitabel stories
by Don Marquis.
English variations: **Mehetabel,
Mehitabelle.**
English nicknames: **Hetty,
Hitty.**

MELANIE—Greek: **Melanos.**
"Black or dark." An epithet
for Demeter in Greek myths;
she wore dark clothing as the
earth goddess of winter.

English nicknames: **Mel,
Mellie.**
English variations: **Melanie,
Melani, Meloni, Melany,
Melony.**

MELANTHA—Greek: **Melan-
thos.** "Dark flower."

MELBA—See **Malva.**

MELICENT—See **Millicent.**

MELINA—Latin: **Melinus.**
"Canary-yellow colored." See
Madeline, Malinda, Carmel.

MELINDA—See **Malinda.**
A name used since the 17th
century to complement
Belinda.

MELISSA—Greek: "honey;
a bee." Melissa Gilbert,
actress; Melissa Manches-
ter, singer.
English nicknames: **Mellie,
Melly, Millie, Milly, Lissa.**
English variations: **Melicent,
Melisent, Melitta, Melessa,
Melisse, Millicent, Millisent,
Melita.**

MELODY—Greek: "song,
beautiful music." Also:
Melodie.

MELVA—See **Malva,
Malvina.**

MELVINA—See **Malvina.**

MERCEDES—See **Mercy.**

MERCIA—Old English:
"from the kingdom of
Mercia." From the 6th to
9th centuries Mercia com-
prised central England.

MERCY—Middle English:

Merci. "Compassion, pity."
Primary usage is from the
Spanish "Santa Maria de las
Mercedes," "Our Lady of
Mercy."
Foreign variation: **Mercedes**
(Spanish).

MEREDITH—Old Welsh:
Maredud. "mortal days"; or
Old Welsh: Magnificent,
Meredydd. "Guardian from the
sea." Also a masculine
name.
English nickname: **Merry**.
English variation: **Meridith**.

MERLE—Latin: **Merula**.
"Thrush; blackbird." Also
used as a masculine name.
Merle Oberon, actress.
English variations: **Merl,
Merlina, Merline, Meryl,
Myrlene, Merola, Merrill**.

MERNA—See **Myrna**.

MEROLA—See **Merle**.

MERRY—Middle English:
Merie. "Mirthful; pleasant."
Also: **Merri, Merrie**. See
Meredith.

MERTICE—Old English:
Maertisa. "Famous and
pleasant."
English variation: **Merdyce**.

MERYL—See **Merle**.
Also: **Merrill**. Meryl Streep,
actress.

MESSINA—Latin; **Messena**.
"That which is in the middle;
a middle child."

META—Latin: "the meas-
urer; a goal." See **Margaret**.

METIS—Greek: "wisdom;
skill." Metis was the first wife
of Zeus, the Greek king of
the gods.

MIA—Modern U.S. form
originally a nickname for
Maria or **Michaela**. Mia
Farrow, actress.

MICHAELA—Hebrew: **Mik-
hael**. "Who is like God?" A
feminine form of **Michael**.
English nicknames: **Mickie,
Micky**.
English variations: **Michaelina,
Michaeline, Michelina,
Micheline, Micaela, Mikaela**.
Foreign variations: **Michel,
Michele, Michelle** (French),
Michaella (Italian), **Miguela,
Miguelita** (Spanish).

MICHELLE—See **Micha-
ela**.

MIGNON—French: "dainty,
graceful, darling." Heroine of
the Ambroise Thomas opera
and of Goethe's *Wilhelm
Meister*. Mignon Eberhart,
writer.
Foreign variation: **Mignonette**
(French).

MILADA—Czech: "my love."

MILDRED—Old English:
Mildraed. "Mild counselor";
or Old English: Mild-
thryth. "Mild power." Mil-
dred MacAfee, Navy
WAVE head, World War II,
president, Wellesley College.
English nicknames: **Mil,
Millie, Milly**.
English variation: **Mildrid**.

MILLICENT—Old German: **Amala-sand**. "Industrious and true"; Latin: "sweet singer." Millicent Fenwick, Congresswoman. See **Melissa**.
English nicknames: **Mil, Millie, Milly, Lissa**.
English variations: **Melicent, Mellicent, Milicent, Milissent, Millisent**.
Foreign variations: **Melisande** (French), **Melisenda** (Spanish).

MIMI—See **Miriam**. Mimi is the heroine of the Puccini opera *La Boheme*.

MINA—see **Minna, Wilhelmina**. Mina Ellis, Canadian author and explorer; Mina Loy, poet.

MINDY—See **Minna**.

MINERVA—Greek: **Menos**. "Force, purpose"; or Latin: **Minerva**. "The thinking one." Minerva was the highest goddess of Rome, coupled with Jupiter and Juno.
English nicknames: **Min, Minnie, Minny**.
Foreign variation: **Minette** (French).

MINNA—Old German: **Minne**. "Love." Medieval German Minnesingers were ballad singers of noble birth. See **Wilhelmina**.
English nicknames: **Min, Mina, Minnie, Minda, Mindy**.
English variations: **Minetta, Minette**.

MINNIE—See **Minerva, Wilhelmina**.

MINTA—Greek: **Min**. "The mint plant."
English variation: **Mintha**.

MIRA—Latin: "wonderful one." Modern Israeli for Giriam, "exalted."
English variations: **Mirra, Mirilla, Mirella, Mirelle, Myra, Myrilla**.

MIRABELLE—Spanish: **Mirabella**. "Beautiful-looking one."
English variations: **Mirabel, Mirabella**.

MIRANDA—Latin: "admirable; extraordinary."
English nicknames: **Randi, Randie, Randee, Randa, Randy**.

MIRIAM—Hebrew: **Miryam**. "Rebellious, strong-willed." See **Mary**. The Biblical Miriam was the sister of Moses and Aaron. Miriam Hopkins, Mitzi Green, actresses.
English nicknames: **Mimi, Minnie, Mitzi**.

MIRNA—See **Myrna**.

MITZI—See **Miriam**.

MODESTY—Latin: **Modesta**. "Modest one."
Foreign variations: **Modesta** (Italian), **Modestia** (Spanish), **Modestine** (French).

MOIRA—Greek: **Moirai**. "Merit; or Irish Gaelic: **Moire**. "Great one." Also

of Mary,
Agnes. Moira
ctress. See **Mary**.

—See **Mary**. Molly
, actress; Molly Pitcher,
. revolutionary war
roine.

MONA—Greek: "one, single one"; or Italian: "my lady"; or Irish Gaelic: **Muadhnait**. "Noble one"; or Teutonic: "lonely, far away"; or North American Indian: "gathered of the seed of the jimson weed." Famous from Da Vinci's painting, "Mona Lisa." See **Monica**.

MONICA, MONIKA—Latin: "wise counselor." Honoring St. Monica, 4th century, mother of St. Augustine. English nickname: **Mona**. Foreign variation: **Monca** (Irish).

MOREEN—See **Maureen**.

MORGAN, MORGANA—Old Welsh: **Morgant**. "Shore of the sea." In ancient English legends Morgan Le Fay was the sister of King Arthur.

MORIA—See **Maureen**.

MORNA—See **Myrna**.

MOSELLE—Hebrew: **Mosheh**. "Taken out of the water." A French feminine form of **Moses**.

English variation: **Mozelle**.

MURIEL—Greek: **Myrrha**. "Myrrh; bitter." See **Mary**. Muriel Spark, British novelist.
English variations: **Murial**, **Meriel**.
Foreign variations: **Muireall** (Scottish), **Muirgheal** (Irish).

MUSETTA—Old French: **Musette**. "A quiet, pastoral aria or song." Musetta is a character in Puccini's *La Boheme*.

MUSIDORA—Greek: **Mousadoros**. "Gift of the Muses." The Greek Muses were nine goddesses who presided over songs, art, poetry, and sciences.

MYRA—Greek: **Mirias**. "Abundance." see **Mira**. Myra Hess, noted pianist.

MYRLENE—See **Merle**.

MYRNA—Celtic: "tender, beloved, polite, gentle." Myrna Loy, actress.
English variations: **Merna**, **Mirna**, **Moina**, **Morna**, **Moyna**.

MYRTLE—Greek: **Myrtos**. "The myrtle." Myrtle was the ancient Greek symbol of triumph and victory.
English variations: **Myrta**, **Myrtia**, **Myrtis**, **Mirtle**, **Mertle**, **Mertice**, **Myrtice**, **Myrt**.

N

NADA—Slavic: "hope."
English variation: Nadine.

NADIA—Russian: "hope."
Also Greek: "charming."
Nadia Comaneci, Romanian
gymnast. Also a Russian
nickname for Nadezhda.

NADINE—See Nada. Na-
dine Gordiner, South African
writer.

NAIDA—Latin: Naiadis. "A
water or river nymph."

NAIRNE—Scottish Gaelic:
Amhuinn. "From the alder-
tree river." Used also as a
masculine name.

NAKIA—Modern U.S.
name of unknown origin. Also:
Nakita.

NANCY—An enlargement
of Nan. See Ann. Namesakes
include Nancy Hanks,
mother of Abraham Lincoln;
Nancy Reagan, wife of 40th
U.S. President.

NANETTE—see Ann. A
variation of Nan, meaning
"little, graceful one."
Nanette Fabray, actress.

NAOMI—Hebrew: "the
pleasant one." "And the name
of the man was Elimelech,
and the name of his wife
Naomi."—Ruth 1:2.
English variations: Naoma,
Noami.

NAPEA—Latin: Napaea.
"She of the valleys." In Greek
myths Napaea was a nymph
of the valleys and glens.

NARA—Old English: Nearra.
"Nearer or nearest one."

NARDA—Latin: Nardus.
"Fragrant ointment."

NASTASSIA—Variant of
Natalie. "Nasturtium." Nastassia Kinski, actress. Also: Nas-
tassja, Nastalya.

NATA—Hindustani: Nat.
"A rope-dancer."

NATALIE—Latin: Natalis.
"Birthday or natal day."
Natalie Wood, actress.
English nicknames: Nat,
Nattie, Natty, Nettie,
Netty.
English variations: Natala,
Natalia, Nataline, Nathalia,
Nathalie, Noel, Noelle,
Novella.
Foreign variations: Natalie,
Noelle (French), Natalia
(Spanish), Natasha (Russian).

NATASHA—Russian variant
of Natalie. Also a nickname
for Natalya or Natalia.

NATHANIA—Hebrew: Na-
than. "A gift," or "given of
God." A feminine form of
Nathan.
English variation: Nathene.

NATIVIDAD—Spanish:

...mas, born at Christ-

...ALA—Irish Gaelic: **Niall**. ...hampion." A feminine form of **Neal** and **Neil**.

NEBULA—Latin: **Nebula**. "Mist, vapor, a cloud."

NEDA—Slavic: **Nedjelja**. "Born on Sunday"; or Old English: **Eadweard**. "Prosperous guardian." A feminine form of **Ned** from **Edward**. Nedda is the heroine of the Leoncavallo opera *Pagliacci*. English variation: **Nedda**.

NELDA—Old English: **At-thea-eldre**. "From a home at the elder-tree," or a development of Nell and Nellie from Eleanore.

NELIA—Spanish diminutive of **Cornelia**, "queenly, womanly, enduring."

NELLIE—See **Helen, Cornelia, Eleanore**. Nellie Melba, opera singer; Nellie Taylor Ross, former Wyoming governor, Nellie Bly, journalist. English variations: **Nelly, Nellie, Nelle, Nell, Nela, Nelda, Nelia, Nella, Nelita, Nelina**.

NELLWYN—Greek-Old English: **Helene-wine**. "Light or bright friend."

NEOLA—Greek: **Neos**. "Youthful one."

NEOMA—Greek: **Neomenia**. "The new moon." "What is

there in thee, moon! That, thou shoulds't move my heart so potently."—Keats.

NERINE—Greek: **Nereos**. "A swimmer; one from the sea." A form of Nereis, an ancient sea-nymph. English variations: **Nerice, Nerissa**.

NERISSA—See **Nerine**.

NESSA—A development of **Nessie**. See **Agnes**.

NETTA—A development of **Astonia, Henrietta, Jeannette**.

NEVA—Spanish: **Nieve**. "Snow or extreme whiteness." See **Nevada**.

NEVADA—Spanish: **Nevada**. "White as snow." English nickname: **Neva**.

NEYSA—A development of **Agnes**.

NICOLE—Greek: **Nikolaos**. "Victorious army, victorious people." A feminine form of **Nicholas**. Nicole Hollander, illustrator. English nicknames: **Nickie, Nicky, Nikki**. English variations: **Nicola, Nichola, Nicolina, Nicoline**.

NIKE—Greek: **Nike**. "Victory."

NIKKI—See **Nicole**.

NILA—Latin: **Nilus**. "The River Nile of Egypt." Also a development of Nela from **Cornelia**.

NINA—Spanish: **Niña**.

"Girl." Nina Cecila Bowes-Lyon, mother of Queen Elizabeth, wife of George VI of England; Nina Foch, actress.
English variations: **Ninetta, Ninette.**

NINON—See **Ann.**

NISSA—Scandinavian: **Nisse** "A friendly elf or brownie."

NITA—See **Ann, Jane.**
Also Choctaw Indian: **Nita.** "A bear."

NIXIE—Old German: **Nichus.** "A little water-sprite."

NOAMI—See **Naomi.**

NOELLE—See **Natalie.**

NOKOMIS—Chippewa Indian: "grandmother."

NOLA—Latin: **Nola.** "A small bell"; or Irish Gaelic: **Nuallan.** "Famous."
English variation: **Nolana.**
See **Olivia.**

NOLANA—see **Nola.**

NOLETA—Latin: **Nolentis.** "Unwilling."
English variation: **Nolita.**

NONA—Latin: **Nona.** "Ninth child."
English nickname: **Nonie.**

NORA—See **Eleanore, Honoria.** Nora Ephron, essayist; Nora Hellmer,

heroine of Ibsen's *A Doll's House.*

NORBERTA—Old German: **Nor-beraht.** "Brilliant heroine"; or Old Norse: **Njorth-r-biart-r.** "Brilliance of Njord." Njord was the ancient Norse deity of the winds and of seafarers. A feminine form of **Norbert.**

NORDICA—German: **Nordisch.** "From the north."

NORMA—Latin: "a rule, pattern or precept." Popularized by Bellini's opera *Norma.* Norma Shearer, Norma Talmadge, actresses.

NORNA—Old Norse: **Norn.** "A Norn or Viking goddess of fate."

NOVIA—Latin: **Nova.** "Young person"; or Latin: **Novicius.** "Newcomer."
English variation: **Nova.**

NUALA—Irish Gaelic: **Nuala** from Fionnghuala. "Fair-shouldered one."

NYDIA—Latin: **Nida.** "From the nest."

NYSSA—Greek: "starting point"; or Latin: **Nisus.** "Striver toward a goal."

NYX—Greek: "night"; or Latin: **Nix.** "Snowy or white-haired." A Greek goddess who personified the night.

O

OBELIA—Greek: **Obelos**. "A pointed pillar."

OCTAVIA—Latin: "eighth child. "The feminine of **Octavius**.
English nicknames: **Tavie, Tavy**.
Foreign variations: **Ottavia** (Italian), **Octavie** (French).

ODELE—Greek: "melody, song." Also: **Odell**.

ODELETTE—French: "a little ode or lyric song."
English variation: **Odelet**.

ODELIA—Old Anglo-French: **Odel**. "Little wealthy one." A feminine form of **Odell**. Odette Myrtil, actress.
English variations: **Odella, Odelinda, Odilia, Otha, Othilia, Odette, Ottilie**.

ODESSA—Greek: **Odysseia**. "The Odyssey, a long journey." A form from the ancient Greek epic poem of the travels of Odysseus. The Russian city of Odessa, founded by Catherine the Great in 1794, was a namesake.

ODETTE—See **Odelia**.

OLA—See **Olga**.

OLENA—Russian, from the Greek: "Light." Also: **Alena**.

OLGA—Old Norse: **Halag**.

Russian: "holy one." A saintly woman dedicated to God. Olga was a favorite name in the imperial Russian family. St. Olga, 10th-century duchess of Kiev; Olga Korbut, Russian champion gymnast.
English variations: **Olva, Olivia, Olive, Elga**.

OLINDA—Latin: **Olid**. "Fragrant." This child was compared to a sweet-smelling herb.

OLIVE—Latin: **Olivia**. "Olive tree or olive branch." The olive branch was symbolic of peace. St. Olivia was a virgin Christian martyr of Carthage.
English nicknames: **Ollie, Olly, Livia, Nollie, Nola, Livvie, Liv**.
English variations: **Olivette, Olva, Olga**.

OLIVIA—See **Olive**. Actresses Olivia de Havilland, Olivia Hussey.

OLYMPIA—Greek: **Olympia**. "Of Olympus; heavenly one." Foreign variations: **Olympe** (French), **Olympie** (German), **Olimpia** (Italian).

OMA—Arabic: **Amir**. "Commander." Feminine of **Omar**.

ONA—Latin and Irish Gaelic: **Una**. "Unity." See

Una. Ona Munson, actress; Oona Chaplin, wife of comedian Charlie Chaplin; Oona White, choreographer. Foreign variations: **Oonagh, Oona** (Irish).

ONAWA—American Indian: "wide-awake one."

ONIDA—American Indian: "the looked-for one, the desired."

OPAL—Sanskrit: **Upala**. "A precious stone."
English variations: **Opalina, Opaline**.

OPHELIA—Greek: **Ophis**. "Serpent"; or Greek: **Ophelos**. "Help"; The serpent was an ancient insignia for wisdom. A serpent with its tail in its mouth symbolized eternity, that is, no beginning or end. Ophelia is a famous character in Shakespeare's *Hamlet*.
English variations: **Ofelia, Ofilia, Oprah**.
Foreign variation: **Ophélie** (French).

ORA—Latin and Old English: "shore or seacoast"; or Latin: **Aurum**. "Gold."
English variations: **Orabel, Orabelle**.

ORALIA—Latin: **Aurelia**. "Golden."

English variations: **Oriel, Orielda**. **Oriole, Oriola, Orielle, Orlena, Orlene, Oralie**.

ORDELLA—Old German: **Ordalf**. "Elfin spike or spear."

OREA—Greek: "of the mountain."

ORELA—Latin: **Oracula**. "A divine announcement."

ORENDA—Iroquois Indian: "magic power."

ORIANA—Latin: "the dawning"; or Celtic: "golden one." In the medieval story *Amadis of Gaul*, Oriana was the beloved of Amadis.

ORIEL—See **Oralia**.

ORLENA—See **Oralis**.

ORNA—Irish Gaelic: **Odharnait**. "Pale or olive color."

ORPAH—Hebrew: "a fawn." "My beloved is like a roe or a young hart."—The Song of Solomon, 2:9.

ORSA—See **Ursula**.

ORVA—Old English: **Ordwine**. "Spear friend." Feminine of **Orvin**.

OTTILIE—See **Odelia**.

OZORA—Hebrew: **Uzziye**. "strength of the Lord."

P

PAGE—Greek: "child." An Anglo-Saxon occupational name for a youth training for knighthood. Modern U.S. Also: **Paige**.

PALLAS—Greek: "wisdom; knowledge." Pallas was a name for the Greek Athena, who represented wisdom.

PALMA—Latin: "a palm." Used for a child born on Palm Sunday.
English variations: **Palmira, Palmyra.**

PALOMA—Spanish: "a dove."
English variations: **Palometa, Palomita.**

PAMELA—Greek: **Pammeli.** "All-honey." Pamela was invented by Sir Philip Sidney in 1590 for a character in *Arcadia.* Namesakes: Pam Dawber, Pamela Mason, actresses.
English nicknames: **Pam, Pammy.**
English variations: **Pamella, Pamelina.**

PANDORA—Greek: **Pandoron.** "The all-gifted one." Pandora in the Greek myth was given a sealed box that contained all human ills, and hope, which escaped when she opened it.

PANPHILA—Greek: **Panphilos.** "The all-loving one." "Love can neither be bought nor sold; its only price being love"—Proverb.

PANSY—French: **Pensée.** "A thought." "There's rosemary, that's for remembrance; . . . and there is pansies, that's for thoughts." —Shakespeare, *Hamlet.*

PANTHEA—Greek: **Pantheios.** "Of all the gods." The Roman Pantheon was built to honor all the ancient gods.

PARNELLA—Old French: **Pernel.** "Little rock." A feminine form of **Parnell** from **Peter.**
English variation: **Pernella.**

PARTHENIA—Greek: **Parthenos.** "Maidenly."

PATIENCE—French: "endurance with fortitude." This name was eulogized by our perseverant Pilgrim Fathers.

PATRICIA—Latin: **Patricius.** "Noble one." Feminine form of **Patrick.** St. Patricia, 7th century, is one of the patrons of Naples, Italy. Patrice Munsel, opera singer; Pat McCormick, champion diver; Patty Berg, champion golfer; singers Pat Benatar, Patti Page.
English nicknames: **Pat, Patti, Pattie, Patsy, Patty.**
Foreign variations: **Patrice** (French), **Patrizia** (Italian).

PAULA—Latin: **Paulus.** "Little." Small in stature but big in love and constancy. Used in honor of St. Paul the Apostle, and St. Paula, a 3rd-century Nicomedian martyr. Paula Prentiss, Paulette Goddard, actresses.
English nicknames: **Pauly, Polly.**
English variations: **Paulette, Pauline, Paulita.**
Foreign variations: **Paule,**

Paulette, Pauline (French), **Paola, Paolina** (Italian), **Paula, Paulina** (Spanish).

PAULINE—See **Paula.**

PAZIA—Hebrew: "golden." Also, **Pazice, Pazit.**

PEACE—Latin: **Pacis.** "Tranquillity." "Let us therefore follow after the things that make for peace." Philippians.

PEARL—Late Latin: **Perla.** "A pearl." Pearl Buck, writer. English variations: **Pearla, Pearle, Pearline.**

PEGGY—See **Margaret.** Peggy Ashcroft, Peggy Wood, actresses.

PELACIA—Greek: **Pelagos.** "From the sea."

PENELOPE—Greek: "worker of the web; weaver." In Greek myths Penelope, wife of Odysseus, wove each day and unraveled the cloth at night. Namesake: Penny Russianoff, psychologist-author. English nicknames: **Pen, Penny, Penina, Penine.**

PENTHEA—Greek: **Pentheus.** "Mourner"; or Greek: **Penta.** "Fifth child."

PEONY—Latin: **Paeonia.** "The god of healing." Sacred to Pan, the Greek god, and also to Apollo. A flower name.

PEPITA—Spanish, from Hebrew: "she shall be fruitful."

PERDITA—Latin: "the lost."

The king's daughter in Shakespeare's *The Winter's Tale.*

PERFECTA—Spanish: "perfect, accomplished one."

PERNELLA—See **Parnella.**

PERRY—Modern U.S. name, originally a nickname of **Pearl.** Also: **Perri.**

PERSEPHONE—Greek: **Persephonia.** "Sacred to the goddess Persephone." Persephone was the Greek deity of the underworld.

PERSIS—Latin: **Persis.** "A woman from Persia." St. Paul honored Persis in the Bible.

PETRA—Latin: "rock." One strong and everlasting. English variations: **Petronia, Petronella, Petronilla.** Foreign variations: **Pierette, Perrine** (French), **Petronille** (German), **Pietra** (Italian).

PETUNIA—Tupi Indian: **Petum.** "Reddish-purple flowered petunia." A flower name.

PHEBE—See **Phoebe.**

PHEDRA—Greek: **Phaidra.** "Bright one." Phaidra was a daughter of King Minos and the wife of Theseus in ancient Crete.

PHILANA—Greek: **Philein.** "Loving." English variations: **Philene, Philina, Philida.**

PHILANTHA—Greek: **Philanthos.** "Flower lover."

PHILBERTA—Old English: "**Fela-beorht.** "Very brilliant one."

PHILIPPA—Greek: **Philippos.** "Lover of horses." Feminine version of **Phillip.** Famed in history from Philippa of Hainault, queen of England's 13th-century King Edward III.
English nicknames: **Phil, Phillie.**
Foreign variations: **Filippa,** (Italian), **Felipa** (Spanish), **Philippine** (German).

PHILOMELA—Greek: **Philomelos.** "Lover of song." A name for the nightingale.

PHILOMENA—Greek: **Philomene.** "Lover of the moon."

PHOEBE—Greek: **Phoibe.** "Bright one, brilliant one." The feminine of **Phoebus,** a name for the sun god Apollo. St. Phoebe of Corinth, 1st century; Phoebe Cary, poet.
English variation: **Phebe.**

PHOENIX—Greek: **Phoinix.** Egyptian: **Bennu.** "The heron or eagle," or "the rejuvenated and reincarnated one." The legendary bird that lived 500 years, was consumed by fire and rose in youthful freshness from its ashes.

PHYLLIS—Greek: "a green branch." A mythological princess changed into an almond tree. Author Phyllis Whitney.

English variations: **Phillis, Phyllys.**
Foreign variation: **Filide** (Italian).

PIA—Italian: "pious."

PIERETTE—French: "little steadfast one." Feminine of **Pierre (Peter).**

PILAR—Spanish: a foundation or pillar. Refers to Mary as the foundation of the church. Pilar Wayne, wife of John Wayne, actor.

PIPER—Old English: **Pipere.** "A pipe player." Piper Laurie, actress.

PLACIDA—Latin: **Placidus.** "Gentle, peaceful one."

PLATONA—Greek: **Platos.** "Broad-shouldered." A feminine form of **Plato,** the great Greek philosopher.

POLLY—See **Mary, Paula.** Polly Bergen, singer, actress.

POLLYANNA—Compound of **Polly** and **Anne.**

POMONA—Latin: "fruitful." Pomona was the Roman goddess of fruit.

POPPY—Latin: **Papaver.** "A poppy flower."

PORTIA—Latin: **Portio.** "An offering." Also the title of an ancient Roman clan, Porcius. Portia was the heroine of Shakespeare's *Merchant of Venice.*

PRIMA—Latin: **Prinaus.** "First child."

PRIMAVERA—Spanish: "springtime."

PRIMROSE—Latin: **Primula.** "Little first one."

PRISCILLA—Latin: "from past or primitive times; of ancient birth." St. Priscilla was a 1st-century hostess to St. Peter at Rome. Priscilla Mullins, wife of John Alden, famous in New England history. Also: **Prisca.** English nicknames: **Pris, Prissie.**

PROSPERA—Latin: **Prosperus.** "Favorable, auspicious."

PRUDENCE—Latin: **Prudentia.** "Foresight; intelligence." Prudence Penny, home economics columnist. English nicknames: **Pru, Prue.**

PRUNELLA—French: **Prunelle.** "Prune-colored; the color of sloe plums."

PSYCHE—Greek: "soul or mind." In mythology, Psyche was the mortal loved by Cupid.

PYRENA—Greek: **Pyrene.** "Fiery one," or "fruit kernel." Pyrene was loved by Hercules; her grave is in the Pyrenees. Fire means "of the light." The kernel could signify the heart or hearth of the home.

PYTHIA—Greek: **Python.** "A prophet or diviner." Pythia was the name of the priestesses of the old Greek oracle of Apollo at Delphi.

Q

QUEENA—Old English: **Cwen.** "A queen." "Grace was in her steps, heaven in her eye, in every gesture dignity and love."—Milton. English nickname: **Queenie.**

QUERIDA—Spanish: "beloved."

QUINTINA—Latin: **Quinctus.** "Fifth child." A feminine form of **Quintin** and **Quentin.**

R

RABI—Arabic: "spring or harvest."

RACHEL—Hebrew: "A lamb." Rachel was the Biblical wife of Jacob, "beautiful and well-favored." (Genesis.)

English nicknames: **Rae. Ray.** Foreign variations: **Rachele** (Italian), **Raquel** (Spanish), **Rachelle** (French), **Rahel** (German), **Raoghnailt** (Scottish).

RADELLA—Old English: **Raedself.** "Elfin counselor."

RADINKA—Slavic: **Radinka.** "Active one."

RADMILLA—Slavic: **Radmilu.** "Worker for the people."

RAE—Old English: **Ra.** "A doe deer." "Make haste, my beloved, and be thou like to a roe or to a young hart upon the mountains of spices." —The Song of Solomon. See **Rachel.**

RAINA—See **Regina.**

RAISSA—Old French: **Raison.** "Thinker, believer."

RAMONA—Spanish or Teutonic: "Mighty or wise protector." A feminine form of **Ramon** or **Raymond**, celebrated from the Helen Hunt Jackson novel *Ramona.* English variations: **Ramonda, Ramonde.** English nickname. **Mona.**

RANI—Hindu: "a queen." English variations: **Ranee, Rania, Rana.**

RANITA—Modern Israeli: "joyful song."

RAPHAELA—Hebrew: **Raphael.** "Healed by God." Foreign variations: **Rafaela** (Spanish), **Rafaella** (Italian).

RASHEDA, RASHIDA— Popular modern U.S. name. Feminine of **Rashid.** Possibly of African origin.

RASIA—see **Rose.**

RAVEN—Middle English: "black, dark-haired."

RAY—See **Rachel.**

REBA—See **Rebecca.**

REBECCA—Hebrew: **Ribqah.** "Bound; yoke." In the Old Testament, Rebecca was the wife of Isaac. English nicknames: **Reba, Rheba, Beckie, Becky, Bekki, Becca.** English variations: **Rebekah, Rebeka.** Foreign variations: **Rébecca** (French), **Rebekka** (German, Swedish), **Rebeca** (Spanish).

REGINA—Latin: "a queen; queenly, royal." English nicknames: **Reggie, Rina, Gina.** English variations: **Regan, Raina, Reyna, Regine.** Foreign variations: **Reine** (French), **Reina** (Spanish), **Rioghnach** (Irish).

RENATA—Latin: "born again." Renata Tebaldi, opera singer; Renata Adler, writer. English nicknames: **Rene, Renee, Rennie.** Foreign variations: **Renée** (French), **Renate** (German).

RENE—See **Irene, Renata.**

RENÉE—See **Renata.** Popular U.S. version of **Renata.**

RENITA—Latin: **Reniti.** "Resister." A rebel.

RESEDA—Latin: "the mignonette flower."

REVA—Latin: **Revalesco.** "To regain strength."

REXANA—Latin-English: **Rex-Anne.** "Regally graceful."

RHEA—Greek: "a stream; literally, a flow"; or Latin: **Rhaea.** "A poppy." Rhea was the mother of the gods in the old Greek religion. English variation: **Rea.**

RHETA—Greek: **Rhetor.** "An orator."

RHODA—Greek: **Rhodon.** "The rose." This name goes back to an unknown Oriental source. The rose is queen of flowers.

RHODANTHE—Greek: "rose flower."

RHODIA—See Rose.

RIA—Spanish: "a river mouth."

RICADONNA—English-Italian: **Rica-donna.** "Ruling lady."

RICARDA—Old English: **Richard.** "Powerful ruler." Feminine of **Richard.** English nicknames: **Rickie, Ricky, Dickie.**

RILLA—Low German: **Rillie.** "A stream or brook." English variation: **Rillette.**

RINA—See Regina.

RISA—Latin: "laughter." Risë Stevens, opera singer.

RITA—A shortened form of **Margherita** (Italian). See **Margaret.** Rita Hayworth, Rita Moreno, actresses.

RIVA—French: **Rive.** "Riverbank, shore." Also, from **Rebecca.** English nicknames: **Rivy, Rivi, Ree, Reevabel.** Also, **Reeva.**

ROANNA—Compound of **Rose** and **Anne.**

ROBERTA—Old English: **Hroth-beorht.** "Shining with fame." Roberta Peters, opera singer. English nicknames: **Bobbie, Bobby, Bertie.** English variations: **Robina, Robinia, Robinette, Bobbette.** Foreign variations: **Robine** (French), **Rupetta** (German).

ROBIN—Anglo-Saxon, originally a form of **Robert,** "bright fame." Popular modern U.S. name. Also: **Robyn, Robina, Robena, Robinia.**

ROCHELLE—French: "from the little rock." An old French directional landmark. English variations: **Rochella, Rochette.** English nickname: **Shelley.**

RODERICA—Old German: **Ruod-rik.** "Famous ruler." A feminine form of **Roderick.** English nicknames: **Roddie, Roddy, Rickie.**

ROHANA—Hindu: **Rohan.** "Sandalwood."

ROLANDA—Old German:

Ruod-lant. "From the famous land." A feminine form of **Roland.**
Foreign variations: **Rolande** (French), **Orlanda** (Italian).

ROMILDA—Old German: **Ruom-hildi.** "Glorious battle maid."

ROMOLA—Latin: **Romula.** "Lady of Rome." The title and heroine of a George Elliot novel.
English variations: **Romella, Romelle.**

RONALDA—Old Norse: **Rognuald.** "Mighty power." Feminine form of **Ronald.**

ROSABEL—Compound of **Rose** and **Belle.** Latin: "Beautiful Rose."
English variations: **Rosabelle, Rosabella.**

ROSALIE—Poetic Irish form; See **Rose.** Also: **Rosaleen.**
English nickname: **Rosy.**

ROSALINDA—Spanish: "beautiful rose"; Irish: "little rose." Rosalind Russell, actress.
English variations: **Rosalind, Roslyn, Rosalynd, Rosaline, Roseline, Rosaleen, Rosina.**

ROSAMOND—Old German: **Rozo-mund.** "Famous protectress." New Latin: "rose of the world."
English variations: **Rosamund, Rosamonde**
Foreign variations: **Rosmunda** (Italian), **Rosemonde** (French),

Rosamunda (Spanish), **Rozamond** (Dutch).

ROSANNA—English: **Rose-anne.** "Graceful rose." Also: **Roseann, Rose-Ann, Roseanne.**

ROSE—Greek: **Rhodos.** "A rose." St. Rose of Lima, died 1617; The favorite of the floral names, for the queen of flowers.
English nicknames: **Rosie, Rosy, Zita.**
English variations: **Rosalie, Rosalia, Rosella, Roselle, Rosetta, Rosette, Rosina, Rasia, Rozella, Rhoda, Rhodia.**
Foreign variations: **Rosa** (Italian, Spanish, Danish, Dutch, Swedish), **Rois** (Irish), **Rosette** (French), **Rosita** (Spanish).

ROSELLEN—Compound of **Rose** and **Helen.**

ROSEMARY—English: **Rose-Mary.** "The rose of St. Mary"; or Latin: **Rosmarinus.** "Dew of the sea," for the rosemary herb. Rosemary Clooney, singer, entertainer.
English variation: **Rose Marie.**

ROSETTA—See **Rose.**

ROSLYN—See **Rosalinda.**

ROUX—See **La Roux.**

ROWENA—Old English: **Hroth-wine.** "Famous friend"; Celtic: "white-clad, light-haired."
Rowena was a heroine of ancient British legends.

ROXANNE—Persian: **Raok-hshna.** "Brilliant one, the new dawning." Roxana is famous as the wife of Alexander the Great. Roxanne is heroine of Rostand's classic, *Cyrano de Bergerac*.
English nicknames: **Roxie, Roxy.**
English variations: **Roxana, Roxanna, Roxine, Roxene, Roxine, Roxann, Roxane.**

ROYALE—Old French: **Roial.** "Regal one." A feminine form of **Roy.**

RUBY—Old French: **Rubi.** "The ruby gem." Ruby Keeler, actress.
English variations: **Rubie, Rubia, Rubina.**

RUDELLE—Old German: **Ruod.** "Famous one."

RUELLA—Compound of **Ruth** and **Ella.**

RUFINA—Latin: **Rufus.** "Red-haired." A feminine form of **Rufus.**

RULA—Latin: **Regula.** "A ruler." A sovereign of her country.

RUPERTA—See **Roberta.**

RUTH—Hebrew: "compassionate, beautiful." "And Ruth said, entreat me not to leave thee or to return from following after thee: for whither thou goest, I will go." —Ruth 1:16. Ruth Gordon, actress.

S

SABA—Greek: "woman of Saba or Sheba." A name glamorized by the vibrant Queen of Sheba, who visited the fabulously rich King Solomon.

SABINA—Latin: "a Sabine lady." The ancient Sabine country was near Rome. St. Sabina was a 1st-century Roman martyr.
English variation: **Savina.**
English nickname: **Bina.**
Foreign variations: **Sabine** (French, German, Dutch), **Saidhbhin** (Irish).

SABRA—Hebrew: "to rest."

SABRINA—Latin: "from the boundary line." Famous from the play *Sabrina Fair* by Samuel Taylor, and the film *Sabrina*.

SADIE—see **Sarah.**

SADIRA—Persian: **Sadar.** "The lotus tree." Dreamy one, like the legendary lotus eaters.

SAGE—Latin: "whole, healthy, wise, knowing."

SALINA—Latin: "from the salty place."

SALLY—See **Sarah.** Sally Ride, astronaut.

SALOME—Hebrew: **Shalom.** "Peace." Salome was the daughter of Herodias in the New Testament.
English variations: **Saloma, Salomi.**
Foreign variation: **Salomé** (French).

SALVIA—Latin: "sage." A fragrant herb used for cooking.
English variation: **Salvina.**

SAMANTHA—Aramaic: "a listener." Samantha Eggar, actress.

SAMARA—Hebrew: **Shemariah.** "Guarded by God."

SAMUELA—Hebrew: **Shemuel.** "His name is God." A feminine form of **Samuel.**
English variations: **Samella, Samelle, Samuelle.**

SANCIA—Latin: "Sacred; inviolable."
Foreign variations: **Sancha, Sanchia** (Spanish).

SANDI—See **Alexandra.**

SANDRA—See **Alexandra.**

SANURA—Swahili: "Like a kitten."

SAPPHIRA—Greek: **Sappheiros.** "Sapphire gem or sapphire-blue color." Modern usage from the Willa Cather novel, *Sapphira and the Slave Girl.*
English variations: **Saphira, Sapphire.**

SARAH, SARA—Hebrew: "princess." Sarah was the wife of Abraham and the mother of Isaac in the Bible. She was first named Sarai meaning "quarrelsome," but when Sarai was changed to Sarah it became "princess" and "one who laughed." Namesakes: Sara Teasdale, poet; actress Sarah Bernhardt.
English nicknames: **Sal, Sallie, Sally, Sadie, Sadye.**
English variations: **Sari, Sarene, Sarine, Sarette, Sadella, Zara, Zarah, Zaria.**
Foreign variations: **Sara** (French, German, Italian, Spanish), **Sorcha** (Irish), **Salaidh, Morag** (Scottish), **Serita** (Italian).

SASHA—Russian nickname for **Alexandra.** Also: **Sacha, Sascha, Sashenka.**

SAVANNA—Old Spanish: **Sabana.** "An open plain." Also, a U.S. place name, for the city in Georgia.
English variation: **Savannah.**

SAVINA—See **Sabina.**

SAXONA—Old English: **Saxan.** "A Saxon: one of the sword-people." The Roman conquerors of Germany applied this name to the natives because they battled with short swords; now applied to persons of English descent.

SCARLETT—Middle English: "scarlet-colored." Famous from Scarlett O'Hara, heroine of the novel, *Gone with the Wind.*

SEASON—Latin: "sowing." Season Hubley, actress.

SEBASTIANE—Latin: **Sebastianus.** "August, reverenced one." A feminine form of **Sebastian.**
English variation: **Sebastiana.**

SECUNDA—Latin: "second child."

SELENA—Greek: "the moon or moonlight"; or Latin: **Coelina.** "Heavenly." Selena Royle, actress.
English nicknames: **Sela, Selie, Celie, Sena, Selia.**
English variations: **Selene, Selina, Selinda, Celene, Celina, Celinda.**

SELIA—See **Selena.**

SELIMA—Hebrew: "peaceful." Also: **Selmah.**

SELINDA—See **Selena.**

SELMA—See **Anselma.** Selma Lagerlöf, Swedish novelist.

SEMELE—Latin: "once; a single time." Semele was the Greek earth goddess, daughter of Cadmus and mother of Dionysus.

SEMIRA—Hebrew: **Shemiramoth.** "The height of the heavens." Semiramis, the older form of Semira, was famous from an ancient Assyrian queen.

SENA—See **Selena.**

SEPTIMA—Latin: "seventh child."

SERAPHINA—Hebrew: **Seraphin.** "Burning or ardent one." The Biblical Seraphim were fiery, purifying ministers of Jehovah. St. Seraphina was a 15th-century Italian abbess.
English variations: **Serafina, Serafine, Seraphine.**

SERENA—Latin: "fair, bright, serene one."

SERILDA—Old German: **Saro-hildi.** "Armored battle-maid."

SHAKA—Modern U.S.: "a warrior."

SHARISSA—Modern U.S. name. Also: **Sherissa.**

SHARLEEN—See **Caroline.**

SHARON—Hebrew: **Sharai.** "A princess"; or from place-name usage, Hebrew: **Sharon.** "A plain."
English nicknames: **Sherry, Shari, Sharry.**

SHAUNA—Modern U.S. name. Feminine of **Shaun** or **Sean.** Also: **Shawna, Shana, Shanna.**

SHEBA—See **Saba.**

SHEENA—Irish Gaelic: **Sine.** "God is gracious." A form of **Jane.**

SHEILA—Irish Gaelic: **Sile.** An Irish spelling of **Cecilia, Sabina.**
English variations: **Sheela, Sheelah, Sheilah, Seila, Shayla, Shelagh.**

SHELLEY—Old English: **Scelfleah.** "From the meadow on the ledge." Also: **Shelly.** Shelley Winters, actress.

SHEREE—See Charlotte.

SHERRILL—See Charlotte.

SHERRY—Popular U.S. name, either a variant of **Sharon, Sarah,** or **Shirley** or a respelling of **Chérie,** French: "cherished one." English variation: **Sheri, Shari, Sherrie, Sheree, Sherge, Sherilyn.**

SHERYL—See Charlotte, Shirley.

SHIRLEY—Old English: **Scirleah.** "From the bright meadow." Shirley MacLaine, Shirley Jones, Shirley Knight, actresses.
English nicknames: **Shir, Shirl.**
English variations: **Shirlee, Shirlie, Shirleen, Shirlene, Sheryl.**

SHOSHANA—See Susan.

SHULAMITH—Hebrew: "peace." Also: **Shula, Sula, Sulamith.**

SIBYL—Greek: **Sibylla.** "A prophetess." There were 10 Sibyls in the classical myths, prophetesses located in various Mediterranean countries. Sybil Thorndike, English actress.
English nicknames: **Sib, Sibbie, Sibby.**
English variations: **Sybil, Sybilla, Sybille, Sibilla, Sibille, Sibyll, Sibelle.**

Foreign variations: **Cybèle, Sibylle** (French, German), **Sibylla** (Dutch), **Sibeal** (Irish).

SIDNEY—See Sydney.

SIDONIA—See Sydney.

SIDRA—Latin: **Sidera.** "Belonging to the stars; glittering."

SIGFREDA—Old German: **Sigifrith.** "Victorious and peaceful." A feminine form of **Siegfried.**

SIGNA—Latin: "a signer." Also: **Signe.** Signe Hasso, actress.

SIGRID—Old Norse: **Sigrath.** "Victorious counselor, beautiful conqueror."

SILVIA—See Sylvia.

SIMONE—Hebrew: **Shim'on.** "Hearer; one who hears, obedient." A feminine form of **Simeon** and **Simon.** Simone Signoret, French actress.
Foreign variations: **Simona, Simonette** (French).

SIOBHAN—Irish variant of **Jane.**

SIRENA—Greek: **Seiren.** "A sweetly singing mermaid siren." Refers to the mythical Greek sirens, whose fatal beauty and songs lured men to their death.

SISSY—Modern U.S.; originally a nickname for "sister." Sissy Spacek, actress.

SKYE—Dutch: "sheltering." Also: **Skyla, Schyler, Skylar.**

SOLVIG—Old German: **Sigilwig.** "Victorious battle-maid."

SONIA, SONYA—Greek: "the wise one."
English variation: **Sona.**
Sonja Henie, Norwegian actress, ice skater.

SOPHIA—Greek: "wisdom." St. Sophia, a lst-century martyr; Sophia Smith, founder of Smith College; Sophia Loren, actress.
English variations: **Sophie, Sophy.**
Foreign variations: **Sofie** (French, Danish, Dutch), **Sofia** (Italian, Spanish), **Sonja, Sonya** (Slavic, Scandinavian), **Sadhbh, Sadhbba** (Irish), **Beathag** (Scottish).

SOPHRONIA—Greek: "sensible one."
Foreign variations: **Sonja, Sonya** (Scandinavian, Slavic).

SORCHA—Irish Gaelic: "bright one."

SPRING—Old English: **Springan,** "The springtime of the year." Spring Byington, actress.

STACEY—See **Anastasia.**

STACIA—See **Anastasia.**

STAR—Old English: **Steorts.** "A star." See **Esther.** Also: **Starr, Starla.**

STELLA—See **Estelle.**
Stella Stevens, actress.

STEPHANIE—Greek: **Stephanos.** "Crowned one." A feminine form of **Stephen.** St. Stephana of Italy (1457–1530); Princess Stephanie of Monaco.
English nicknames: **Stefa, Steffie, Stepha.**
English variations: **Stephania, Stephana, Stevana, Stevena.**
Foreign variations: **Stéphanie** (French), **Stephanie** (German).

STOCKARD—Old English: **Stock-hart.** "Hardy tree stump." Stockard Channing, actress.

STORM—Old English: "a tempest or storm." Also: **Stormi, Stormie, Stormy.**

SUMMER—Middle English: **Sumar.** "Summer." Summer Bartholomew, actress.

SUNNY—English: "bright, cheerful, genial."

SUSAN—Hebrew: **Shoshannah.** "Lily or graceful lily"; or Modern Israeli: "rose." St. Susanna was a 3rd-century Roman martyr. Susan B. Anthony, American reformer; Susan Glaspell, writer; Susan Hayward, Susan Strasberg, Zsa Zsa Gabor, actresses.
English nicknames: **Sue, Susie, Susy, Suze, Suzie, Suzy, Suki, Sukey.**
English variations: **Susanna, Susannah, Suzanna, Suzannah, Susanne, Susette, Suzette.**
Foreign variations: **Susanne** (French, German), **Susanna** (Italian), **Shoshana, Susana**

(Spanish), **Zsa Zsa** (Hungarian nickname), **Sosanna** (Irish), **Siusan** (Scottish).

SYBIL—See **Sibyl.**

SYDNEY—Old French: **Saint-Denis.** "From St. Denis, France"; or Phoenician: **Sidon.** "From the city of Sidon." A feminine form of **Sidney.**

SYLVIA—Latin: "girl from the forest." Sylvia Porter, columnist; Sylvia Sidney, actress.
English variations: **Silva, Sylva, Silvana, Sylvana, Zilvia.**
Foreign variations: **Silvie** (French), **Silvia** (Italian, Spanish).

SYNA—Greek: Syn. "Together." Companionship for two like minds and hearts.

T

TABITHA—Greek: "gazelle; a child of grace."
English nicknames: **Tabby, Tabbi, Tabbie.**

TACITA—Latin: "silent."

TALIA—Hebrew: "the gentle dew from heaven." Also: **Talya.**

TALITHA—Aramaic: "maiden."

TALLULAH—Choctaw Indian: "leaping water." Tallulah Bankhead, actress.
English nicknames: **Tallie, Tally.**

TAMARA—Hebrew: "palm tree."
English nicknames: **Tammie, Tammy.**
English variation: **Tamar.**

TAMIKA—Popular modern U.S. name. From Japanese "tami," meaning "people."
English variations: **Tamike, Tomika, Tamiko.**

TAMMY—Hebrew: **Tema.** "Perfection." A feminine form of **Thomas.** See **Tamara, Thomasa.** Tammy Grimes, actress.

TANGERINE—English: "girl from the city of Tangier, Morocco."

TANIA—Russian: "the fairy queen." Russian diminutive for **Tatiana.** Also: **Tanya.**

TANISHA—Modern U.S. name, linked to a Hausa day name, used for children born on Monday.

TANSY—Middle Latin: **Tanacetum.** "Tenacious one."

TARA—Irish Gaelic: **Torra.** "Rocky pinnacle or crag." Tara was the ancient capital of the Irish kings.

TASHA—Pet form of **Natasha.** Tasha Tudor, children's book author and illustrator.

TATIANA—Russian. Origin unknown. Russian nicknames: **Tania, Tanya, Tati**.

TATUM—Modern U.S. name, gaining in popularity. Possibly Middle English: **Tayt-um**. "She who brings cheer to others." Tatum O'Neal, actress.

TECLA—Greek: "divine fame." St. Tecla was the first woman martyr. Also, Swedish: **Tekla**. "Fresh-water pearl." See **Thecla**.
English variations: **Thecla, Telca, Telka**.

TEMPEST—Old French: Tempeste. "Stormy one."

TENLEY—of unknown origin, probably family name. Tenley Albright, Olympic skating champion.

TERENTIA—Greek: Tereus. "Guardian"; or Irish Gaelic: **Toirdealbach**. "Shaped like the god Thor." A feminine form of **Terence**. Characterized as like the Norse thunder god Thor.
English nicknames: **Teri, Terri, Terrie, Terry**.

TERESA—See **Theresa**.

TERI—See **Terentia, Theresa**.

TERRY—See **Terentia, Theresa**. Terry Moore, actress.

TERTIA—Latin: "third child."

TESSA—Greek: **Tessares**. "Fourth child." See **Theresa**.

English nicknames: **Tess, Tessie**.

THADDEA—Greek: **Thaddaios**. "Courageous one." A feminine form of **Thaddeus**. English variations: **Thada, Thadda**.

THALASSA—Greek: "from the sea." Thalassa Cruso, herbalist and gardener.

THALIA—Greek: **Thaleia**. "Blooming; luxuriant." In Greek myths Thalia was one of the three Graces and the Muse of Comedy.

THEA—Greek: "goddess."

THEANO—Greek: **Theanoma**. "Divine name." Theano was the wife of Pythagoras.

THECLA—Greek: **Thekla**. "Divinely famous." St. Thecla was a follower of St. Paul. English variations: **Tecla, Thekla**.

THEDA—See **Theodora, Theodosia**. Theda Bara, actress, 1890–1955.

THELMA—Greek: **Thele**. "A nursling." Thelma Ritter, actress.

THEODORA—Greek: **Theodoros**. "Gift of God." A feminine form of **Theodore**. See **Dorothy**. Famous from Theodora, 6th-century Roman Empress of the East. English nicknames: **Theda, Dora, Teddy**. Foreign variations: **Teodora** (Italian, Spanish), **Fedora, Feodora**, (Slavic).

THEODOSIA—Greek: "God-given."
English nicknames: **Theda, Dosia, Dosie.**
Foreign variations: **Teodosia** (Italian), **Feodosia** (Slavic).

THEOLA—Greek: **Theologos.** "Speaker with God."

THEONE—Greek: **Theonoma.** "God's name."

THEOPHANIA—Greek: **Theophaneia.** "Appearance of God."

THEOPHILA—Greek: **Theophilos.** "Beloved of God."

THEORA—Greek: **Theoro.** "Watcher, contemplater."

THERA—Greek: "wild, untamed."

THERESA—Greek: **Theriso.** "Reaper." St. Theresa of Avila in Castile, 1515–1582, Spanish nun, mystic, and writer, was one of the most admired women in religious history. Teresa Wright, actress.
English nicknames: **Teri, Terri, Terrie, Terry, Tessa, Tessie, Tessy, Tracie, Tracy, Zita.**
English variations: **Teresa, Terese, Teressa, Teresita.**
Foreign variations: **Thérèse** (French), **Therese** (German), **Teresa** (Italian, Spanish), **Toireasa** (Irish).

THETIS—Greek: "positive, determined one." In Greek myths she was the mother of Achilles.

THIRZA—Hebrew: **Tirzah.** "Pleasantness."

THOMASA—Greek: **Thomas.** "A twin." A feminine form of **Thomas.**
English nicknames: **Tommie, Tommy, Tammy.**
English variations: **Thomasina, Thomasine, Tomasina, Tomasine.**

THORA—Old Norse: **Thori-r.** "Thunder." A name for the old Norse god Thor.

THORBERTA—Old Norse: **Thor-biartr.** "Brilliance of Thor." A feminine form of **Thorbert.**

THORDIS—Old Norse: **Thoridyss.** "Thor-spirit." English variation: **Thordia.**

THYRA—Greek: **Thyreos.** "Shield-bearer."

TIBELDA—Old German: **Theudo-bald.** "Boldest of the people."

TIBERIA—Latin: "of the River Tiber."
English nicknames: **Tibbie, Tibby.**

TIFFANY—Popular modern U.S. name; a form of **Theophania**, Greek: "manifestation of God." The Theophania was an ancient spring festival celebrating the appearance of Apollo.

TILDA—See **Mathilda.**

TIMMY—Modern U.S. from Hebrew **Timothea**: "she fears God."

English variations: **Timmi,
Timi.**

TIMOTHEA—Greek: **Timotheos.** "Honoring God." A
feminine form of Timothy.
English nicknames: **Timmie,
Timmy.**

TINA—See **Christine.** Also
used independently.

TITA—Latin: **Titulus.** "A
title of honor."

TITANIA—Greek: **Titan.**
"Giant." The Titans were
primordial Greek deities of
gigantic size. Titania was the
Queen of the Fairies in
Shakespeare's *A Midsummer
Night's Dream.*

TOBY—Hebrew: **Tobhiyah.**
"The Lord is good." A
feminine form of **Tobias.**
Toby Wing, actress.

TONIA—See **Antonia.** Also:
Tonya, Toni.

TOPAZ—Latin: **Topazos.**
"A topaz gem."

TOURMALINE—Singhalese:
Tormalli. "A carnelian or
tourmaline gem."

TOYA—Modern U.S.:
"Toy," with a feminine
ending. Also: **Latoya.**

TRACY—Latin: **Thrasius.**
"Bold or courageous"; or Irish
Gaelic: **Treasach.** "Battler."
Also: **Traci, Tracee.** See
Theresa.

TRAVIATA—Italian: "one

who goes astray." Made
famous by the Verdi opera
La Traviata.

TRILBY—Italian: **Trillare.**
"To sing with trills." A name
coined by George du
Maurier for the heroine of the
novel *Trilby,* who became a
beautiful singer.

TRINITY—Latin: "Triad."
from the Holy Trinity. Also:
Trini, Trinidad, Tini.

TRISTA—Latin: **Triste.**
"Melancholy."

TRIXIE—See **Beatrice.**
Trixie Friganza, entertainer
(1870–1955). Also: **Trixi,
Trixy.**

TRUDA—Old German:
"loved one"; Polish: "spearmaiden."
English nickname: **Trudie.**

TRYPHENA—Latin: **Tryphaena.** "Delicate one."

TUESDAY—Old English:
Tiwesdaeg. "Born on Tuesday." Tuesday Weld,
actress.

TULLIA—Irish Gaelic:
Taith-leach. "Peaceful, quiet
one." A feminine form of
the Irish "Tully."

TWYLA—Middle English:
"woven of double thread."
Twyla Tharp, choreographer.

TYNE—Old English: "river."
Tyne Daly, actress.

TZIGANE—Hungarian: **Czigany.** "A gypsy."

U

UDA—Old German: **Udo.**
"Prosperous one."
English variation: **Udelle.**

ULA—Old German: "owner
of an inherited estate." Also a
varient of **Eula** or **Ulla.**

ULIMA—Arabic: **Alim.**
"Wise, learned one."

ULRICA—Old German:
Alh-ric. "All-ruler." Feminine
form of **Ulric.**

ULTIMA—Latin: "the most
distant, aloof one."

ULVA—Gothic: **Wulfila.**
"Wolf." The wolf was a
medieval symbol of courage.

UNA—Latin: "one, unity;
everything in one"; or Hopi:
"memory." Also: **Unity.**

Una Merkel, Una O'Connor,
actresses.

UNDINE—Latin: **Unda.**
"Of the waves." Undine was a
water sprite in classical myths.

URANIA—Greek: **Ourania.**
"Heavenly." Urania was the
Greek Muse of Astronomy.

URSULA—Latin: **Ursa.** "A
she-bear." St. Ursuline;
Ursula LeGuin, novelist.
English nicknames: **Ursa,
Ursie, Ursy, Orsa.**
English variations: **Ursuline,
Ursola, Orsola.**
Foreign variations: **Ursule**
(French), **Orsola** (Italian),
Ursola (Spanish).

UTA—Diminutive form of
Ottalie: "the rich one." Uta
Hagen, actress.

V

VALA—Gothic: **Waljan.**
"Chosen one."

VALBORGA—Old German:
Waldburga. "Protecting ruler."

VALDA—Old Norse: **Uald.**
"Governor, ruler"; or Teutonic:
"battle-heroine."
English variation: **Velda.**

VALENTINA—Latin: **Valentis.**
"Strong, healthy one." St.

Valentina was a 4th-century
virgin martyr.
English nicknames: **Val,
Vallie.**
English variations: **Valentine,
Valentia, Valeda, Valida,
Velora.**

VALERIE—Old French:
Valeriane. "Strong." St.
Valerie was a 3rd-century
martyr. Valerie Harper,

actress; Valerie Brisco-Hooks, Olympic runner. English nicknames: **Val, Vallie,** English variations: **Valeria, Valery, Valoree, Valencia.** Foreign variations: **Valérie** (French), **Valeria** (Italian).

VALESKA—Old Slavic: **Valdislava.** "Glorious ruler." A feminine form of **Vladislav.**

VALONIA—Latin: **Valles.** "From the vale or hollow."

VANESSA—Greek: "butterflies." Used by Jonathan Swift for Esther Vanhomrigh. Vanessa Redgrave, actress. English nicknames: **Van, Vannie, Vanny, Vanna, Vania.**

VANNA—See **Vanessa.**

VANORA—Old Welsh: **Gwenhwyvar.** "White wave." A development of **Guinevere.**

VARINA—Slavic: **Varvara.** "Stranger." A Slavic development of **Barbara.** Varina Davis, "first lady" of the U.S. Confederacy.

VASHTI—Persian: "beautiful one," or "thread of life." Vashti was the queen of King Ahasuerus in the Biblical Book of Esther.

VEDA—Sanskrit: "knowledge." English variation: **Vedis.**

VEDETTE—Italian: **Vedetta.** "Guardian or sentinel."

VEGA—Arabic: **Waqi.** "The falling one." Referring to the bright star Vega when it sinks below the horizon.

VELDA—Teutonic: "wise."

VELIKA—Old Slavic: "great one."

VELMA—See **Wilhelmina.**

VELVET—Middle English. **Velouette.** "Velvety." Also: **Velvor, Velvina,** in modern U.S. usage.

VENTURA—Spanish: "happiness and good luck."

VENUS—Latin: "loveliness, beauty." Venus, the name for the goddess of beauty and love, personified feminine perfection. English variations: **Venita, Vinita, Vinny, Vinnie.**

VERA—Latin: **Verus:** "True." Vera Miles, actress. English variations: **Vere, Verena, Verene, Verina, Verine, Verla.**

VERBENA—Latin: **Verbenae.** "Sacred boughs."

VERDA—See **Verna.**

VERENA—Old German: **Varin.** "Defender; protector." See **Verna.**

VERNA—Latin: "springlike." English variations: **Verne, Verneta, Vernita, Verda, Verena, Vernis, Virna, Virina.**

VERONICA—See **Bernice.** St. Veronica wiped the face of Jesus Christ as he was on

his way to Calvary. Name-
sakes: Veronica Lake,
Veronica Cartwright, actresses.
English nicknames: **Vonnie,
Vonny, Ronnie.**

VESPERA—Latin: **Vesper.**
"The evening star."

VESTA—Latin: "she who
dwells or lingers." Vesta was
the Roman goddess of the
household and of flocks and
herds.

VEVAY—See **Vivian.**

VEVILA—Irish Gaelic:
Bebhinn. "Melodious harmonious lady."

VICKI—See **Victoria.**

VICTORIA—Latin: "vic-
tory." Famous from Queen
Victoria of England (1819–1901);
Queen Victoria of Spain, wife
of Alphonso XIII; Vicki
Baum, author.
English nicknames: **Vic,
Vickie, Vicki, Vicky.**
English variation: **Victorine.**
Foreign variations: **Vitoria**
(Spanish), **Vittoria** (Italian),
Victoire (French).

VIDA—Hebrew: **Dawid.**
"Beloved one." A feminine
form of **David.**

VIDONIA—Portuguese:
Vidonho. "A vine branch."

VIGILIA—Latin: **Vigilis.**
"Awake and alert."

VIGNETTE—French: "little vine."

VILLETTE—French: **Ville.**
"From the country estate."

VIÑA—Spanish: "from the
vineyard." Vina Delmar,
author.

VINCENTIA—Latin:
Vincentius. "Conquering one."
A feminine form of **Vincent.**

VINITA—See **Venus.**

VIOLA—See **Violet.**

VIOLET—Old French:
Violete. "A violet flower."
Violet Kemble Cooper,
Violet Heming, actresses,
English variations: **Viola,
Violetta, Violette, Iolanthe,
Yolanda, Yolande, Yolanthe.**
Foreign variations: **Viola,
Viole, Violette** (French),
Violetta (Italian), **Violante**
(Spanish, Portuguese.)

VIRGILIA—Latin: **Virgilius.**
"Rod or staff bearer."

VIRGINIA—Latin: "maid-
enly." Virginia Dare, born at
Roanoke, Virginia, in 1587,
was the first white child born
in America of English
parents. Virginia Woolf,
novelist and diarist.
English nicknames: **Virgie,
Virgy, Ginger, Ginnie,
Ginny.**
Foreign variations: **Virginie**
(French, Dutch), **Virginia**
(Italian, German).

VIRIDIS—Latin: **Viridis.**
"Fresh blooming, green."

VITA—Latin: "life."
English variations: **Veta, Vitia.**

VIVECA—Scandinavian
form of Viva. "Also, **Viveka.**
Viveca Lindfors, actress.

VIVIAN—Latin: **Viva.**
"Alive." Saint Vivian or
Vibiana was an early martyr.
Actresses Vivien Leigh,
Vivian Vance, Vivian Blaine.
English nicknames: **Viv,
Vivie.**
English variations: **Viviana,
Vivien, Vivienne, Vivyan.**

Foreign variations: **Vivienne**
(French), **Viviana** (Italian).

VOLANTE—Italian: "flying
one."

VOLETA—Old French:
Volet. "A flowing veil."

VONNY—See **Veronica.**

W

WALDA—Old German:
Waldo. "Ruler."
English variation: **Welda.**

WALLIS—Old English:
Waleis. "One from Wales,
Welshman." Feminine form
of **Wallace.** Wallis Warfield,
Duchess of Windsor.
English nicknames: **Wallie,
Wally.**

WANDA—Old German:
Wando, Wendi. "Wanderer";
Slavic: "shepherdess, wan-
dering one." Wanda Hendrix,
actress.
English nicknames: **Wandie,
Wendy.**
English variations: **Wandis,
Wenda, Wendeline.**

WANETTA—Old English:
Wann. "Pale one."

WARDA—Old German:
Warto. "Guardian." A feminine form of **Ward.**

WELDA—See **Walda.**

WENDY—See **Wanda.**
Wendy Hiller, actress.

WENONA—American In-
dian: "first-born daughter."

WILDA—Old German:
"Untamed." Also: **Wylda.**

WILHELMINA—Old Ger-
man: **Willi-helm.** "Resolute
protector." A feminine form
of **William.** Famous from
Wilhelmina, Queen of
Holland. Willa Cather,
novelist; Wilma Rudolph,
track champion.
English nicknames: **Willie,
Willy, Minnie, Minny,
Billie, Billy, Helma.**
English variations: **Wilhelma,
Wilhelmine, Willamina,
Willa, Willete, Wilmette,
Wilma, Wylma, Vilma,
Willabelle.**
Foreign variations: **Guillelmine,
Guillemette** (French),
Wilhelmine (German, Dan-
ish), **Guglielma** (Italian),
Guillelmina (Spanish), **Vilhel-
mina** (Swedish).

WILLA—See **Wilhelmina.**

WILLABELLE—See
Wilhelmina.

WILLOW—Modern U.S.
name, after the graceful tree.

WILMA—See **Wilhelmina.**

WILVA—Teutonic: "determined."

WINEMA—Modoc Indian: "woman chief."

WINIFRED—Old German: Wini-frid. "Peaceful friend." English nicknames: **Winnie, Winny.**

WINOLA—Old German:

Wini-holdo. "Gracious friend."

WINONA—Sioux Indian: **Winona.** "First-born daughter." Winona Judd, country singer. English variations: **Winonah, Wenona, Wyomia.**

WYNNE—Old Welsh: Wyn. "Fair, White."

X

XANTHE—Greek: **Xanthos.** "Yellow."

XAVIERA—Spanish Basque: **Javerri; Xaver.** "Owner of the new house." A feminine form of **Xavier.**

XENIA—Greek: "hospitable one, guest." English variations: **Xena, Xene, Zenia.**

XYLONA—Greek: **Xylon.** "From the forest."

Y

YASMIN—See **Jasmine.**

YEDDA—Old English: **Giddian.** "To sing; singer." English variation: **Yetta.**

YETTA—Old English: **Geatan.** "To give; giver." See **Henrietta, Yedda.**

YNEZ—See **Agnes, Inez.**

YOLANDA—Greek: **Iolanthe.** "Violet flower." See **Violet, Iolanthe.** Yolande, queen of

Scotland's King Alexander III, 1249–1286. English variations: **Eolande, Iolande, Iolanda.** Foreign variations: **Yolande** (French), **Yolanda** (Italian).

YVETTE—See **Yvonne.** Yvette Mimieux, actress.

YVONNE—Old French: **Yves.** "Yew-bow." Yvonne de Carlo, actress. English variations: **Yvette, Yevette.**

Z

ZADA—Arabic: **S'ad.**
"Lucky one." Also: **Zayda,
Zaida.**

ZANDRA—See **Alexandra.**

ZANETA—See **Jane.**

ZARA—Hebrew: **Zarah.**
"East; dawn brightness." Also,
an Arabic royal name:
"princess."

ZEA—Latin: "a kind of
grain." Also: **Zia.**

ZELDA—See **Griselda.**
Zelda Fitzgerald, novelist.
and wife of F. Scott Fitzgerald.

ZELIA—Greek: **Zelos.** "Zeal."
Zelia Nuttall, Ameri-
can archaeologist.
English variations: **Zele,
Zelie, Zelina.**

ZELMA—See **Anselma.**

ZENA—See **Xenia, Zenobia.**

ZENAIDA—See **Zenobia.**

ZENDA—See **Zenobia.**

ZENIA—See **Xenia, Zenobia.**

ZENINA—See **Zenobia.**

ZENNA—See **Zenobia.**

ZENOBIA—Greek: **Zenbios.**
"Given life by Jupiter or
Zeus." Jupiter or Zeus was
the head of the gods of
antiquity. Zenobia was the
3rd-century A.D. ruler of the
Syrian city-state of Palmyra.

English variations: **Zena,
Zenaida, Zenda, Zenna,
Zenia.**
Foreign variation: **Zénobie**
(French).

ZERA—Hebrew: **Zera'im.**
"Seeds."

ZERLINDA—Hebrew-Spanish:
Zarah-linda. "Dawn-beautiful."
English variation: **Zerlinda.**

ZETA—Greek: "the letter
'Z,' sixth letter of the Greek
alphabet."

ZEVA—Greek: **Siphos.**
"Sword."

ZILLA—Hebrew: **Zillah.**
"Shadow." Protective shade.

ZINNIA—New Latin: "the
zinnia flower." Named for
German Prof. J. G. Zinn,
18th century.
English variation: **Zinia.**

ZIPPORA—Hebrew: **Zipporah.**
"Beauty; trumpet; or spar-
row." Zipporah was the
Biblical wife of Moses.

ZITA—See **Rosita, Theresa.**

ZOË—Greek: "Life." Zoë
Caldwell, actress.

ZONA—Latin: "a girdle."
Zona was applied as a name
for the belt of Orion in the
great constellation. Zona Gale,
author.

ZORA—Slavic: "Aurora or dawn."
English variations: **Zorina, Zorine.** Zora Neale Hurston, author.

ZSA ZSA—Hungarian form of **Susan.**

ZULEIKA—Arabic: "fair and bright." *Zuleika Dobson*, a novel by Max Beerbohm.

Names for Boys

●

A

AARON—Hebrew: **Aharon.** "Lofty or exalted," Aaron, brother of Moses, qualified and enlightened, was exalted as the first high priest of the Hebrews. Aaron Burr, 3rd Vice-President of the U.S.
English variation: **Aron.**
Foreign variation: **Haroun** (Arabic).

ABBOT—Old English: **Abod,** from Arabic: **Abba.** "Abbey father." Abbott Thayer, American painter (1849-1921); Abbot Kinney, creator of Venice, California. Also: **Abbott.**
Foreign variations: **Abboid** (Gaelic), **Abott, Abbe** (French), **Abad** (Spanish).

ABDUL—Arabic: "servant of Allah." Also: **Abdullah.** Kareem Abdul-Jabbar, basketball player and author.

ABEL—Hebrew: **Heb-hel.** "Breath, evanescence." Abel was the second son of Adam and Eve.

ABELARD—Old German: **Adelhard.** "Nobly resolute." Pierre Abelard, 12th-century French philosopher, renowned for his romance with Heloise.

ABNER—Hebrew: **Abhner.** "Father of Light." Abner Doubleday, inventor of baseball.

ABRAHAM—Hebrew: "father of the multitude." The most exalted founder of the Hebrew people. Abraham Lincoln, 16th President of the U.S.
English nicknames: **Abe, Abie, Bram.**
Foreign variations: **Abramo, Abrahamo** (Italian), **Abrahán** (Spanish), **Ibrahim** (Arabic).

ABRAM—Hebrew: "the lofty one is father." Abram Newkirk, American Episcopal bishop, 1824-1901,
English nicknames: **Abe, Abie.**
Foreign variations: **Abramo** (Italian), **Bram** (Dutch).

ACE—Latin: **As.** "Unity," that is, "first in luck or accomplishment." English nickname: **Acey.**

ACKERLEY—Old English: **Aecer-leah.** "Dweller at the oak-tree meadow." Also: **Ackley.** English nickname: **Ack.**

ADAIR—Scottish Gaelic: **Athdara.** "From the oak-tree ford." James Adair (1710-1780), American writer. Scottish ballad: "Robin Adair."

ADALARD—Old German: **Adal-hard.** "Noble and brave." St. Adalard, c. 751-827, abbey founder in Saxony. Also: **Adelard.**

ADAM—Hebrew: **Adham.** "Man of the red earth." And God created Adam of the red dust of the earth, and breathed into his nostrils life." Adam may be the oldest remembered name. English nicknames: **Ad, Ade.** Foreign variations: **Adan** (Spanish), **Adamo** (Italian) **Adao** (Portuguese), **Adhamh** (Irish and Scottish).

ADDISON—Old English: **Addison.** "Son of Adam." Addison Verrill, American zoologist.

ADEL, ADAL—teutonic: "noble."

ADELBERT—See **Albert.**

ADLAI—Hebrew: "my witness, my ornament." Adlai E. Stevenson, statesman.

ADLER—Old German: **Adlar.** "Eagle." Keen of mind and vision. Alfred Adler (1870-1937), Austrian psychiatrist and psychologist. Also: **Adlar.**

ADNEY—Old English: **Addan-eye.** "Dweller on the noble-one's island."

ADOLPH—Old German: **Adal-wolf.** "Noble wolf," or "noble hero." Adolph Zukor, noted motion picture pioneer; Adolphe Menjou, noted actor; Adolpho Lopez Mateos, President of Mexico. English nicknames: **Ad, Dolf, Dolph** Foreign variations: **Adolf** (German, Swedish, Dutch, Danish), **Adolphus** (Swedish), **Adolfo** (Spanish, Italian), **Adolphe** (French).

ADON—Phoenician: "lord." Adon was a sacred Hebrew name for God. Foreign variation: **Adonis** (Greek).

ADRIAN—Latin: **Ater.** "Dark one," or "from Adna"; Adria was an ancient town in central Italy. Adrian Stokes, British painter (1854–1935); Adrian, motion picture costume designer. English variation: **Hadrian.** Foreign variation: **Adriano** (Italian), **Adrien** (French), **Adrián** (Spanish).

ADRIEL—Hebrew: **Adriyel.** "From God's congregation."

AENEAS—Greek: **Aineias.**
"The praised one." The
legendary defender of Troy,
memorialized in Greek song
and story.
English variation: **Eneas.**
Foreign variation: **Enne**
(French), **Eneas** (Spanish).

AHERN—Irish Gaelic:
Each-thighearn. "Horse-lord"
or "Owner of many horses."
Brian Aherne, noted actor.
Foreign variations: **Ahearn,
Aherin, Aherne, Hearne,
Hearn.** (English and Irish).

AHMED—Arabic: "highly
praised." Also: **Ahmad.**

AHREN—Old Low German: "eagle."

AIDAN—Irish Gaelic:
Aodhan. "Little fiery one." St.
Aidan, famous Irish monk,
died A.D. 651; Aidan Quinn,
actor.
English variation: **Eden.**

AIKEN—Old North English: **Ad-ken.** "Little Adam,"
or "oaken." The oak is a
symbol of strength. Conrad
Aiken, American poet.
English variations: **Aikin,
Aickin.**

AINSLEY—Old English:
Ainesleah. "Meadow."

ALAN—Irish Gaelic: **Alain.**
"Handsome, cheerful, harmonious one." Alan B.
Shepard, first American
astronaut; Alan Paton,
author; Alan Jay Lerner,
lyricist and librettist.

English variations: **Allan,
Allen, Allyn, Aland.**
Foreign variations: **Alain**
(French), **Alano** (Italian,
Spanish), **Ailean** (Scottish),
Ailin (Irish).

ALARIC—Old German:
Alh-ric: "Ruler of all" or Old
German: **Adal-ric:** "Noble
ruler." Famous as a 4th-
century king of the
Visigoths. Alaric Watts,
English poet and journalist,
1797–1864.
Foreign variations: **Alarico**
(Spanish), **Alrik** (Swedish).

ALASTAIR—Greek: **Alastor.**
"The avenger"; or Scottish
Gaelic: **Alasdair,** a form of
Alexander. "Defender of
men." Alastair Cooke,
author and TV commentator.
English variations: **Allister,
Alister, Alaster.**

ALBEN—Latin: **Albinus.**
"Fair-complexioned one."
Alben Barkley, Vice-President of the U.S. St. Alban,
English martyr, died A.D
303.
English variations: **Albin,
Alban.**
Foreign variations: **Aubin**
(French), **Alban** (Irish) **Alva**
(Spanish).

ALBERN—Old English:
Aethelbeorn. "Noble warrior."

ALBERT—Old English:
Aethelberht. "Noble and
brilliant or illustrious."
Albert Einstein, scientist
(1879-1955); King Albert of
Belgium, ruled 1909-1934.

English nicknames: **Al, Albie, Bert.**
English variations: **Elbert, Adelbert.**
Foreign variations: **Albrecht, Adalbert** (German), **Aubert** (French), **Alberto** (Italian, Spanish), **Ailbert** (Scottish).

ALBIN—See **Alben.**

ALCOTT—Old English: **Aldcott.** "Dweller at the old cottage."

ALDEN—Old English: **Aldwine.** "Old, wise protector or friend." John Alden, Pilgrim settler in 1620 at Plymouth, Massachusetts. English variations: **Aldin, Aldwin, Aldwyn, Elden, Eldin.**

ALDER—Old English: **Aler.** "At the alder-tree."

ALDIS—Old English: **Aldhus.** "From the old house." Aldous Huxley, writer. English variations: **Aldous, Aldus.**

ALDO—Old German: **Ald.** "Old and wise." Aldo Ray, American actor; Aldo Manutius, Italian printer (1449-1515).

ALDRICH—Old English: **Aldric.** "Old, wise ruler." Thomas Bailey Aldrich (1836-1907), American writer, poet, novelist. English variations: **Aldric, Eldric.** Foreign variation: **Audric** (French).

ALDWIN—Old English: **Aldwine.** "Old friend or protector." English variation: **Eldwin.**

ALEK—Russian variant of Alexander. Greek: "he helps people." Also: **Alik.**

ALERON—Middle Latin: **Alerio.** "Eagle."

ALEXANDER—Greek: **Alexandros.** "Helper and defender of mankind." Alexander the Great, Macedonian world conqueror, died 323 B.C.; Alexander Hamilton, American statesman; Sir Alec Guinness, actor. English nicknames: **Alex, Alexis, Alec, Sandy, Sander, Saunders.** Foreign variations: **Alister, Alasdair** (Scottish), **Alsandair** (Irish), **Alessandro** (Italian), **Alejandro** (Spanish), **Alexio** (Portuguese), **Alexandre** (French, Portuguese), **Aleksandr** (Russian).

ALEXIS—See **Alexander.** Foreign variation: **Alejo** (Spanish).

ALFONSO—See **Alphonso.**

ALFORD—Old English: **Aldford.** "The old ford or river-crossing."

ALFRED—Old English: **Aelfraed.** "Good or elfin counselor." King Alfred the Great of England; Alfred, Lord Tennyson, poet; Alfred Hitchcock, director, producer.

English nicknames: **Al, Alf, Alfie.**
Foreign variations: **Alfredo** (Italian, Spanish), **Ailfrid** (Irish).

ALGER—Old German: **Adalgar.** "Noble spearman." Horatio Alger, American writer.
English variation: **Algar.**

ALGERNON—Old French: **Algrenon.** "Man with a mustache or beard." Algernon Swinburne, famous 19th-century English poet.
English nicknames: **Algie, Algy.**

ALI—Arabic: "lion of God." Muhammed Ali, boxer.

ALISON—Old English: **Adalson:** "Noble one's son." Also English: **Alice-son;** Old German-French: **Alh-som.** "Holy or sacred fame." Sir Archibald Alison, British historian (1792-1867).
English nickname: **Al.**
English variation: **Allison.**

ALLAN—See Alan.

ALLARD—Old English: **Alhhard.** "Sacred and brave", or Old English: **Aethelhard.** "Noble, brave." Allard Lowenstein, civil rights activist.
Foreign variation: **Alard** (French).

ALLEN—See Alan.

ALLISON—See Alison.

ALLISTER—See Alastair.

ALMO—Old English:

Aethelmaer. "Noble and famous."

ALONZO—See Alphonso.

ALOYSIUS—Late Latin: **Aloisius.** "Famous warrior." See Lewis. St. Aloysius, 1568-1591, a Jesuit of Lombardy.
English variations: **Aloys, Lewis, Louis.**
Foreign variations: **Louis** (French), **Ludwig** (German), **Alabhaois** (Irish).

ALPHONSO—Old German: **Adal-funs.** "Noble and ready." Alphonso Taft, U.S. Secretary of War, 1876; Alphonso XIII, King of Spain, 1886-1931; Alphouse Daudet, famous 19th-century French writer; Alonzo Stagg, football coach.
English variations: **Alfonso, Alonso, Alonzo.**
Foreign variations: **Alfonso** (Spanish, Italian, Swedish), **Alonso** (Spanish), **Alphonse** (French), **Alfons** (German, Swedish), **Alphonsus** (Irish), **Affonso** (Portuguese).

ALPIN—From Latin: **Albinus.** Pictish-Scottish: "blond one." Clan MacAlpin, descendants of Kenneth MacAlpin, claim to be the oldest Scottish clan.

ALROY—Irish Gaelic: **Giollaruaidh.** "Red-haired youth."

ALSTON—Old English: **Aethelstun.** "Noble one's estate."

ALTMAN—Old German:
Altmann. "Old, wise man."
St. Altman, founder of
Benedictine Abbey, Austria
(1020-1091).

ALTON—Old English:
Ald-tun. "Dweller at the old
town or estate."

ALVA—Latin: **Albinus.**
"Blond one. Thomas Alva
Edison, American inventor
(1847-1931).
Foreign variation: **Alba**
(Spanish).

ALVAH—Hebrew: "exalted
one."

ALVIN—Old German: **Alh-
win.** "Friend of all"; or
Adal-win: "noble friend."
English variations: **Alwin,
Alwyn, Alvan.**
Foreign variations: **Aloin,
Aluin** (French), **Aluino**
(Spanish), **Alwin** (German).

ALVIS—Old Norse: **Alviss.**
"All-wise." The dwarf Alviss
in Nordic mythology
demanded the daughter of the
god Thor in marriage.

AMADEO—Italian: "one
who loves God." Also:
Amadeus. Wolfang Amadeus
Mozart, composer.

AMASA—Hebrew: "burden
bearer." Amasa Walker,
American political econo-
mist. (1799-1875).

AMBROSE—Greek: **Ambro-
tos.** "Divine, immortal
one." St. Ambrose, 4th-
century Bishop of Milan,

Italy; Ambrose Bierce, noted
American writer.
Foreign variations: **Ambrogio,
Ambrosi** (Italian), **Ambroise**
(French), **Ambrosio** (Spanish),
Ambrosius (German, Swe-
dish, Dutch), **Ambros** (Irish).

AMERIGO—See **Emery.**
Amerigo Vespucci, Italian
explorer after whom Amer-
ica was named.

AMERY—See **Amory.**

AMMON—Egyptian: **Amen.**
"The hidden." "No man shall
see the face of God." St.
Ammon the Great, one of the
earliest and greatest hermit-
monks, died A.D. 350.

AMORY—Old German:
Alh-mar-ric. "Divine, famous
ruler." An ancestor who
seemed endowed with wisdom
from on high.
English variation: **Amery.**

AMOS—Hebrew: "a bur-
den, borne by God." Amos
was an 8th-century Biblical
prophet. Amos Bronson Alcott
(1799-1888), American
teacher, philosopher.

ANATOLE—Greek: **Anatolios.**
"Man from the East." Anatole
France, French writer
(1844-1924).
Foreign variations: **Anatol**
(Slavic), **Anatolio** (Spanish).

ANDERS—See **Andrew.**

ANDREW—Greek: **Andreas.**
"Strong, manly." St. Andrew
the Apostle is the patron
saint of Scotland. St. Andrew's

"X" shaped cross appears on the British flag and on innumerable coats-of-arms of Scottish and English families. Andrew Jackson, 7th President of United States; Andrew Carnegie (1837-1919), steel magnate and philanthropist; André Maurois, French writer.
English nicknames: **Andie, Andy.**
Foreign variations: **Andreas** (German, Dutch, Swedish), **André** (French), **Andrés** (Spanish), **Andrea** (Italian), **Andrej** (Slavic), **Aindreas** (Scottish and Irish), **Anders** (Swedish).

ANGELO—Greek: "angel or messenger." Pope John XXIII (Angelo Roncalli).
English variations: **Angel, Angell.**
English nickname: **Angie.**

ANGUS—Scottish Gaelic: **Aonghus.** "Unique strength; the choice." Angus or Aonghus, grandson of Niall of the Nine Hostages, 10th-century Irish ruler, was ancestor of many Irish and Scottish clans. Angus is a popular Scottish name. Angus Wilson, author.

ANNAN—Celtic: **Anant.** "From the stream."

ANSCOM—Old English: **Aenescumb.** "Dweller in the valley of the awe-inspiring one."
English variations: **Anscomb.**

ANSEL—Old French:

Ancel. "Adherent of a nobleman." See **Anselm.** Ansel Adams, photographer.
English variations: **Ansell.**

ANSELM—Old German: **Anshelm.** "With divine protection." St. Anselm, the Father of Scholasticism, died A.D. 1109.
English nicknames: **Anse, Ansel.**
Foreign variations: **Anselme** (French), **Anselmi** (Italian), **Anselmo** (Spanish, Portuguese), **Anshelm** (German).

ANSLEY—Old English: **Aene's-leah.** "From the awe-inspiring one's pasture meadow."

ANSON—Old English: **Aene's-son.** "Awe-inspiring one's son." Anson Williams, actor.

ANSTICE—Greek: **Anastasios.** "Resurrected one."
English variation: **Anstiss.**

ANTHONY—Latin: **Antonius.** "Inestimable, priceless one." St. Anthony the Great, died A.D. 356, early Christian hermit; St. Anthony of Padua, died A.D. 1231, patron saint of the poor; Anthony Wayne, American Revolutionary War general; Anthony Eden, British Prime Minister; actors include Anthony Quinn, Anthony Quayle, Tony Randall, Tony Curtis.
English nicknames: **Tony.**
Foreign variations: **Antonio** (Spanish, Italian, Portuguese), **Antoine** (French),

Anton, Antonius (German, Swedish), **Anntoin** (Irish).

ANTOINE—Popular modern U.S. form of **Anthony**. Originally French.

ANWELL—Welsh-Celtic: **Anwyl**. "Beloved or dear one."
English variations: **Anwyl, Anwyll**.

ANYON—Welsh-Celtic: **Einion**. "Anvil."

ARCHARD—Anglo-French-German: **Erchan-hardt**. "Sacred, powerful."
English variation: **Archerd**.

ARCHER—Old English: **Archere**. "Bowman, archer."

ARCHIBALD—Anglo-French-German: **Erchan-bold**. "Sacred, noble, and bold."
Archibald MacLeish, American poet and dramatist.
English nicknames: **Arch, Archie**.
Foreign variations: **Archaimbaud, Archambault** (French), **Archibaldo** (Spanish), **Gilleasbuig** (Scottish), **Archimbald** (German).

ARDEN—Latin: **Ardens**. "Ardent, fiery."
English variation: **Ardin**.

ARDLEY—Old English: **Ardaleah**. "From the home-lover's meadow."

ARDMORE—Latin and Teutonic: "more ardent, more fervent."

ARDOLPH—Old English: **Ardwolf**. "Home-loving wolf."

ARGUS—Greek: **Argos**. "Watchful guardian." Argus in Greek mythology was the giant with a hundred eyes. Legend says that these eyes later ornamented the peacock's tail feathers.

ARGYLE—Scottish Gaelic: **Arregaithel**. "From the Land of the Gaels, an Irishman."

ARIC—Old English: **Alhric**. "Sacred ruler."
English nicknames: **Ric, Rick, Ricky**.

ARIEL—Hebrew: "lion of God."

ARIES—Latin: "a ram."

ARISTOTLE—Greek: "best of the thinkers." Aristotle, Greek philosopher; Aristotle Onassis.
Foreign variation: **Ari** (Israeli).

ARLEDGE—Old English: **Harelache**. "Dweller at the hare or rabbit lake." Roone Arledge, broadcasting executive.

ARLEN—Irish Gaelic: **Airleas**. "Pledge." Michael Arlen, English writer; Richard Arlen, American actor.
Foreign variation: **Arles** (Scandinavian).

ARLEY—Old English: **Hara-leah**. "From the rabbit meadow."
English variation: **Harley**.

ARLO—Spanish: "the barberry." Arlo Guthrie, singer.

ARMAND—Old German:

Hariman. "Armed, protective one." Armand was patron saint of the Netherlands. English variations: **Armin, Ormond, Armond.** Foreign variations: **Armando** (Spanish, Italian), **Arman** (Russian).

ARMSTRONG—Old English: **Arm-strang.** "Strong of arm (in battle)."

ARNALL—Old German: **Arn-hold.** "Eagle-gracious." English variation: **Arnell.**

ARNETT—Old Franco-English: **Arnet.** "Little eagle." English variations: **Arnatt, Arnott.**

ARNEY—Old German: **Arni.** "Eagle." English variation: **Arnie.** Foreign variation: **Arne** (Norwegian).

ARNO—Old German: **Arn-wulf.** "Eagle-wolf." Peter Arno, American cartoonist. Foreign variations: **Arnou, Arnoux** (French).

ARNOLD—Old German: **Arn-wald.** "Eagle-ruler" or "strong as an eagle." Arnold Bennett, famous English novelist (1867–1931). Foreign variations: **Arnaldo** (Spanish), **Arnoldo** (Italian), **Arnaud** (French).

ARNOT—Old Franco-German: "little eagle." English variation: **Arnott.**

ARTEMAS—Greek: "gift of Artemis." St. Artemas, 1st century, was one of St. Paul's disciples. Artemas Ward, American Revolutionary War general (1727-1800).

ARTHUR—Cymric-Welsh: **Arth-wr.** "Noble one" or "bear-man." King Arthur, semi-legendary 6th-century English ruler was the subject of many romantic tales. Arthur Balfour, British statesman (1848-1930); Art Linkletter, television personality. English nicknames: **Art, Artie.** Foreign variations: **Arturo** (Spanish, Italian), **Artair** (Scottish), **Artur** (Irish), **Artus** (French).

ARUNDEL—Old English: **Arndell.** "Dweller at the eagle dell."

ARVAD—Hebrew: "wanderer." Arpad, who died in A.D. 907, was the national hero of Hungary. Foreign variation: **Arpad** (Hungarian).

ARVAL—Latin: **Arvalis.** "Cultivated land." Welsh: **Arvel.** "Wept-over." English variation: **Arvel.**

ARVIN—Old German: **Hariwin.** "Friend of the people."

ASA—Hebrew: "physician." The Biblical Asa was a Judean king. Asa Gray, American botanist (1810-1888).

ASCOT—Old English: **Est-**

cot. "Dweller at the east cottage."
English variation: **Ascott.**

ASHBURN—Old English: **Aesoburne.** "Ash-tree brook."

ASHBY—Old English: **Aesc-by.** "Ash-tree farm."

ASHER—Hebrew: "happy one."

ASHFORD—Old English: **Aesc-ford.** "Dweller at the ash-tree ford."

ASHLEY—Old English: **Aesc-leah.** "Dweller at the ash-tree meadow." Also used for women.

ASHLIN—Old English: **Aesc-lin** "Dweller at the ash-tree pool."

ASHTON—Old English: **Aesc-tun.** "Dweller at the ash-tree farm." Sir Frederick Ashton, choreographer.

ASHUR—East Semitic: "warlike one." Ashur-banipal and Ashur-nasirpal were ancient Assyrian kings.

ASWIN—Old English: **Aesc-wine.** "Spear-friend or protector."

ATHERTON—Old English: **Aethre-tun** "Dweller at the spring-farm."

ATLEY—Old English: **Atte-leah.** "Dweller at the meadow."

ATWATER—Old English: **Atte-water.** "Dweller at the

water." Wilbur Atwater, American chemist (1844-1907).

ATWELL—Old English: **Atte-welle.** "Dweller at the spring."

ATWOOD—Old English: **Atte-wode.** "At the forest." George Atwood, English mathematician (1746-1807).

ATWORTH—Old English: **Atte-worthe.** "At the farmstead."

AUBERT—See **Albert.**

AUBIN—Old French: "fair, blond one."

AUBREY—Old French: **Albaric.** "Blond ruler, elf ruler, spirit ruler." Aubrey Beardsley, 19th-century English painter.
Foreign variation: **Alberik** (Swedish).

AUDRIC—Old German: **Adalric.** "Noble ruler."

AUDWIN—Old German: **Adalwine.** "Noble friend."

AUGUST—Latin: **Augustus.** "Imperial, exalted, revered." Augustus Caesar, 63 B.C.-A.D. 14, first Roman emperor; Auguste Rodin, sculptor; Auguste Renoir, Augustus John, painters.
English nickname: **Gus.**
English variations: **Augustus, Augustine, Austin.**
Foreign variations: **Agosto** (Italian), **Auguste,** (French), **Augusto** (Spanish), **Aguistin** (Irish).

AUGUSTINE—Latin: **Augustinus.** "Belonging to Augustus." St. Augustine, Oracle of the Western Church, A.D. 354-430. English variations: **Austin, Austen.**

AUSTIN—See **Augustine.**

AVENALL—Old French: **Avenelle.** "Dweller at the oat field. English variations: **Avenel, Aveneil.**

AVERELL—Middle English: **Averil.** "Born in the month of April"; or Old English: **Efer-hild.** "Boar-warrior." Averell Harriman, American statesman. English variations: **Averil, Averill.**

AVERY—Old English: **Aelfric.** "Elf-ruler." Legendary, mischievous elfin ruler of primeval Britain. Avery Brundage, Olympics administrator. Also: **Aubrey.**

AXEL—Old German: **Apsel.** "Father of peace." Scandinavian form of the Hebrew **Absalom.**

AXTON—Old English: **Aecce's-stanc.** "Sword-wielder's stone."

AYLMER—Old English: **Aethel-maere.** "Noble-famous one"; or Old English: **Aegel-maere.** "Awe-inspiring, famous." John Aylmer, bishop of London (1521-1594).

AYLWARD—Old English: **Aegel-weard.** "Awe-inspiring guardian"; or Old English: **Aethel-weard.** "Noble guardian."

B

BAILEY—Old French: **Bailli.** "Bailiff or steward." English variations: **Baillie, Baily, Bayley.**

BAINBRIDGE—Old English: **Ban-brigge.** "Bridge over white water." Commodore William Bainbridge (1774-1833), American naval officer.

BAIRD—Irish Gaelic: **Bhaird.** "Ballad singer, bard, minstrel." Baird, a 13th-century chieftain, founded the Scottish clan Baird.

English variation: **Bard.**

BALBO—Latin: **Balbus.** "The indistinct speaker." General Italo Balbo, prominent in World War II. Foreign variations: **Bailby** (French), **Balbi** (Italian).

BALDEMAR—Old German: "bold or princely and famous." Foreign variation: **Baumer** (French).

BALDER—Old English: **Bald-here.** "Bold army." An extremely brave army leader;

or Old Norse: **Baldr.**
"Prince." Balder was the god
of peace in old Norse
mythology.
Foreign variation: **Baldur**
(Norse), **Baudier** (French).

BALDRIC—Old German:
"bold or princely ruler." St.
Baldric was a 7th-century
French religious leader;
Baldric, a landowner, is
listed in the 11th-century
English Domesday Book.
Foreign variation: **Baudric**
(French).

BALDWIN—Old German:
"bold friend or protector."
Baldwin of Flanders was a
famous 11th-century King of
Jerusalem;
Foreign variations: **Balduin**
(German, Swedish, Danish),
Baudoin (French), **Baldovino**
(Italian).

BALFOUR—Gaelic-Pictish:
Baile-four. "From the pasture
place." Balfour, a noted
Scottish name, is from a town
in Fifeshire.

BALLARD—Old German:
Baldhardt. "Bold, strong."

BALTHASAR—Greek:
Baltasaros. "May the Lord
protect the king." Balthasar
was one of the Three Wise
Men or Magi who brought
gifts to the Christ Child.
Foreign variations: **Belshazzar**
(Hebrew), **Baltasar** (Ger-
man, Swedish), **Balthasar**
(French), **Baldassare** (Italian).

BANCROFT—Old English:

Benecroft. "From the bean
field." A medieval place name
and family name.

BANNING—Irish Gaelic:
Ban-ain. "Little blond one."
Old English: **Bana-ing.**
"Son of the slayer." An
Anglo-Saxon family name,
probably occupational, for one
who read the banns in
church.

BARCLAY—Old English:
Berc-leah. "Dweller at the
birch-tree meadow." Bar-
clay is a famous clan name.
English variation: **Berkeley.**

BARD—Irish Gaelic: "poet
and singer."
Foreign variations: **Baird**
(Scottish), **Barde** (French).

BARDOLF—Old English:
Barda-wulf. "Axe-wolf."
Bardolfus is listed in the
English Curia Regis Rolls,
A.D. 1205.
English variations: **Bardolph,**
Bardulf, Bardulph.
Foreign variations: **Bardoul,**
Bardou (French).

BARDRICK—Old English:
Barda-ric. "Axe-ruler."

BARLOW—Old English:
Baer-hloew. "Dweller at the
bare hill." Alternate origin,
Old English: **Bar-hloew.**
"Boar-hill."

BARNABAS—Greek, He-
brew: "Son of prophecy or
consolation." An heir of his
father who taught spiritual
truths. St. Barnabas was a
companion of St. Paul;

Barnaby Rudge, a character
in Dickens' writings.
English nicknames: **Barnaby,
Barney, Barny.**
Foreign variations: **Barnabé**
(French), **Barnaba, Barna**
(Italian), **Bernabé, Barnebás**
(Spanish).

BARNABY—See **Barnabas.**

BARNARD—See **Bernard.**
St. Barnard, 9th-century
French archbishop.

BARNETT—Old English:
Boern-et. "Nobleman; leader."

BARNUM—Old English:
Beorn's-ham. "Nobleman's
home." Phineas T. Barnum,
famous American circus owner
and showman (1810-1891).

BARON—Old English:
"nobleman, warrior." James
Barron, American Navy
Commodore (1769-1851).
English variation: **Barron.**

BARR—Old English: **Barre.**
"A gateway." Alternate origin,
Old German: **Ber.** "Bear."

BARRET—Old German:
Bero-walt. "Bear-mighty."
Baret was a landowner in
the English Domesday Book,
11th century; Barrett
Wendell, American author-
educator.
English variation: **Barrett.**

BARRIE—See **Barry.**

BARRIS—Old Welsh: **Ab-
Harry.** "Son of Harry."

BARRY—Irish Gaelic:
Bearach. "Spearlike or

pointed." Alternate origin,
Old French: **Bari.** "Barrier or
farm." American actors
include Barry Sullivan and
Barry Bostwick.

BARTHOLOMEW—Hebrew:
Bar-Talmai. "Son of the
furrows; a farmer." St.
Bartholomew was one of the
twelve Apostles; Bartholomew
Dias, Portuguese explorer.
English nicknames: **Bart,
Bartel, Barth, Bat.**
Foreign variations: **Barthélemy,
Bartholomé** (French),
Bartholomaus, Barthel (Ger-
man), **Bartolomeo** (Italian),
Bartolome (Spanish), **Parlan**
(Scottish), **Bartholomeus** (Swe-
dish, Dutch).

BARTLEY—Old English:
Bart-leah. "Bart's meadow."
Foreign variation: **Beartlaidh**
(Irish).

BARTON—Old English:
Beretun. "He holds the land
or farmstead." Barton
MacLane, American actor.
English nickname: **Bart.**

BARTRAM—Old English:
Beorht-hramm. "Glorious
raven." The raven was the
Viking armorial symbol. John
Bartram, American botanist
(1699-1777).
English variation: **Barthram.**

BASIL—Latin: **Basileolus.**
"Kingly, magnificent." St.
Basil the Great, A.D.
329-379, was founder of the
Greek Orthodox Church;
Basil Rathbone, actor.
Foreign variations: **Basile**

(French), **Basilio** (Italian, Spanish, Portuguese), **Basilius** (German, Swedish, Dutch), **Vassily** (Russian).

BAXTER—Old English: **Backstere.** "Bread-baker." Baxter Ward, American television commentator. English nickname: **Bax.**

BAYARD—Old English: **Bayhard.** "Reddish-brown haired and powerful." The Chevalier Bayard, medieval French knight, was renowned for courage and honor; Bayard Taylor, 19th-century American essayist. English nickname: **Bay.** Foreign variations: **Biaiardo, Baiardo** (Italian).

BEACHER—Old English: **Bece-ere.** "Dweller by the beech tree." An old locality name. English nicknames: **Beach, Beachy, Beech, Beechy.** English variations: **Beecher.**

BEAGAN—Irish Gaelic: **Beagan.** "Little one." English variation: **Beagen.**

BEAL—Old French: **Bel.** "Handsome one." William J. Beal (1838–1924), American botanist. English variations: **Beale, Beall.**

BEAMAN—Old English: **Beomann.** "Beekeeper."

BEAMER—Old English: **Bemeere.** "Trumpeter."

BEATTIE—Irish Gaelic:

Biadhtaiche. "Public victualer." Masculine form of Beatrice, thus: "he who blesses." Warren Beatty, actor-director. English variations: **Beatie, Beaty, Beatty.**

BEAU—Old French: "handsome one." Beau Brummell, admired by women and envied by men, a 19th-century English dandy; Beau Bridges, actor.

BEAUFORT—Old French: "from the beautiful stronghold." Henry Beaufort, English 15th-century cardinal.

BEAUMONT—Old French: "from the beautiful mountain." Francis Beaumont, English dramatist (1584-1616).

BECK—Middle English: **Bek.** "A brook."

BEECHER—See **Beacher.** Henry Ward Beecher, 19th-century American clergyman.

BELDEN—Old English: **Bel-dene.** "Dweller in the beautiful glen." English variation: **Beldon.**

BELLAMY—Old French: "handsome friend." Ralph Bellamy, American actor.

BEN—Hebrew: "son." Also a nickname for **Benjamin.** Ben Jonson, 17th-century English dramatist, Ben-Hur, fictional character. English variation: **Benn.**

BENDIX—See **Benedict.**

BENEDICT—Latin:

Benedictus. "Blessed one."
St. Benedict, A.D. 490-542,
founder of Benedictine Order
of monks; Benito Juarez,
19th-century President of
Mexico; Benedict Arnold,
American Revolutionary War
general.
English nicknames: **Ben,
Benedick, Bennet, Bendix,
Dick.**
Foreign variations: **Benedikt**
(German, Swedish), **Benoit**
(French), **Benedetto** (Italian),
Benedicto, Benito (Span-
ish), **Bengt** (Swedish).

BENITO—See **Benedict.**

BENJAMIN—Hebrew: **Binya-
min.** "Son of the right hand."
The Biblical Benjamin was
Jacob's youngest son, who
carried out his father's
wishes; Benjamin Franklin,
American statesman (1706-
1790); Benjamin Spock,
American pediatrician; Benny
Goodman, orchestra leader.
English nicknames: **Ben,
Bennie, Benjy, Benny.**
Foreign variations: **Beniamino**
(Italian), **Benjamin** (French,
Spanish), **Beathan** (Scottish).

BENNETT—French-Latin:
Benet. "Little blessed one."
Bennett Cerf, American
publisher.

BENONI—Hebrew: "son of
my sorrow." Jacob's youngest
son in the Bible was named
Benoni by Rachel, who died
at his birth. He was
renamed Benjamin by his
father.

BENSON—Hebrew-English:
"son of Benjamin." Also
shortened from **Benedict-
son.** Benson Fong, actor.

BENTLEY—Old English:
Beonet-leah. "From the
bent-grass meadow." Rich-
ard Bentley, 18th-century
English critic.

BENTON—Old English:
Beonet-tun. "From the bent-
grass farm." Thomas Hart
Benton, American statesman
(1782-1858).

BERESFORD—Old En-
glish: "from the barley-ford."
Charles Beresford, English
admiral.

BERG—German: "from the
mountain."

BERGEN—Scandinavian:
"hill or mountain dweller."
Also: **Bergin.**

BERGER—French:
"shepherd."

BERGREN—Scandinavian:
"mountain branch." Also:
Berggren.

BERK—See **Burke.**

BERKELEY—See **Barclay.**

BERN—Old German: **Berin.**
"Bear."
English variations: **Berne,
Bernie, Berny.**

BERNARD—Old German:
Berin-hard. "Brave as a
bear." St. Bernard of
Clairvaux, 12th century; St.
Bernard of Menthon, patron
saint of mountaineers; Ber-

nard Baruch, American financier, economist, statesman. English nicknames: **Barney, Barny, Bernie, Berny.** English variation: **Burnard.** Foreign variations: **Bernhard** (German, Swedish), **Bernardo** (Italian, Spanish), **Barnard** (French), **Bearnard** (Scottish, Irish), **Bjorn** (Swedish).

BERT—Old English: **Beorht.** "Shining, glorious one." See also **Albert, Herbert.** Bert Parks, entertainer; Bert Lahr, comedian; Burt Lancaster, actor.

BERTHOLD—Old German: **Bercht-wald.** "Brilliant ruler." St. Berthold of France founded the Carmelite Order, 12th century; Bertold Brecht, dramatist. English nicknames: **Bert, Bertie.** English variation: **Bertold.** Foreign variations: **Berthoud** (French), **Bertoldi** (Italian).

BERTON—Old English: **Beorhttun.** "Brilliant one's estate"; or Old English: **Burh-tun.** "Fortified town." Also: **Burton.** English nicknames: **Bert, Bertie.**

BERTRAM—Old English: **Beorht-hram.** "Brilliant raven, he shall be famous." The raven was symbolic of wisdom. Also: **Bertrand.** St. Bertrand, 7th-century evangelizer of France and Flanders; Bertrand Russell, English writer and philosopher.

Foreign variations: **Bertrand** (French), **Beltrán** (Spanish), **Bertrando** (Italian).

BEVAN—Welsh: **Ab-Evan.** "Son of the well-born or youthful one." English variations: **Beaven, Beavan, Beven.**

BEVIS—Old French: **Beaveis.** "Fair view." Foreign variation: **Beauvais** (French).

BICKFORD—Old English: **Bieca-ford.** "Hewer's ford." Charles Bickford, American actor. English nickname: **Bick.**

BILL—See **William.**

BING—Old German: **Binge.** "From the kettle-shaped hollow." Bing Crosby, noted actor and singer.

BINK—North English: **Bink.** "Dweller at the bank or slope."

BIRCH—Old English: **Beore.** "At the birch tree." Birch Bayh, U.S. Senator. English variation: **Birk.**

BIRKETT—Middle English: **Birk-hed.** "Dweller at the birch headland." Birket Foster, English painter (1825–1899).

BIRKEY—North English: "from the birch-tree island."

BIRLEY—Old English: **Byre-leah.** "Cattle shed on the meadow."

BIRNEY—Old English: **Burneig.** "Dweller on the brook-island." David Birncy, actor.
English variation: **Burney.**

BIRTLE—Old English: **Bird-hil.** "From the bird hill."

BISHOP—Old English: **Biscop.** "The bishop." Sir Henry Bishop, English composer (1786-1855).

BJORN—Scandinavian form of **Bernard.** Bjorn Borg, tennis player.

BLACK—Old English: **Blaec.** "Dark complected." James Black, American lawyer and prohibition leader (1823-1893).

BLADE—Old English: **Blaed.** "Prosperity, glory."

BLAGDEN—Old English: **Blaec-dene.** "From the dark valley."

BLAINE—Irish Gaelic: **Blian.** "Thin, lean one." St. Blane, 6th-century Scottish bishop; James G. Blaine, 19th-century American statesman.
English variation: **Blayne.**

BLAIR—Irish Gaelic: **Blar.** "From the plain or field." Francis Blair, American politician, Civil War general (1821-1875).

BLAISE—See **Blaze.**

BLAKE—Old English: **Blac.** "Fair haired and fair complexioned"; or Old

English: **Blaec.** "Dark one." Blake Edwards, film director.

BLAKELEY—Old English: **Blaec-leah.** "From the black meadow."

BLAKEY—Old English: **Blac-ey.** "Little fair-haired one."

BLANCO—Spanish: "blond, white." A strange mutation, beloved by his race.

BLAND—Latin: **Blandus.** "Mild, gentle one."

BLANE—See **Blaine.**

BLANFORD—Old English: **Bland-ford.** "Gray-haired one's river crossing."

BLASE—See **Blaze.**

BLAYNE—See **Blaine.**

BLAZE—Latin: **Blasius.** "Stammerer." Some philologists say, "Torch or firebrand," from Old German: **Blas.** St. Blaze, world-renowned 4th-century Armenian bishop, patron of physicians; Blaise Pascal, French scientist and philosopher.
English variations: **Blaise, Blase, Blayze.**
Foreign variations: **Blaise** (French), **Blasien** (German), **Biagio** (Italian), **Blas** (Spanish), **Blasius** (Swedish).

BLISS—Old English: "joyful one." Bliss Perry, American author, editor.

BLYTHE—Old English: "merry one."

BOAZ—Hebrew: "in the Lord is strength." In the Bible Boaz was a pillar of wisdom in the Temple of the Lord. Boaz was the husband of Ruth.
English variations: **Boas, Boase.**

BODEN—Old French: **Bodin.** "Herald, messenger."

BOGART—Old German: **Bogo-hardt.** "Bow-strong." Humphrey Bogart, actor.

BONAR—Old French: **Bonaire.** "Kind, gentle, good." Bonar Law, British statesman (1858-1923).
English variation: **Bonner.**

BOND—English, Icelandic: "he stays with the soil."

BONIFACE—Latin: **Boni-facius.** "Doer of good, of good fate." St. Boniface, the Apostle of Germany, born in England, A.D. 675.
Foreign variations: **Bonifacius** (German, Swedish, Dutch), **Bonifacio** (Italian, Spanish).

BOOKER—Origin uncertain. Probably a reference to the Bible, the "Book." Booker T. Washington, educator.

BOONE—Old French: **Bone.** "Good one." Daniel Boone, American explorer (1735-1820).

BOOTH—Old Norse: **Bothi.** "Herald"; or Middle English:

Bothe. "Dweller in a hut." A place name. Booth Tarkington, American novelist (1869-1946).
English variations: **Both, Boothe, Boot, Boote.**

BORDEN—Old English: **Bardene.** "From the boar-valley."

BORG—Norse: "castle dweller."

BORIS—Slavic: "fighter, or stranger." St. Boris, King of Bulgaria, died A.D. 907; Boris Godunov, 17th-century Russian czar; Boris Karloff, noted actor; Boris Pasternak, author.

BOSWELL—Old French: **Bosvile.** "Forest-town." St. Boswell, 7th-century abbot of Melrose, Scotland; James Boswell, 18th-century Scottish biographer.

BOSWORTH—Old English: "at the cattle-enclosure." A place name. Joseph Bosworth, 19th-century English clergyman.

BOTOLF—Old English: **Bote-wolf.** "Herald-wolf." St. Botolph, famous 7th-century English abbot, for whom Boston, England, and Boston, Massachusetts, were named.

BOURKE—See **Burke.**

BOURNE—Old English: "from the brook." See also **Burne.**

BOWEN—Old Welsh: **Ab-**

Owen. "Son of the well-born or youthful one"; or Gaelic: **Buad-hachan.** "Little victorious one." Francis Bowen, 19th-century American author.

BOWIE—Irish Gaelic: **Buidhe.** "Yellow-haired." Col. James Bowie, American scout, died 1836.

BOYCE—Old French: **Bois.** "From the forest." A woodland dweller whose contact with the town was rare. Willian Boyce, English composer (1710-1799).

BOYD—Irish Gaelic: **Buidhe.** "Blond one." E. Boyd Smith, American artist, illustrator; William Boyd, actor.

BOYNE—Irish Gaelic: **Bofind.** "White cow." Famous Battle of the Boyne, Ireland, 1690.

BOYNTON—Irish Gaelic: "from the Boyne, or white cold river."

BRAD Old English: "broad, wide place." See also **Bradley, Bradford.**

BRADBURN—Old English: **Brad-bourne.** "Broad brook."

BRADEN—Old English: **Brad-dene.** "From the wide valley."

BRADFORD—Old English: "from the broad river crossing." William Bradford, famous 17th-century New England governor; Bradford Dillman, actor.

BRADLEY—Old English: **Brad-leah.** "From the broad meadow."
English nicknames: **Brad, Lee.**

BRADY—Irish Gaelic: **Bradach.** "Spirited one"; or Old English: **Brad-ig.** "From the broad-island." "Diamond Jim" Brady. English nickname: **Brad.**

BRAINARD—Old English: **Bran-hard.** "Bold raven." The raven was symbolic of bravery. David Brainerd, American missionary to the Indians (1718-1747).
English variation: **Brainerd.**

BRAM—See **Bran, Abraham.** Bram Stoker, English writer of *Dracula* (1847-1912).

BRAMWELL—Old English: **Braem-wiella.** "From the bramble-bush spring." Bramwell Brontë, painter.

BRAN—Old Celtic: **Brann.** "Raven." The dove, the raven and the phoenix bird are symbols of continued life or rebirth. Prince Bran, Gaelic Irish legends say, sailed to a sunny land in the southern seas, returning after a hundred years, still a young man.
English variation: **Bram.**

BRAND—Old English: "firebrand." In Norse myths Brand was the grandson of Woden, king of the gods.

BRANDER—Old Norse: **Brandr.** "Sword; firebrand."

BRANDON—Old English:
Brand-dun. "From the beacon
hill." Brandon Peters,
Brandon de Wilde, actors.

BRANT—Old English:
"proud one"; or Old English:
Brand. "Firebrand." Joseph
Brant (1742-1807), Mohawk
Indian war chief.

BRAWLEY—Old English:
Bra-leah. "From the hillslope
meadow."

BRENDAN—Irish Gaelic:
Breandan. "A brave, bold
man, even in his youth."
Also: **Brennan, Brendon.** St.
Brendan, famous 6th-
century Irish leader, patron
of sailors; Brendan Behan,
Irish playwright.

BRENT—Old English:
Brent. "Steep hill." George
Brent, actor.

BRETT—Celtic: **Bret.**
"Briton." A native of the isle
the Romans called Brittania.
Bret Harte, famed 19th-
century American writer.
English variation: **Bret.**

BREWSTER—Old English:
Brewstere. "Brewer." William
Brewster, American Pilgrim
leader.

BRIAN—Celtic: "strength,
virtue, honor." Brian Boru,
most famous of all Irish
kings, A.D. 926-1014; actors
include Brian Aherne, Brian
Keith, Brian Dennehy.
English variations: **Briant;
Brien, Brion, Bryan,
Bryant, Bryon.**

Foreign variation: **Briano**
(Italian).

BRICE—Celtic-Welsh: **Brys.**
"Quick one, awake, ambitious."
English variation: **Bryce.**

BRIDGER—Old English:
Brigge-ere. "Dweller at the
bridge; bridge-builder." Jim
Bridger, American explorer,
frontier scout, 19th century.

BRIGHAM—Middle En-
glish: **Brigge-ham.** "Dweller
at the bridge enclosure." A
bridge fringed by heliotrope
and heather. Brigham
Young, American religious
leader (1801-1877).

BROCK—Old English:
Brok. "Badger." Brock Peters,
actor.
English nicknames: **Broc,
Brockie, Brok.**

BROCKLEY—Old English:
Broc-leah. "From the badger
meadow."

BRODERICK—Middle En-
glish: **Brod-rig.** "From the
broad ridge"; or Welsh:
Ab-Roderick. "Son of famous
ruler." Broderick Crawford,
actor.

BRODIE—Irish Gaelic:
Broth. "A ditch." An
individual who built a canal
to irrigate his land. Brodie is a
famous Scottish clan name.
Sir Benjamin Brodie was
surgeon to the British royal
family in the mid-1800s.
English variation: **Brody.**

BROMLEY—Old English:

Brom-leah. "Dweller at the broom-meadow."

BRONSON—Old English: **Brunson.** "Son of the brown one." Bronson Howard, American dramatist, journalist (1842-1908).

BROOK—Middle English: **Brok.** "Dweller at the brook." English variation: **Brooke.**

BROOKS—Middle English: **Broks.** "Dweller at the brooks." Brooks Atkinson, American drama critic.

BROUGHER—Old English: **Burghere.** "Fortress resident."

BROUGHTON—Old English: **Burg-tun.** "From the fortress town."

BROWN—Middle English: **Brun.** "Dark, reddish complexion." John Brown, 19th-century American abolitionist.

BRUCE—Old French. **Bruis.** "Dweller at the thicket." Robert the Bruce, Scotland's famous king, liberated his land from England in the 1300s. Bruce Springsteen, singer-songwriter.

BRUNO—Italian: "brown-haired one." St. Bruno, founder of the Carthusian Order of monks, died A.D. 1101. Bruno Walter, orchestra conductor.

BRYAN—See **Brian.** William Jennings Bryan, American lawyer and politician.

BRYANT—See **Brian.** Bryant Gumbel, commentator.

BRYCE—See **Brice.**

BUCK—Old English: **Boc.** "Buck deer." Buck Rogers, science fiction hero.

BUCKLEY—Old English: **Boc-leah.** "Dweller at the buck-deer meadow." William F. Buckley, author and publisher.

BUDD—Old English: **Boda.** "Herald or messenger." The messenger of kings, the herald of the town. Also a nickname from Richard. Budd Schulberg, American novelist.
English variations: **Bud, Budde, Buddie, Buddy.**

BUNDY—Old English: **Bondig.** "Free man."

BURBANK—Old English: **Burh-bank.** "Dweller on the castle hillslope." Luther Burbank, famous American horticulturist.

BURCH—Middle English: **Birche.** "Birch tree."

BURCHARD—Old English: **Burgh-hard.** "Strong as a castle." Burchard was a famous 12th-century French abbot.
Foreign variations: **Burckhardt, Burkhart** (German), **Burgard, Burgaud** (French).

BURDETT—Old French: **Bordet.** "Little shield."

BURDON—Old English:

Burh-don. "Dweller at the castle hill."

BURFORD—Old English: **Burh-ford.** "Dweller at the castle-ford."

BURGESS—Middle English: **Burgeis.** "Citizen of a borough or town." Burgess Meredith, actor.

BURKE—Old French: **Burc.** "Dweller at the fortress or stronghold." Sir John Burke, famous English genealogist and heraldic expert, 19th century. English variations: **Berk, Berke, Bourke, Burk.**

BURKETT—Old French: **Burcet.** "From the little stronghold."

BURL—Old English: **Byrle.** "Cup-bearer." A server of wine to the lord of a medieval castle. Burl Ives, folk singer and actor.

BURLEY—Old English: **Burh-leah.** "Dweller at the castle meadow." English variation: **Burleigh.**

BURNABY—Old Norse: **Biorn-byr.** "Warrior's estate." Frederick Burnaby, 19th-century English traveler.

BURNARD—See **Bernard.**

BURNE—Old English: **Bourne.** "Brook." English variations: **Bourn, Bourne, Burn, Byrne.**

BURNELL—Old French: **Brunel.** "Little brown-haired one."

BURNETT—Middle English: **Burnet.** Whit Burnett, editor.

BURNEY—Old English: **Bureig.** "Dweller at the brook island."

BURR—Old Norse: **Burr.** "Youth." Burr Tillstrom, actor.

BURRELL—Old French: **Burel.** "Reddish-brown complexion."

BURT—See **Bert.**

BURTON—Old English: **Burhtun.** "Dweller at the fortified town." Burton Holmes, noted American traveler, lecturer.

BUSBY—Scottish-Norse: **Busbyr.** "Dweller at the village in the thicket." Busby Berkeley, choreographer.

BYFORD—Old English: **Bi-ford.** "Dweller by the river crossing."

BYRAM—Old English: **Byreham.** "Dweller at the cattle-shed place."

BYRD—Old English: "birdlike." Admiral Richard E. Byrd, American Antarctic explorer.

BYRLE—See **Burl.**

BYRNE—See **Bourne.**

BYRON—Old French: **Buiron.** "From the cottage or country estate." George, Lord Byron, famous English poet (1788-1824). Byron Nelson, golf champion.

C

CADBY—Old Norse-English: Cada's-byr. "Warrior's settlement."

CADDOCK—Old Welsh: Cad-awg. "Battle keenness."

CADELL—Old Welsh: Cad-el. "Battle spirit." St. Cadell of Wales, 7th century.

CADMAN—Old Anglo-Welsh: "battle-man." Charles Wakefield Cadman, American composer.

CADMUS—Greek: Kadmos. "Man from the East." Legendary hero, founder of Grecian Thebes, who brought the alphabet to his people.

CAESAR—Latin: "long-haired or hairy"; through usage, "emperor." Cesar Romero, actor.
Foreign variations: Cäsar (German), Cesare (Italian), César (French, Spanish, Portuguese), Caesar (Swedish, Danish).

CAIN—Hebrew: "possession or possessed"; or Gaelic: "tribute." The first son of Adam and Eve, who murdered his brother Abel.

CALDER—Old English: Call-dwr. "The brook."

CALDWELL—Old English: Cald-wiella. "Cold spring."

CALEB—Hebrew: Kaleb. "Bold one", or "dog." A name that symbolizes affection and fidelity. Caleb Young Rick, American poet (1872-1943).
English nicknames: Cale, Cal.

CALEY—Irish Gaelic: Caolaidhe. "Thin, slender."

CALHOUN—Irish Gaelic: Coill-cumhann. "From the narrow forest." John C. Calhoun, American statesman (1782–1850).

CALVERT—Old English: Calf-hierde. "Calf-herder." George Calvert, founder of Maryland (1580-1632).

CALVIN—Late Latin: Calvinus. "Bald one." Calvin Coolidge, 30th U.S. President; Calvin Peete, golfer.
English nickname: Cal.
Foreign variation: Calvino (Italian, Spanish).

CAMDEN—Anglo-Gaelic: Camdene. "From the crooked or winding valley." William Camden, English scholar (1551-1623).

CAMERON—Scottish Gaelic: Cam-shron. "Wry or crooked nose." A Scottish clan name, originally from a nickname. Cameron Mitchell, actor.
English nickname: Cam.

CAMPBELL—Scottish Gaelic:

Cam-beul. "Wry or crooked mouth." A Scottish clan name.
English nicknames: **Cam, Camp.**

CANUTE—Old Norse: **Knut-r.** "Knot." Canute or Knut was King of England and Denmark, A.D. 1017-1035; Knute Rockne, famous American football coach (1888-1931); Knut Hamsum, novelist.
Foreign variation: **Knut** (Scandinavian).

CAREY—Old Welsh: **Caerau.** "Dweller at the castles." Cary Grant, actor.
English variation: **Cary.**

CARL—See **Charles.** Also, Old German: **Karl.** "Farmer." Carl Sandburg, noted American poet, author; Carl Hayden, U.S. Senator; Carl Reiner, actor.

CARLETON—Old English: **Carla-tun.** "From Charles's homestead." Carleton Carpenter, actor; Carlton Chapman, American painter (1860-1925).
English variation: **Carlton.**

CARLIN—Old Gaelic Irish: **Cearbhallan.** "Little champion."
English variation: **Carling.**

CARLISLE—Old English: **Caer-luel.** "Castle tower." John G. Carlisle, American statesman (1835-1910).

CARLOS—Spanish form of **Charles,** "Manly."

CARMICHAEL—Scottish Gaelic: **Cara-michil.** "Friend of St. Michael"; or Scottish Gaelic: **Kermichil.** "From Michael's stronghold."

CARMINE—Middle Latin: "crimson or purplish-red."

CARNEY—Irish Gaelic: **Cearnach.** "Victorious."
English variation: **Carny.**

CAROL—See **Carroll.**

CAROLLAN—Irish Gaelic: **Cearbhallain.** "Little champion."

CARR—Old Norse: **Kiarr.** "Dweller at a marsh."
English variations: **Karr, Kerr.**

CARRICK—Irish Gaelic: **Carraig.** "Rocky headland."

CARROLL—Irish Gaelic: **Cearbhall.** "Champion." Lewis Carroll, famous author (1832-1898); Sir Carol Reed, actor.

CARSON—Middle English: "son of the dweller at a marsh." Jack Carson, actor; Johnny Carson, comedian.

CARSWELL—Old English: **Caerse-wiella.** "Dweller at the watercress spring."

CARTER—Old English: **Cartere.** "Cart driver." Carter Glass, U.S. Senator; Carter Dickson, English author.

CARTLAND—Scottish-English: **Caraid-land.** "Land between the streams."

CARVELL—Old French:
Cara-ville. "Spearman's es-
tate, marshy estate."
English variation: **Carvel.**

CARVEY—Gaelic Irish:
Cearrbhach.

CARY—See **Carey.**

CASEY—Irish Gaelic:
Cathasach. "Valorous, brave,
watchful." Casey Stengel,
baseball manager.

CASH—Latin: **Cassius.**
"Vain one."
English variation: **Cass.**

CASIMIR—Old Slavic:
Kazatimiru. "He who commands peace." A leader at
peace with himself and the
world. Casimir the Pacific
was Poland's great 11th-
century king.
Foreign variations: **Casimiro**
(Spanish), **Kasimir** (German, Slavic).

CASPAR—Persian: **Kansbar.**
"Treasure-master." See **Gaspar.**
English nickname: **Cass.**
English variations: **Casper,
Gaspar, Gasper.**

CASS—See **Cash, Caspar.**

Cassidy—Irish Gaelic:
Casidhe. "Ingenious, clever
one; curly-haired one."

CASTOR—Greek: **Kastor.**
"Beaver." A nickname first
applied to a man of diligence
and determination. Castor
was one of the Greco-Roman
"Heavenly Twins" known as
"The Gemini."

CATHMOR—Irish Gaelic:
Cathaoir-mor. "Great warrior."

CATO—Latin: **Catus.** "Sa
gacious, wise one." Cato the
Elder and Younger were
famous ancient Roman patriots.

CAVAN—Irish Gaelic:
Caomhan. "Handsome one."
English and Irish variation:
Kavan.

CAVELL—Old French:
Cavel. "Little active one."

CAWLEY—Scottish-Norse:
MacAmhlaidh. "Ancestral
relic."

CECIL—Latin: **Caecilius.**
"Dim-sighted or blind."
Notables include Cecil
Rhodes, English South African
administrator (1853-1902);
Cecil B. De Mille, famous
film director-producer.
English nickname: **Cece.**
Foreign variations: **Cécile**
(French), **Cecilius** (Dutch).

CEDRIC—Old English:
Caddaric. "Battle chieftain."
A character in Scott's
Ivanhoe. Sir Cedric Hard-
wicke, noted English actor.

CHAD—Old English:
Cadda. "Warlike." St. Chad,
English bishop, 7th cen-
tury; Chad Everett, actor.

CHADWICK—Old En-
glish: **Cadda-wic.** "Warrior's
estate or town." Sir Edwin
Chadwick, English social
reformer (1800-1890).

CHAIM—Hebrew: **Chai.**
"Life." Chaim Weizmann,

Israeli statesman; Chaim Potok, author. Also, **Hyam.**

CHALMER—Old Scottish. "Head of household." English variation: **Chalmers.**

CHANCE—Middle English: "good fortune." See **Chauncey.**

CHANCELLOR—Middle English: **Chaunceler.** "King's secretary." English nicknames: **Chance, Chaunce.**

CHANDLER—Middle English: **Chaundler;** Old French: **Chandelier.** "Candle maker, he provides light." Howard Chandler Christy, noted illustrator (1873-1952).

CHANNING—Old French: **Chanoine.** "Canon; church dignitary." Channing Pollock, American dramatist. English nickname: **Chan.**

CHAPMAN—Old English: **Ceapmann.** "Merchant." Chapman Revercomb, U.S. Senator; Roy Chapman Andrews, noted explorer.

CHARLES—Old German: **Karl;** Latin: **Carolus.** "Strong, manly." Charles I, King of England, 1600–1649; Charles Darwin, English naturalist, 1809-1882; Charles de Gaulle, President of France; actors Charles Boyer, Charles Laughton. English nicknames: **Charley, Charlie, Chick, Chuck.** Foreign variations: **Karl, Carl** (German, Swedish), **Carlo**

(Italian), **Carlos** (Spanish), **Karel** (Dutch), **Teàrlach** (Scottish).

CHARLTON—Old English: **Carla-tun.** "From Charles's homestead." Charlton Heston, actor. English variations: **Charleton, Carlton, Carleton.**

CHASE—Old French: **Chacier.** "Hunter." W. M. Chase, American painter (1849-1916); Salmon P. Chase, former U.S. Secretary of the Treasury.

CHATHAM—Old English: **Cadda-hamm.** "Soldier's land." Named for a royal land grant.

CHAUNCEY—Middle English: **Chanceler.** "Chancellor church official." A diligent man who earned his good fortune. Chauncey Depew, American lawyer. English nicknames: **Chance, Chancey, Chaunce.**

CHENEY—Old French: **Chesne.** "Dweller at the oak forest." John Vance Cheney, American author (1848-1922). English variation: **Cheyney.**

CHESTER—Old English: **Ceaster.** "Dweller at the fortified army camp." Chester A. Arthur, 21st U.S. President; Chester Bowles, American diplomat. English nicknames: **Ches, Chet.**

CHETWIN—Old English:

Cete-wind. "From the cottage on the winding path."

CHEYNEY—See **Cheney.**

CHILTON—Old English: **Celdtun.** "From the spring farm."

CHRISTIAN—Greek: **Christos.** "Believer in Christ, anointed one." A follower of Christ's teachings. St. Christian, 12th-century bishop of Clogher; a long line of Danish kings named Christian, beginning in 1448; Christian Dior, designer. English nicknames: **Chris, Chrissy, Christie, Christy.** Foreign variations: **Kristian** (Swedish), **Chrétien** (French), **Christiano** (Italian, Spanish).

CHRISTOPHER—Greek: **Christoforos.** "Christ-bearer." Used in honor of St. Christopher, 3rd-century martyr, protector of travelers; Christopher Columbus, discoverer of America, known as Cristoforo Colombo in Italy and Cristóbal Colon in Spain; Christopher Fry, English dramatist. English nicknames: **Chris, Chrissy, Kit.** Foreign variations: **Cristóbal** (Spanish), **Christophe** (French), **Cristoforo** (Italian), **Christoph, Christophorus** (German), **Kristofor** (Swedish), **Christoffer** (Danish), **Gillecriosd** (Scottish).

CHURCHILL—Old English: **Circe-hyll.** "Dweller at the church-hill." Sir Winston Churchill, English statesman, writer.

CIAN—Irish Gaelic: **Céin.** "Ancient." The most famous Cian was the son-in-law of Ireland's celebrated 11th-century king, Brian Boru.

CICERO—Latin: "vetch or chick-pea." Named for his field of bright chick-peas, Cicero, died 43 B.C., was a noted Roman orator and statesman.

CLARE—Latin: **Clarius.** "Famous, illustrious one." Clair Engle, U.S. Senator. English variation: **Clair.**

CLARENCE—Latin: **Clarensis.** "Famous one." Clarence Darrow, famous attorney;

CLARK—Old French: **Clerc.** "Scholar." Clark Gable, actor (1901-1961).

CLAUDE—Latin: **Claudius.** "The lame one." A handicap may become a stimulus for great achievements. Famous from two Roman emperors in the 1st and 3rd centuries A.D.; Claudian, 5th-century Roman poet; Shakespearean characters named Claudio; Claude Debussy, French composer, Claude Pepper, U.S. Senator; Claude Rains, actor. Foreign variations: **Claude** (French), **Claudio** (Italian, Spanish), **Claudius** (German, Dutch).

CLAUS—See **Nicholas.**

CLAY—Old English: **Claeg.**
"From the earth; mortal."
Henry Clay, American
statesman (1777-1852).

CLAYBORNE—Old English: **Claeg-borne.** "From
the clay-brook."
English nickname: **Clay.**
English variations: **Claiborn,
Claybourne.**

CLAYTON—Old English:
Claegtun. "From the clay
estate; mortal."

CLEARY—Irish Gaelic:
Cleirach. "Scholar."

CLEMENT—Latin:
Clementis. "Gentle, merciful,
kind one." St. Clement, 1st
century; six medieval Popes;
Clément Delibes, French
operatic composer (1836-1891);
Clement Attlee, British
statesman; Clement Moore,
American author of *The
Night Before Christmas*.
English nicknames: **Clem,
Clemmy, Clim.**
Foreign variations: **Clemente**
(Italian, Spanish), **Klemens**
(German), **Clément** (French),
Clemens (Danish), **Clementius**
(Dutch).

CLEVE—See **Clive,
Cleveland.**

CLEVELAND—Old English: **Clif-land.** "From the
cliff-land." Cleveland Amory,
American author.
English nicknames: **Cleve,
Clevie.**
English variations: **Clevon,
Cleon.**

CLIFF—Old English: **Clif.**
"From the steep rock or cliff."
See **Clifford.** Cliff Robert-
son, actor; Cliff Arquette
(Charley Weaver), Ameri-
can comedian.

CLIFFORD—Old English:
"from the cliff-ford." Clifford
Case, U.S. Senator; Clifford
Odets, dramatist.
English nicknames: **Clif, Cliff.**

CLIFTON—Old English:
Cliftun. "From the cliff-estate
or town." Clifton Webb,
actor; Clifton Fadiman,
literary critic.

CLINTON—Old English:
Clinttun. "From the headland-
estate or town." Clinton
Anderson, U.S. Senator; Clint
Walker, American actor.
English nickname: **Clint.**

CLIVE—Old English: **Clif.**
"From the cliff." An ancestor
who took his name from his
home on a precipice. Clive
Brook, English actor; Clive
Barnes, American critic.
English variations: **Cleve,
Clyve.**

CLOVIS—Old German: **Chlod-
wig.** "Famous warrior." An
early spelling of Ludwig or
Lewis. Clovis, A.D. 481-511,
founded the Frankish dynasty
of French kings.
Foreign variation: **Clodoveo**
(Spanish).

CLUNY—Irish Gaelic:
Cluainach. "From the
meadow."

CLYDE—Welsh: **Clywd.**
"Warm"; or Scottish Gaelic:
Cleit. "Rocky eminence;
heard from afar." From the
famous River Clyde in
Scotland. Clyde Cessna,
American aircraft pioneer;
Clyde Reed, U.S. Senator.

COBB—See **Jacob.**

CODY—Old English: "a
cushion." Historic use: honors
Wild Bill Cody. Also: **Codi,
Codie.**

COLAN—See **Colin.**

COLBERT—Old English:
Ceol-beorht. "Brilliant sea-
farer"; or Old German:
Kuhl-berht. "Cool, calm,
brilliant."
English variations: **Colvert,
Culbert.**

COLBY—Old Anglo-Norse:
Kolbyr. "From the black or
dark settlement." Bainbridge
Colby, U.S. Secretary of
State.

COLE—See **Nicholas.** Also:
Colin. Cole Porter, American
composer.

COLEMAN—Old English:
Colomann. "Adherent of
Nicholas"; or Irish Gaelic:
Column-an. "Little dove." St.
Colman, patron of Austria,
died 1012; Ronald Colman,
actor.
English variation: **Colman.**

COLIN—Irish Gaelic:
Coilin. "Young and virile"; or
French-Greek: **Nicolin.**
"Victorious army."

English variations: **Colan,
Cole.**
Foreign variation: **Cailean**
(Scottish).

COLLIER—Old English:
Colier. "Charcoal merchant;
miner." Collier Young,
American film and television
executive.
English variations: **Coller,
Colis, Collyer, Colyer.**

COLTER—Old English:
Coltere. "Colt herder."

COLTON—Old English:
Coletun. "From the dark
estate or town." Walter
Colton, American editor,
writer (1797-1851).

COLVER—See **Culver.**

CONAN—Celtic: **Kunagnos.**
"Intelligence, wisdom"; or
Irish Gaelic: "high, ex-
alted." St. Conan, Irish
bishop on the Isle of Man,
died 648; Sir Arthur Conan
Doyle, English writer,
creator of Sherlock Holmes.

CONLAN—Irish Gaelic:
Connlan. "Hero."
English variations: **Conlin,
Conlon.**

CONRAD—Old German:
Kuon-raet. "Bold counselor."
St. Conrad of Hildesheim,
12th-century follower of St.
Francis; Konrad Adenauer,
German Chancellor; Conrad
Hilton, American hotel
executive.
English nicknames: **Con,
Connie, Cort, Curt.**
Foreign variations: **Konrad,**

Kort, Kurt (German),
Konrad (Swedish), **Conrade**
(French), **Conrado** (Italian,
Spanish), **Koenraad** (Dutch).

CONROY—Irish Gaelic:
Con-aire. "Wise one"; or
Celtic: "persistent."

CONSTANTINE—Latin:
Constantinus. "Firm, constant
one." Constantine the
Great, 4th-century Roman
emperor; Constantine, King
of Greece (1868–1923).
Foreign variations: **Costantino**
(Italian), **Constantin** (French,
German, Danish), **Constantino**
(Spanish), **Konstantin**
(Swedish).

CONWAY—Irish Gaelic:
Conmhaighe. "Hound of the
plain." Conway Twitty,
singer.

COOPER—Old English:
Cupere. "Barrel maker." A
skilled artisan who fash-
ioned barrels for commerce.
English nickname: **Coop.**

CORBETT—Old French:
Corbet. "Raven." The raven
symbolized wisdom and was
used on flags and shields of
the Norse Viking conquer-
ors of Normandy and
northwest France. Harvey
W. Corbett, noted American
architect.
English variations: **Corbet,
Corbin, Corby.**

CORBIN—See **Corbett.**

CORCORAN—Irish Gaelic:
Corcurachan. "Of reddish
complexion." W. W.

Corcoran, American financier,
art collector (1798–1888).

CORDELL—Old French:
Cordel. "Little rope-maker,"
or "little rope"; or Celtic:
"of the sea." Cordell Hull,
U.S. Secretary of State.

COREY—Irish and Scottish
Gaelic: **Coire.** "Dweller by a
hollow or by a seething
pool"; or Anglo-Saxon: "the
chosen."
English variation: **Cory.**

CORMICK—Irish Gaelic:
Corbmac. "Charioteer."
English and Irish variations:
Cormac, Cormack.

CORNELIUS—Latin: "horn-
colored; hornlike"; or Late
Latin, Greek: **Cornolium.**
"Cornel-cherry tree." St.
Cornelius, 1st century A.D.;
Cornelius Vanderbilt, 19th-
century American capitalist;
Cornelius Ryan, author.
Foreign variations: **Cornelio**
(Italian, Spanish, Portu-
guese), **Cornélius** (French).

CORNELL—See **Cornelius.**
Cornel Wilde, actor.
English variations: **Cornall,
Cornel.**

CORT—Old Norse: **Kort-r.**
"Short"; or Old German:
Kort. "Bold." See **Conrad.**

CORWIN—Old Franco-
English: **Cor-wine.** "Heart
friend." "Greater love hath
no man than this, that a man
lay down his life for his
friends."—John 15:13.

CORYDON—Greek: **Korudon.** "Helmeted, ready for battle." English variation: **Coryell.**

COSMO—Greek: **Kosmos.** "Order, harmony; the universe." St. Cosmos, 3rd-century Christian martyr, patron of physicians; Cosmo the Elder and Cosmo the Great, medieval de' Medici rulers of Florence, Italy. Foreign variations: **Cosme** (French), **Cosimo** (Italian, Spanish).

COURTLAND—Old English: **Court-land.** "Dweller at the farmstead or court land." English nickname: **Court.**

COURTNEY—Old French: **Courtenay.** "Dweller at the farmstead or court."

COVELL—Old English: **Cofa-healh.** "Dweller at the cave slope." Place name from a descriptive landmark.

COWAN—Irish Gaelic: **Cobhan.** "Hillside hollow." Alternate source, Irish Gaelic: **Comhghan.** "A twin."

COYLE—Irish Gaelic: **Cathmaol.** "Battle follower."

CRADDOCK—Old Welsh: **Caradoc.** "Abounding in love; beloved." Renowned from Caradoc, heroic 1st-century King of Wales.

CRAIG—Scottish Gaelic: **Creag.** "Dweller at the crag." Craig Stevens, American actor.

CRANDELL—Old English: **Cran-dell.** "Dweller at the crane valley." English variation: **Crandall.**

CRANLEY—Old English: **Cran-leah.** "From the crane meadow."

CRANSTON—Old English: **Crans-tun.** "From the crane estate or town." The cranes owned the large estate and the people were their tenants. Senator Alan Cranston.

CRAWFORD—Old English: **Crawe-ford.** "From the crow-ford." Crawford Long, American scientist (1815-1878).

CREIGHTON—Middle English: **Creke-tun.** "Dweller at the creek estate or town."

CRISPIN—Latin: **Crispus.** "Curly-haired." St. Crispin, 3rd century, patron of shoemakers; Crispus Attuchs, first man killed in the American Revolution. U.S. variation: **Crispus.** Foreign variations: **Crispino** (Italian), **Crépin** (French), **Crispus** (German), **Crispo** (Spanish), **Krispijn** (Dutch).

CROMWELL—Old English: **Cromb-wiella.** "Dweller at the crooked or winding spring." Oliver Cromwell, English ruler (1653-1658).

CROSBY—Old Norse: **Krossby-r.** "Dweller at the shrine of the Cross." Bing Crosby, singer. English variations: **Crosbey, Crosbie.**

CROSLEY—Old English:
Cros-leah. "From the cross-meadow." Place name from a directional landmark on the meadow.

CULBERT—See **Colbert.**

CULLEN—Irish Gaelic:
Cuil-thinn. "Handsome one."
William Cullen Bryant, American poet (1794-1878).
English variations: **Cullan, Cullin.**

CULLEY—Irish Gaelic:
Coille. "At the woodland."
English variation: **Cully.**

CULVER—Old English:
Colfre. "The dove, peace-loving." A symbol of peace to all nations.
English variation: **Colver.**

CURRAN—Irish Gaelic:
Curadhan. "Champion or hero."
English nicknames: **Currey, Currie, Curry.**

CURTIS—Old French:
Curteis. "Courteous one."
General Curtis LeMay, U.S. Air Force Chief of Staff; Curtis Wilbur, U.S. Secretary of the Navy.
English nickname: **Curt.**

CUTHBERT—Old English:
Cuth-beorht. "Famous, brilliant." St. Cuthbert of England, died A.D. 687.

CYNRIC—Old English:
Cyneric. "Powerful and

royal." A very old Anglo-Saxon name.

CYPRIAN—Greek: **Kupris.**
"Man from the island of Cyprus." Cyprus was the mythical birthplace of Venus; its name means "Place of Venus." St. Cyprian. 3rd century.
Foreign variation: **Cipriano** (Spanish).

CYRANO—Greek: **Kurene.**
"From Cyrene." Cyrene was the capital city of Cyrenaica in ancient North Africa. Famous from *Cyrano de Bergerac*, hero of classical drama by Rostand, modeled on a 17th-century soldier-poet.

CYRIL—Greek: **Kyrillos.**
"Lordly one." St. Cyril of Alexandria, A.D. 376-444; Cyril Ritchard, actor.
Foreign variations: **Cyrille** (French), **Cirillo** (Italian), **Cyrill** (German), **Cirilo** (Spanish), **Cyrillus** (Danish, Swedish, Dutch).

CYRUS—Old Persian:
Kurush. "The sun." Named for the old pagan sun god, portrayed in medieval plays. Cyrus the Great was the 5th-century B.C. founder of the Persian Empire; Cyrus McCormick, American inventor; Cyrus Vance, U.S. Secretary of State.
English nickname: **Cy.**
Foreign variation: **Ciro** (Spanish).

D

DACEY—Irish Gaelic:
Deasach. "Southerner."
English variation: **Dacy.**

DAG—Old Norse: **Dag-r.**
"Day or brightness." The
Norse god Dag was born of
light and love, while night
(Nott) was born of chaos.
Dag Hammarskjold (1903–
1961), UN Secretary General.

DAGAN—East Semitic:
"the earth," or "little fish."
Dagan, the Babylonian god
of earth was once called the
god of water and fish, and
later the god of the earth and
agriculture.
Foreign (West Semitic),
variation: **Dagon**

DAGWOOD—Old English:
Daegga's wode. "Bright one's
forest." Made famous from
the comic strip character
Dagwood.

DALBERT—Old English:
Deal-beorht. "Proud, brilliant
one"; or Old English:
Dael-beorht. "Shining valley."
Delbert Mann, stage and
motion picture director.
English variation: **Delbert.**

DALE—Old English: **Dael.**
"Dweller in the valley." Dale
Carnegie, writer and
lecturer; Dale Robertson,
actor: Also, **Daley.**

DALEY—See **Dale.** Daley

Thompson, British decathlon
champion.

DALLAS—Scottish Gaelic:
Daileass. "From the waterfall-
field or ravine-field," from a
Scottish place. George Dallas
(1792-1804), American statesman after whom Dallas,
Texas, was named.

DALTON—Old English:
Daeltun. "From the valley
estate or town." Dalton
Trumbo, writer.

DALY—Irish Gaelic: **Dalach.**
"Counselor." Arnold Daly,
actor; John Daly, radio and
TV personality.

DALZIEL—Scottish Gaelic:
Dalyell. "From the little
field."

DAMEK—Czech: form of
Adam: "man of the red
earth."

DAMIAN—Greek: "tam-
ing; he makes men gentle."
Also: **Damien.**

DAMON—Greek: "constant
one"; or Greek: **Damas.**
"Tamer." Damon and
Pythias, ancient Pythagorean
scholars, valued friendship
more than life. Damon was
truly the "constant one."
Damon Runyon, American
writer.
Foreign variations: **Damien**

(French), **Damiano** (Italian), **Damian** (German).

DAN—Hebrew: "judge." See **Daniel**.

DANA—Old English: **Dane**. "Man from Denmark." Also short for Hebrew **Daniel**: "judged by God." Dana Clark, Dana Andrews, actors; Richard Henry Dana, novelist.

DANBY—Old Norse: **Dan-r-by-r**. "From the Dane's settlement." Francis Danby, English painter (1793-1861).

DANIEL—Hebrew: **Daniyel**. "God is my judge." Daniel, the Biblical Hebrew prophet; Daniel Boone, American explorer; Daniel Defoe, 18th-century English author of *Robinson Crusoe;* Daniel Taradash, film writer; actors Dan Dailey, Danny Thomas, Danny Kaye, Dan Duryea. English nicknames: **Dan, Dannie, Danny**. Foreign variations: **Danielle** (Italian), **Dane** (Dutch), **Daniel** (German, French, Spanish, Swedish), **Dàniel** (Scottish).

DANTE—Latin: "lasting." From the medieval Italian poet, Dante Aligheri.

DARBY—Irish Gaelic: **Diarmaid**. "Free man"; or Old Norse: **Dyr-by-r**. "From the deer estate." John Nelson Darby, founder of Plymouth Brethren; George Derby, American humorist. English variation: **Derby**.

DARCY—Old French: **D'Arcy**. "From the fortress"; or Irish Gaelic: **Dorchaidhe**. "Dark man." Baron Thomas Darcy, English statesman, religious rebel (1467-1537). English variations: **Darsey, Darsy**.

DARIUS—Greek: **Dareious**. "Wealthy one." Original usage in honor of Darius the Great, ancient Persian king; St. Darius, early Christian martyr.

DARNELL—Old English: **Derne-healh**. "From the hidden nook."

DARRELL—Old French: **Darel**. "Little dear or beloved one." Darryl Zanuck, noted film producer; Darryl Strawberry, baseball player. English variations: **Daryl, Darryl**.

DARREN—Irish Gaelic: **Dearan**. "Little great one." Darren McGavin, actor.

DARRICK—See **Derrick**.

DARSEY—See **Darcy**.

DARTON—Old English: **Deortun**. "Deer park or estate."

DAVID—Hebrew: "beloved one." Famous from the Biblical David, King of Israel, and St. David, 6th century, patron saint of Wales; David Livingstone, British explorer; David Ben-Gurion, Premier of Israel; David Brinkley,

commentator; actors David
Niven, David Wayne.
English nicknames: **Dave,
Davie, Davy.**
Foreign variations: **Davide**
(French), **Davidde** (Italian),
Daibidh (Scottish).

DAVIN—Old Scandinavian:
Dagfinn-r. "Brightness of
the Finns."

DAVIS—Old English:
Davidsone. "Son of the
beloved one." Old English
and Scottish contraction of
"David's son." Davis
Phinney, Olympic cyclist.

DEAN—Old English: **Dene.**
"Dweller in the valley." Also,
from the last name. Dean
Acheson, American statesman;
Dean Rusk, U.S. Secretary
of State; Dean Martin, actor.

DEARBORN—Old English: **Dere-bourne.** "From
the deer-brook." Walter F.
Dearborn, American educator.

DEDRICK—Old German:
Dietrich. "Ruler of the
people." See **Theodoric.**

DEEMS—Old English:
Demasone. "Son of the
judge." Deems Taylor,
American composer, writer.

DELANO—Old French:
De la Noye. "From the place
of the nut trees." Franklin
Delano Roosevelt, 32nd U.S.
President.

DELBERT—Old English:
Daegel-beorht. "Day-bright."
See **Dalbert.** Delbert
Mann, director.

English nicknames: **Del, Bert.**

DELLING—Old Norse:
Delling-r. "Very shining one."

DELMAR—Latin: "from
the sea." Also: **Delmer,
Delmore.** Delmore Schwartz,
poet.

DELWYN—Old English:
Deal-wine. "Proud friend"; or
Old English: **Daegel-wine.**
"Bright friend"; or Old
English: **Dael-wine.** "Valley-
friend."
English variations: **Delwin,
Delevan.**

DEMAS—Greek: "Popular
one."

DEMETRIUS—Greek:
Demetrios. "Belonging to
Demeter, Greek fertility
goddess." Demetrius, a
silversmith of Ephesus,
fomented disturbances against
St. Paul.
Foreign variations: **Demetre**
(French), **Demetrio** (Italian),
Dmitri (Russian).

DEMOS—Greek: "the people." A shortened form of
Demosthenes, after the
orator.

DEMPSEY—Irish Gaelic:
Diomasach. "Proud one." Jack
Dempsey, American boxing
champion.

DEMPSTER—Old English:
Dema-stere. "The judge."
Arthur J. Dempster,
American physicist (1885-1950).

DENBY—Old Norse; **Dan-**

r-by-r. "From the Dane's settlement."

DENIS—See **Dennis.**

DENLEY—Old English: **Dene.** "Dweller in the valley meadow."

DENMAN—Old English: **Deneman.** "Valley resident." Denman Thompson, American actor.

DENNIS—Greek: **Dionys-os.** "God of wine." Dennis Day, singer; actors Dennis O'Keefe, Dennis Morgan, Dennis Weaver.
English nicknames: **Den, Denney, Denny.**
English variations: **Denis, Denys, Dion, Deon.**
Foreign variations: **Dionisio** (Italian, Spanish), **Dionysus** (German), **Denis** (Irish).

DENNISON—Old English: **Dennis-sone.** "Son of Dennis." Denison Clift, author, director.

DENTON—Old English: **Denetun.** "From the valley estate or town."

DENVER—Old English: **Deneofer.** "Dweller at the valley edge." James W. Denver, U.S. Congressman and Territorial Governor (1812-1892).

DEON—See **Dennis.** Pet form of **Dionysus,** from the Greek God. Also: **Dion.**

DERBY—See **Darby.**

DEREK—See **Derrick.**

DERMOT—Irish Gaelic: **Diar-maid.** "Free man." English variation: **Dermott.**

DERRICK—Old German: **Dietrich.** "Ruler of the people." Derek Bond, Dirk Bogarde, actors; Dirk Bouts, 15th-century Dutch painter. English variations: **Derek, Dirk.**

DERRY—Irish Gaelic: **Dearg.** "The red one."

DERWARD—Old English: **Deor-ward.** "Deer warden or guardian."

DERWIN—Old English: **Deora-wine.** "Beloved friend."

DESHAWN—New name based on **Shawn.** See **John.**

DESMOND—Irish Gaelic: **Deas-mumhan.** "Man from south Munster." Munster, now a south Irish province, was an ancient kingdom. Also, French: "of the world, sophisticated."

DEVERELL—Old Welsh-English: **Dufr-healh.** "From the riverbank."

DEVIN—Irish Gaelic: **Daimhin.** "Poet, savant."

DEVLIN—Irish Gaelic: **Dob-hailen.** "Fierce valor."

DEWEY—Old Welsh: **Dewi.** "Beloved one." A Welsh form of the Biblical **David.** Admiral George Dewey, hero of Spanish-American War; Thomas E. Dewey, American lawyer, politician.

DE WITT—Old Flemish: "blond one." De Witt Clinton, American statesman (1769-1828).

DEXTER—Latin: "dexterous one." Timothy Dexter, 18th-century American merchant; Anthony Dexter, actor. English nicknames: **Deck, Dex.**

DIAMOND—Old English: **Daeg-mund.** "Bright protector"; or Old French: **Diamant.** "A diamond."

DIEGO—Spanish form of **James.**

DIGBY—Old Norse: **Diki-by-r.** "From the dike settlement." Digby Diehl, book critic.

DILLON—Irish Gaelic: **Diolmhain.** "Faithful one."

DION—See **Dennis.**

DIRK—See **Derrick.**

DIXON—Old English: **Dikkesone.** "Son of Richard." See **Richard.** Joseph Dixon, American inventor (1799-1869); Maynard Dixon, American Western painter.

DOANE—Old English: **Doune.** "From the down or hill." G. W. Doane, 19th-century U.S. clergyman.

DOLAN—Irish Gaelic: **Dubhlachan.** "Black-haired." Robert E. Dolan, composer, conductor.

DOMINIC—Latin: **Dominicus.** "Born on Sunday, the Lord's Day," or "belonging to the Lord." St. Dominic (1170-1221), Spanish founder of Dominican Order; Dominick Dunne, author.
English nicknames: **Dom, Dommie, Nick.**
English variations: **Dominick.**
Foreign variations: **Domenico, Dominico** (Italian), **Domingo** (Spanish), **Dominique** (French), **Dominik** (Slavic).

DONAHUE—Irish Gaelic: **Donn-chadh.** "Brown warrior." English nicknames: **Don, Donn.**

DONALD—Scottish Gaelic: **Domhnall.** "World-mighty, world-ruler." Donald of the Isles, famous chief of clan MacDonald, died 1289; actors Donald Sutherland, Don Ameche, Donald O'Connor.
English nicknames: **Don, Donnie, Donny.**

DONATO—Latin: **Donatio.** "A gift." "God has given some gifts to the whole human race, from which no one is excluded"—Seneca. St. Donatian, 4th-century bishop of Rheims.

DONOVAN—Celtic: "Dark warrior."

DOOLEY—Irish Gaelic: **Dubh-laoch.** "Dark hero." Dr. Tom Dooley, famous medical pioneer; Dooley Wilson, pianist-actor.

DORAN—Greek: "a gift." Celtic: "a stranger."

DORIAN—Greek: **Dorios.** "From the sea, from Doria." The Dorians were ancient Hellenic settlers of Greece. From the fictional hero of Oscar Wilde's *The Picture of Dorian Gray.*

DORY—French: **Doré.** "Golden-haired."

DOUGAL—Celtic: "dark stranger." English variations: **Doyle, Dugald.**

DOUGLAS—Scottish Gaelic: **Dubh-glas.** "From the black or dark water." A famous clan name. General Douglas MacArthur; Douglas Dillon, U.S. Secretary of the Treasury; Douglas Fairbanks, Jr., actor. English nickname: **Doug.** English variations: **Douglass, Dugald.**

DOW—Irish Gaelic: **Dubh.** "Black-haired." Neal Dow, 19th-century American reformer. English variation: **Dowie.**

DOYLE—Irish Gaelic: **Dubhg-hall.** "Dark stranger."

DRAKE—Middle English: **Draca.** "Owner of the 'Sign of the Dragon' Inn." The picture of a Draca or Dragon was a familiar English medieval trademark on shops and hostelries, Sir Francis Drake, 16th-century English navigator.

DREW—Old Welsh: **Dryw.** "Wise one"; or Old German:

Drugi. "Vision, phantom"; or Old German: **Drud.** "Strength." Also shortening of **Andrew,** "manly." Drew Pearson, noted columnist.

DRUCE—Old Anglo-Welsh: **Dryw-sone.** "Son of the wise man."

DRUMMOND—Celtic: "he lives on the hilltop."

DRURY—Old French: **Druerie.** "Sweetheart; darling."

DRYDEN—Old English: **Drygedene.** "From the dry valley." John Dryden, 17th-century English poet.

DUANE—See **Dwayne.**

DUDLEY—Old English: **Dudda-leah.** "From the people's meadow." Dudley Field Malone, noted American attorney; Dudley Moore, actor; Dudley Beck, American cyclotron inventor. English nicknames: **Dud, Dudd.**

DUFF—Irish Gaelic: **Dubh-thach.** "Dark-complexioned one." Dubh-thach was the Arch-Poet of King Laeghaire of Ireland, whom St. Patrick converted in A.D. 433. English variation: **Duffy.**

DUGALD—See **Douglas.**

DUGAN—Irish Gaelic: **Dubh-gan.** "Dark-complexioned."

DUKE—Old French: **Duc.** "Leader." Duke Ellington, composer and musician.

DUNCAN—Scottish Gaelic: **Donn-chadh.** "Brown warrior, swarthy chief." Duncan, King of Scotland, 1034-1040, was murdered by Macbeth; Duncan Phyfe, furniture designer; Duncan Hines, international gourmet. English nickname: **Dunc.**

DUNLEY—Old English: **Dunleah.** "From the hill meadow."

DUNMORE—Scottish Gaelic: **Dun-mor.** "From the great hill fortress."

DUNN—Old English: "dark-complexioned one."

DUNSTAN—Old English: "brown stone, brown fortress." Place name from a locational landmark. St. Dunstan was a 10th-century Archbishop of Canterbury. Also: **Dustin.**

DUNTON—Old English: **Duntun.** "From the hill estate or town."

DURANT—Latin: **Durantis.**

"The enduring one." Will Durant, American writer, educator.

DURWARD—Old English: **Duru-weard.** "Gate keeper, unfailing guard." Durward G. Hall, U.S. Congressman.

DURWIN—Old English: **Deor-wine.** "Beloved friend."

DUSTIN—See **Dunstan.** Dustin Hoffman, actor.

DUTCH—German: **Deutsch.** "The German."

DWAYNE—Irish Gaelic: **Dubhain.** "Little dark one." Dwayne Hickman, actor. English variation: **Duane.**

DWIGHT—Old Dutch: **Wit.** "White or blond one." Dwight D. Eisenhower, 34th U.S. President; Dwight Gooden, baseball player.

DYLAN—Old Welsh: "from the sea." The ancient Welsh deity of the ocean. Dylan Thomas, poet (1914-1953); American singer and composer, Bob Dylan.

E

EACHAN—Irish Gaelic: "A horseman."

EARL—Old English: **Eorl.** "Nobleman; chief"; or Irish Gaelic: **Airleas.** "A pledge." Erle Stanley Gardner, author; Errol Flynn, actor; Earl Warren, Chief Justice of the United

States; Earl Monroe, basketball player.
English variations: **Earle, Erl, Erle, Errol.**

EATON—Old English: **Ea-tun.** "From the riverside estate."

EBENEZER—Hebrew: **Eben-**

haezer. "Stone or rock of help." The stone erected by Samuel in the Bible to commemorate defeat of the Philistines. Ebenezer Horsford, American chemist (1818–1893). English nicknames: **Eb, Eben.**

EBERHARD—Old German: **Ebur-hardt.** "Wild-boar brave." A person compared to a brave boar protecting its young.

EBNER—See **Abner.**

EDBERT—Old English: **Ead-beorht.** "Prosperous, brilliant."

EDEL—Old German: **Adal.** "Noble one."

EDELMAR—Old English: **Aethel-maere.** "Noble, famous."

EDEN—Hebrew: "place of delight and pleasure." Sir Anthony Eden, English statesman.

EDGAR—Old English: **Ead-gar.** "Prosperous spearman." Edgar, 10th-century King of England; Edgar Allan Poe, American writer; Edgar Guest, American poet; Edgar Bergen, entertainer. English nicknames: **Ed, Eddie, Eddy, Ned.** Foreign viriations: **Edgar** (German), **Edgardo** (Italian), **Edgard** (French).

EDISON—Old English: **Eadward-sone.** "Son of Edward." Thomas A. Edison, American inventor.

English variation: **Edson.**

EDMUND—Old English: **Eadmund.** "Prosperous protector." Edmund Halley, English scientist (1656-1742); St. Edmund, 9th-century English ruler; Edmund Spenser, 16th-century English poet; Eamon de Valera, Irish president; Edmund Wilson, critic. English nicknames: **Ed, Eddie, Eddy, Ned.** Foreign variations: **Eamon** (Irish), **Edmundo** (Spanish), **Edmond** (French, Dutch).

EDRIC—Old English: **Eadric.** "Prosperous ruler." English nicknames: **Ed, Ric.**

EDSEL—Old English: **Eadsele.** "A prosperous man's manor house or hall." Edsel Ford, American manufacturer.

EDWALD—Old English: **Eadweald.** "Prosperous ruler."

EDWARD—Old English: **Eadward.** "Prosperous guardian." Name for many kings of England; Edward Steichen, photographer; Edward Villella, ballet dancer; Edward Kennedy, U.S. Senator. English nicknames: **Ed, Eddie, Eddy, Ned, Ted, Teddy.** Foreign variations: **Eduardo** (Italian, Spanish, Portuguese), **Edouard** (French), **Eduard** (German, Dutch), **Edvard** (Swedish, Danish).

EDWIN—Old English: **Ead-wine.** "Prosperous friend."

Sir Edwin Arnold, 19th-century English poet; Edwin Stanton, U.S. Secretary of War; Edwin Booth, famous American actor; Edwin Arlington Robinson, American poet.
English nicknames: **Ed, Eddie, Eddy.**
Foreign variation: **Eduino** (Italian, Spanish).

EFREM— See **Ephraim.**

EGAN—Irish Gaelic: **Aodhagan.** "Ardent, fiery one." Also: **Egon.**

EGBERT—Old English: **Ecg-beorht.** "Bright, shining sword." Egbert the Great, King of the West Saxons and first King of England.

EHREN—Old German: "honorable one."

EINAR—Old Norse: **Ein-her.** "Warrior leader." Also, "non-conformist; he thinks for himself." The Einherjar were kings and heroes of the Norse Valhalla or heaven. Also: **Inar.**
Foreign variation: **Ejnar,** (Danish).

ELBERT—See **Albert.** Elbert Hubbard, American author, editor (1856-1915); Elbert Thomas, U.S. Senator.

ELDEN—Old English: **Aelf-dene.** "Elf valley."

ELDER—Old English: **Aeldra.** "Dweller at the elder tree."

ELDON—Old English:

Ealhdun. "From the holy hill."

ELDRED—Teutonic: "battle counselor." Also: **Eldridge.** Eldridge Cleaver, author.

ELDWIN—See **Aldwin.**

ELEAZAR—Hebrew: **El'azar.** "To whom God is a help." Form of the Hebrew Lazarus. St. Eleazar, follower of St. Francis.
Foreign variations: **Eléazar** (French), **Eleazaro** (Spanish).

ELI—Hebrew: "Jehovah," or "the Highest." A scared name, for the Lord. Eli Whitney, American inventor (1765-1825).
English variations: **Ely, Eloy, Eloi.**

ELIAS—See **Elijah.**

ELIHU—Hebrew: "God, the Lord." Elihu Root, American statesman, Nobel prize winner.

ELIJAH—Hebrew: **Eli-yah.** "Jehovah is my God." Elias Ashmole, 17th-century English antiquarian; Elias Howe, American inventor (1819-1867); Elie Wiesel, writer; Elia Kazan, noted director.
English variations: **Elias, Ellis.**
Foreign variations: **Elia** (Italian), **Elie** (French), **Elias** (German, Dutch), **Elías** (Spanish).

ELISHA—Hebrew: "God, my salvation. "Elisha Grau,

American inventor (1835-1901); Elisha Cook, Jr., actor. Foreign variations: **Eliseo** (Italian, Spanish), **Elisée** (French).

ELLARD—Old English: **Ealh-hard.** "Sacred, brave"; or Old English: **Aethel-hard.** "Noble, brave."

ELLERY—Middle English: "from the elder-tree island." William Ellerey, American Revolutionary patriot; Ellery Queen, fictional detective. English variation: **Ellerey.**

ELLIOT—Hebrew-French: **Eli-yah-ot.** "Jehovah is my God." Elliot Coues, American naturalist (1842-1899); Elliot Gould, actor. English variation: **Elliott.**

ELLIS—See **Elijah.**

ELLISON—Old English: **Elle-sone.** "Son of Ellis."

ELMER—Old English: **Aethel-maere.** "Noble-famous." Elmer Davis, commentator (1890–1958); Elmer Rice, dramatist. English variation: **Aylmer.**

ELMO—Latin, from Greek: "friendly, lovable"; or Italian: "helmet; protector." St. Elmo or Erasmus, patron of seamen.

ELMORE—Old English: **Elm-mor.** "Dweller at the elm-tree moor." Elmore Leonard, author.

ELROY—Old French: **Le roy.** "The king." Elroy is a transposition of **Le Roy.** Elroy Hirsch, athlete, actor.

ELSDON—Old English: **Aethelis-dun.** "Noble one's hill," or "Ellis-hill."

ELSON—See **Ellison.**

ELSTON—Old English: **Aethelis-tun.** "Noble one's estate or town"; or Old English: **Aethel-stan.** "Noble-stone."

ELSWORTH—Old English: **Aethelis-worth.** "Noble one's estate." Also: **Ellsworth.** Ellsworth Kelly, artist.

ELTON—Old English: **Eald-tun.** "From the old estate or town." Elton John, singer.

ELVIN—See **Elwin.**

ELVIS—Old Norse; **Alviss.** "All wise." Elvis Presley, Elvis Costello, singers.

ELVY—Old English: **Aelf-wig.** "Elfin warrior."

ELWELL—Old English: **Ealdwiella.** "From the old spring."

ELWIN—Old English: **Aelf-wise.** "Godly friend." English variations: **Elvin, Elwyn, Wynn.**

ELWOOD—Old English: **Ealdwode.** "From the old forest." English variation: **Ellwood.**

ELY—See **Eli.**

EMANUEL—See **Emmanuel.**

EMERSON—See **Emery.**

EMERY—Old German: **Amalric.** "Industrious ruler"; or Old German: **Ermin-ric.** "Joint or coruler." Emory Upton, U.S. Civil War leader; Emory Parnell, actor. English variations: **Emmery, Emory, Emerson.** Foreign variations: **Emmerich** (German), **Amerigo** (Italian), **Emeri** (French).

EMIL—Gothic: **Amal.** "Industrious one"; or Latin: **Aemilius.** "Flattering, winning one." Emile Zola, 19th-century French writer; Emil Jannings, actor. Foreign variations: **Emile** (French), **Emilio** (Spanish).

EMLYN—Welsh: "waterfall." Emlyn Williams, actor and playwright.

EMMANUEL—Hebrew: **Im-manu-el.** "God with us." Emanuel the Great, Portuguese king (1469-1521); Immanuel Kant, philosopher. English variation: **Immanuel.** English nicknames: **Mannie, Manny.** Foreign variations: **Emanuele** (Italian), **Manuel** (Spanish), **Emanuel** (German).

EMMETT—Old German: **Amal-hardt.** "Industrious-strong"; or Old English: **Aemete.** "An ant." Emmett Kelly, famed American circus clown. English variations: **Emmet, Emmit, Emmott.**

EMORY—See **Emery.**

ENEAS—See **Aeneas.**

ENNIS—Irish Gaelic: **Aonghus.** "One-choice," or "only choice"; or Greek: **Ennea.** "Ninth child."

ENOCH—Hebrew: **Khanok.** "Consecrated, dedicated." Enoch, the Biblical patriarch, was father of Methuselah. Enoch Arden, hero of tale by Tennyson.

ENRICO—Italian form of **Henry.** See **Henry.**

EPHRAIM—Hebrew: "very faithful." Also: **Efrem, Ephream, Ephrim, Ephrem.** Efrem Zimbalist Jr., actor.

ERASMUS—Greek: **Erasmois.** "Lovable; worthy of love." Erasmus or St. Elmo, patron of sailors; Erasmus D. Preston, American astronomer (1851-1906). English nicknames: **Ras, Rasmus.** Foreign variations: **Erasmo** (Italian, Spanish), **Erasme** (French).

ERASTUS—Greek: **Erastos.** "Beloved." A giver of love, beloved in return. English nicknames: **Ras, Rastus.** Foreign variation: **Eraste** (French).

ERIC—Old Norse: **Ei-rik-r.** "Ever powerful; ever-ruler." Eric the Red, Norwegian Viking hero; Eric Ambler, Erich Segal, authors. English nicknames: **Ric, Rick, Ricky.**

Foreign variations: **Erik** (Scandinavian), **Erich** (German).

ERLAND—Old English: **Eorlland.** "Nobleman's land."

ERLING—Old English: **Eorlsone.** "Nobleman's son."

ERMIN—See **Herman.**

ERNEST—Old English: **Earnest.** "Earnest one." Ernest Hemingway, American author; Ernest C. Watson, physicist; actors Ernie Kovacs, Ernest Borgnine. English nicknames: **Ernie, Erny.**
Foreign variations: **Ernst** (German), **Ernesto** (Italian, Spanish), **Ernestus** (Dutch).

ERROL—A variant of **Earl.** Also, Latin: "wandering."

ERSKINE—Scottish Gaelic: **Airdsgainne.** "From the height of the cleft." Erskine Caldwell, novelist.

ERWIN—Old English: **Ear-wine.** "Sea friend." See Irving. Erwin Schroedinger, German physicist.

ESMOND—Old English: **Est-mund.** "Gracious protector, protected by God's grace."

ESTE—Italian. **Est.** "From the East." Estes Kefauver, U.S. Senator.
English variation: **Estes.**

ETHAN—Hebrew: **Eythan.** "Firmness, strength, steadfast; strong and reliable." Ethan Allen, Revolutionary War leader; *Ethan Frome,* novel by Edith Wharton.

EUGENE—Greek: **Eugenios.** "Well-born, noble." There were four Popes named Eugene; Eugene McCarthy, U.S. Senator; Eugene O'Neill, American dramatist. English nickname: **Gene.**
Foreign variations: **Eugenio** (Italian, Spanish, Portuguese), **Eugen** (German), **Eugène** (French), **Eugenius** (Dutch).

EUSTACE—Latin: **Eustathius.** "Stable, tranquill"; Greek: "fruitful, productive." St. Eustace, Roman soldier, was martyred in A.D. 118, and is the patron of hunters.
Foreign variations: **Eustache** (French), **Eustazio** (Italian), **Eustasius** (German), **Eustquio** (Spanish), **Eustatius** (Dutch).

EVAN—Irish Gaelic: **Eoghan;** Old Welsh: **Owein.** "Well-born one; young warrior." Welsh form of **John,** "God is gracious."
English variations: **Ewan, Ewen, Owen.**

EVERARD—Old English: **Efer-hard.** "Strong or brave as a boar; always true." Sir Everard Home, surgeon (1756-1832); Everett Dirksen, U.S. Senator.
English nickname: **Ev.**
English variations: **Evered, Everett.**
Foreign variations: **Eberhard** (German), **Evraud** (French), **Everardo** (Italian), **Everhart** (Dutch).

EVERETT—See Everard.

EVERLEY—Old English: **Efer-leah.** "From Ever's lea," a place name.

EWALD—Old English: **Aew-weald.** "Law-powerful"; or Teutonic: "always powerful."
English variation: **Evald.**

EWERT—Old English: **Ewe-heorde.** "Ewe-herder."

EWING—Old English: **Aew-winc.** "Law-friend." A lawyer who used the law to protect his fellow men.

EZEKIEL—Hebrew: **Yekhezqel.** "Strength of God." Ezekiel, great Hebrew Biblical prophet.
English nickname: **Zeke.**
Foreign variations: **Ezechiel** (French), **Ezechiele** (Italian), **Ezechiel** (German, Dutch), **Ezequiel** (Spanish).

EZRA—Hebrew: "help, helper." Famous Hebrew prophet of the Bible. Ezra Pound, American poet.
Foreign variations: **Esdras** (French, Spanish), **Esra** (German).

F

FABIAN—Latin: **Fabianus.** Originally, "Bean-grower." A medieval agriculturist who knew his husbandry. Fabius, Roman general; Also from Fabius, a dilatory general; hence implies "procrastinating, indecisive." Fabius, Roman general Pope Fabian, 3rd century; Fabian Forte, actor, singer. Foreign variations: **Fabio, Fabiano** (Italian), **Fabien** (French).

FABRON—South French: "little blacksmith." An apprentice who desired to learn the trade.
Foreign variations: **Fabre** (French), **Fabroni** (Italian).

FAGAN—Irish Gaelic: **Faodhagan.** "Little fiery one." English variation: **Fagin.**

FAIRFAX—English: "light haired."

FAIRLEY—See Farley.

FANE—Old English: **Faegen.** "Glad; joyful."

FARLEY—Old English: **Faerr-leah.** "From the bull or sheep meadow." Farley Granger, actor.
English variations: **Fairlie, Fairleigh, Farly.**

FARNELL—Old English: **Fearn-healh.** "From the fern slope."
English variations: **Farnall, Fernald.**

FARNHAM—Old English: **Fearn-hamm.** "From the fern field."

FARNLEY—Old English: **Fearn-leah.** "From the fern meadow."

FAROLD—Old English:
Faer-wald. "Mighty traveler."

FARR—Old English: **Faer.**
"Traveler."

FARRAND—See **Ferrand.**

FARRELL—Irish Gaelic:
Fearghal. "Most valorous
one," or "champion,
warrior."
English variations: **Farrel,**
Ferrell.

FARRIS—See **Ferris.**

FAUST—Latin: **Faustis.**
"Lucky, auspicious." Dr.
Faustus, legendary 15th-
century necromancer, was
used as hero of Gounod's
opera *Faust,* and Goethe's
drama; Faustus Socinus
16th-century Italian reformer.
Foreign variation: **Fausto**
(Italian).

FAY—Irish Gaelic: **Feich.**
"Raven." The raven symbol-
ized wisdom in medieval
Europe. Richard D. Fay,
American educator.
English variation: **Fayette.**

FELIPE—Spanish for
Phillip, from Greek for "lover
of horses."

FELIX—Latin: "fortunate,
lucky one." Felix Adler,
19th-century ethical reformer;
Felix Frankfurter, Supreme
Court Justice. There are over
70 saints named Felix.
Foreign variations: **Felix**
(French), **Felice** (Italian),
Félix (Spanish).

FELTON—Old English:

Feldtun. "From the field
estate or town."

FENTON—Old English:
Fenntun. "From the marsh
farm or estate."

FEODOR—See **Theodore.**

FERDINAND—Gothic:
Fair-honanth. "World-daring;
life-adventuring." Ferdi-
nand the Great, 11th-century
Spanish king; Ferdinand
Magellan, Portuguese naviga-
tor; Hernando Cortez,
conqueror of Mexico; Fer-
nando Lamas, actor.
English nicknames: **Ferd,**
Ferdie.
Foreign variations: **Ferdinando**
(Italian). **Fernando, Hernando**
(Spanish).

FERGUS—Irish Gaelic:
Fearghus. "Very choice one,
strong man." Ten saints
Fergus are listed in the
Martyrology of Donegai.
Feargus O'Connor, Irish
chartist (1794–1855).
English nickname: **Fergie.**

FERNALD—See **Farnall.**

FERRAND—Old French:
Ferrant. "Iron-gray hair."
English variations: **Farrand,**
Farrant, Ferrant.

FERRIS—Irish Gaelic:
Feoras. "Peter, 'The Rock',"
or "very choice one."
English variation: **Farris.**

FIDEL—Latin: **Fidelis.**
"Faithful, sincere." St. Fidelis
of Sigmaringen, "Advocate
of the Poor"; Fidel Castro,
Cuban leader.

Foreign variations: **Fidele**
(French), **Fidelio** (Italian).

FIELDING—Old English:
Felding. "Dweller at the
field."

FILBERT—Old English:
Felabeorht. "Very brilliant
one."
English variation: **Philbert.**
Foreign variations: **Filberto**
(Italian, Spanish), **Filberte**
(French).

FILMER—Old English:
Felamaere. "Very famous
one." Millard Fillmore,
13th U.S. President.
English nickname: **Fil.**
English variations: **Filmore,**
Fillmore.

FILMORE—See **Filmer.**

FINDLAY—See **Finley.**

FINLEY—Irish Gaelic:
Fionn-ghalac. "Little fair-
haired valorous one"; or
Irish Gaelic: **Fionn-laoch.**
"Fair soldier." Finlay
Currie, actor.
English nicknames: **Fin, Lee.**
English variations: **Findlay,**
Findley, Finlay.

FINN—Irish Gaelic: **Fionn.**
"Fair-haired and complex-
ioned"; or Old German:
Fin. "From Finland." Finn
Ronne, Antarctic explorer.

FIORELLO—Italian: "little
flower." Fiorello LaGuardia,
mayor of New York.

FIRMIN—Old French:
"firm, strong one."

FISKE—Middle English:

"fish." Used by an ancestor
from his medieval shop-
sign. Fiske Kimball, American
architect (1888-1955).

FITCH—Middle English:
Fitche. "European marten
or ermine." John Fitch,
American steamboat inven-
tor (1743-1798).

FITZ—Old French: **Filz.**
"Son." Introduced to Britain
by the Normans and altered
from "Filz" to "Fitz."

FITZGERALD—Old En-
glish: "Son of spear-mighty."
See **Gerald.** Fitzgerald
Molloy, historian.

FITZHUGH—Old English:
"son of the intelligent one."
Fitzhugh Lee, Virginia
governor (1835-1905).

FLANN—Irish Gaelic: "red-
haired one."

FLAVIAN—Latin: **Flavius.**
"Golden-yellow haired one."
Flavius Valens, eastern
Roman Emperor, 4th century;
Flavius Josephus, famous
Jewish historian, 1st century.

FLETCHER—Middle En-
glish: **Fleccher.** "Arrow-
maker." From the surname.
A man named for his dexterity
in putting feathers on
arrows.

FLINN—See **Flynn.**

FLINT—Old English: **Flynt.**
"A stream." In America we
call obsidian "flint," but in
Britain it was an ancient word
for a brook.

FLORIAN—Latin: "flowering."

FLOYD—See **Lloyd**.

FLYNN—Irish Gaelic: **Floinn**. "Son of the red-haired man."
English variation: **Flinn**.

FORBES—Irish Gaelic: **Fear-bhirigh**. "Man of prosperity"; or Irish Gaelic: **Forba**. "Owner of fields." Scottish clan name, suggesting "headstrong one."

FORD—Old English: "river crossing." Ford Madox Ford, writer.

FORREST—Old French: "dweller at a forest." Forrest Tucker, actor.
English variation: **Forest**.

FORRESTER—Middle English: **Forester**. "Forest guardian."
English nicknames: **Forrie, Foss**.
English variations: **Forester, Forster, Foster**.

FORSTER—See **Forrester**.

FORTUNE—Old French: "lucky one." St. Fortunatus, 6th-century Bishop of Poitiers, France.
Foreign variations: **Fortunio** (Italian), **Fortuné** (French).

FOSS—See **Forrester**.

FOSTER—See **Forrester**.

FRANCHOT—See **Francis**.

FRANCIS—Latin: **Franciscus**. "Free man," or "Frenchman." St. Francis of Assisi

(1181-1226); Lord Francis Bacon, English philosopher (1561-1626); Francisco Pizarro, 15th-century Spanish conquistador; Franz Josef Haydn, composer; Franchot Tone, actor.
English nicknames: **Fran, Frank**.
Foreign variations: **François, Franchot** (French), **Franciskus, Franz** (German), **Francesco** (Italian), **Francisco** (Spanish, Portuguese), **Frans** (Swedish), **Frants** (Danish).

FRANK—Old French: **Franc**. "Free man." See **Franklin, Francis**. Frank Sinatra, actor, singer.

FRANKLIN—Middle English: **Frankeleyn**. "Free holder of land." Franklin Pierce, 14th U.S. President; Franklin D. Roosevelt, 32nd U.S. President.
English nicknames: **Frank, Frankie**.
English variations: **Franklyn, Francklin, Francklyn**.

FRASER—See **Frazer**.

FRAYNE—Middle English: **Fren**. "Stranger, foreigner"; or Old French: "dweller at the ash-tree."
English variations: **Fraine, Frean, Freen, Freyne**.

FRAZER—Old French: **Frasier**. "Strawberry"; or Old English: **Frisa**. "Curly-haired one; Frisian Dutchman."
English variations: **Fraser, Frasier, Frazier**.

FREDERICK—Old Ger-

man: **Fridu-rik.** "Peaceful ruler." Frederick the Great, Prussian King (1740-1786); Fritz Weaver, Fredric March, actors.
English nicknames: **Fred, Freddie, Freddy.**
English variations: **Frederic, Fredric, Fredrick.**
Foreign variations: **Friedrich, Fritz** (German), **Fréderic** (French), **Federigo** (Italian), **Federico** (Spanish), **Fredrik** (Swedish), **Frederik** (Danish, Dutch).

FREEMAN—Old English: **Freo-man.** "Free man."

FREMONT—Old German: **Fri-munt.** "Free or noble protector." General John C. Fremont (1813–1890).

FREWIN—Old English: **Freo-wine.** "Free, noble friend." **Freo-wine,** descendant of Woden, was ancestor of the early English kings of Wessex.

English variation: **Frewen.**

FREY—Old English: **Fre.** "Lord." Frey was the ancient Norse god of prosperity, peace, and fertility.

FRICK—Old English: **Freca.** "Bold man."

FRIDOLF—Old English: **Fridu-wulf.** "Peaceful wolf."

FRITZ—See **Frederick.**

FULLER—Middle English: **Fullere.** "Cloth-thickener." An occupational name for a man who moistened and pressed cloth.

FULTON—Old English: **Fugeltun.** "Dweller at the fowl-enclosure." From a place name. Alternate, Old English: **Fula-tun.** "People's estate." Bishop Fulton J. Sheen, American clergyman, author.

FYFE—Pictish-Scottish: **Fibh.** "From Fifeshire, Scotland."

G

GABLE—Old French: **Gabel.** "Little Gabriel."

GABRIEL—Hebrew: "hero of God, God gives him strength." The Archangel of the Annunciation.
English nicknames: **Gabe, Gabie, Gabby.**
Foreign variations: **Gabriele, Gabriello** (Italian), **Gabriel** (German, French, Spanish).

GAGE—Old French: "pledge, a pledge of security."

GAIL—See **Gale.**

GAIR—Irish Gaelic: **Gearr.** "Short one."

GALE—Old English: **Gal.** "Gay, lively one." Alternate, Irish Gaelic: **Gall.** "Foreigner." Gale Gordon, actor.

English variations: **Gail,
Gaile, Gayle.**

GALEN—Irish Gaelic:
Gaelan. "Little bright one."

GALLAGHER—Irish Gaelic:
Galchobhar. "Foreign helper
or eager helper."

GALLOWAY—Old Gaelic:
Gallgaidheal. "Man from the
land of the stranger Gaels."
A Scottish Celt of the
Highlands. Galway Kinnell,
poet.
English variations: **Galway,
Gallway.**

GALTON—Old English:
Gafoltun. "Owner of a rented
estate."

GALVIN—Irish Gaelic:
Gael-bhan. "Bright, shining
white"; or Irish Gaelic:
Gealbhan. "Sparrow."
English variations: **Galvan,
Galven.**

GAMALIEL—Hebrew: **Gamal-
yel.** "Recompense of God."
Gamaliel the Elder, 1st-
century teacher of the Apostle
Paul; Gamaliel Bradford,
American biographer (1863-
1932); Warren Gamaliel
Harding, 29th U.S.
President.

GANNON—Irish Gaelic:
Gionnan. "Little fair-
complexioned one."

GARDNER—Middle En-
glish: **Gardiner.** "A gardener." Gardiner Spring,
American clergyman, author
(1785-1873); Gardner McKay,
actor.

English variations: **Gardener,
Gardiner.**

GAREY—See Gary.

GARFIELD—Old English:
Garafeld. "Triangular field";
or Old English: **Gari-feld.**
"War or battle-spear field."
James Garfield, 20th U.S.
President.

GARLAND—Old English:
Gari-land. "From the spear-
land"; or Old French:
Garlande. "Wreath of flowers
or leaves."

GARMAN—Old English:
Garmann. "Spearman."

GARMOND—Old English:
Gar-mund. "Spear-protector."
English variations: **Garmon,
Garmund.**

GARNER—Old French:
Garnier. "Guardian army;
army guard."

GARNETT—Old English:
Gar-nyd. "Armed with a
spear"; or Late Latin:
Granatus. "A seed; pomegran-
ate seed."
English variation: **Garnet.**

GARNOCK—Old Welsh:
Gwer-nach. "Dweller by the
alder-river."

GARRETT—Old English:
Gar-hard. "Spear-brave; firm-
spear." Garrett Hobart,
24th U.S. Vice President;
Garrett Morris, actor.
English variations: **Garrard,
Garrett, Garret, Garritt,
Gerard.**
Foreign variation: **Gearoid**
(Irish).

GARRICK—Old English: **Gar-ric.** "Spear-ruler."

GARROWAY—Old English: **Gar-wig.** "Spear-warrior." Dave Garroway, television personality.
English variation: **Garraway.**

GARSON—Old English: "son of Gar." Garson Kanin, playwright.

GARTH—Old Norse: **Garth-r.** "From the garden."

GARTON—Old English: **Garatun.** "Dweller at the triangular farmstead."

GARVEY—Irish Gaelic: **Gair-bhith.** "Rough peace"; or Irish Gaelic: **Garbhach.** "Rough one." An intricate paradox meaning probably, "Peace after much controversy."

GARVIN—Old English: **Gar-wine.** "Spear-friend." English variation: **Garwin.**

GARWOOD—Old English: **Gyr-wode.** "From the fir forest."

GARY—Old English: **Gari.** "Spear; spearman." Gary Hart, U.S. Senator; Gary Cooper, Gary Merrill, actors.
English variations: **Gari, Garey, Garry.**

CASPAR—Persian: **Kansbar.** "Treasure-master." Gaspar was one of the three Wise Men or Magi in the Bible; Gaspar Cortereal, Portuguese navigator (1450-1501). English variations: **Caspar,**
Casper, Gasper, Kaspar, Kasper, Jasper.
Foreign variations: **Gaspard** (French), **Gasparo** (Italian), **Kaspar** (German).

GASTON—French: **Gascon.** "Man from Gascony, the Land of the Basques." Gaston Plante, French physicist, 19th century.

GAVIN—Old Welsh: **Gwalchmai.** "From the hawk field." Sir Gawain, nephew of King Arthur in the medieval Round Table romances; Gavin McLeod, actor.
English variations: **Gavan, Gaven, Gawen, Gawain.**

GAYLE—See **Gale.**

GAYLORD—Old French: **Gaillard.** "Lively one." English variations: **Gayler, Gaylor, Gallard.**

GAYNOR—Irish Gaelic: **Mac-Fionnbharr.** "Son of the fair-head." English variations: **Gainer, Gainor, Gayner.**

GEARY—Middle English: **Gery.** "Changeable one." English variations: **Gearey, Gery.**

GEOFFREY—See **Jeffrey, Godfrey.**

GEORGE—Latin: **Georgius,** from Greek: "Land-worker; farmer." St. George, patron of England, 4th century; English kings George I to VI; George Washington, 1st

U.S. President; George
Gershwin, composer; actors
George Burns, George
Montgomery, George Raft.
English nicknames: **Georgi,
Georgy, Geordie.**
Foreign variations: **Georg**
(German, Danish, Swedish),
Giorgio (Italian), **Jorge**
(Spanish) **Georges** (French)
Geòras (Scottish).

GERALD—Old German.
Gerwalt. "Spear-mighty,"
or Old German: **Ger-wald.**
"Spear-ruler." Gerald Ford,
38th U.S. President.
English nicknames: **Gerry,
Jerry.**
Foreign variations: **Géralde,
Geraud, Giraud** (French),
Giraldo (Italian), **Gerold**
(German), **Gearalt** (Irish).

GERARD—Old English:
Gar-hard. "Spear-brave; spear-
strong." Gerhart Haupt-
mann, German dramatist;
Gerard Hopkins, English
poet.
English nicknames: **Gerry,
Jerry.**
English variations: **Gerrard,
Gerhard.**
Foreign variations: **Gerhardt,
Gerhard** (German), **Geraud**
(French), **Gerardo, Gherardo**
(Italian), **Gerardo** (Spanish),
Gerhard (Danish, Swedish),
Gerard (Irish).

GERONIMO—See **Jerome.**

GIBSON—Old English:
Gibbesone. "Son of Gilbert." See **Gilbert.**

GIDEON—Hebrew: **Gid-on.**

"Hewer or feller; destroyer."
Gideon in the Bible ruled
Israel for 40 years; Gideon
Granger, U.S. Postmaster
General (1767-1822).

GIFFORD—Old English:
Gifu-hard. "Gift-brave." Gifford
Pinchot, Pennsylvania
governor.
English nicknames: **Giff,
Giffy.**
English variations: **Giffard,
Gifferd.**

GILBERT—Old English:
Gisel-beorht. "Brilliant pledge
or hostage." Gilbert Ches-
terton, English writer; Gil
Gerard, actor.
English nicknames: **Gil, Gill,
Gib, Gibb, Bert.**
Foreign variations: **Giselbert,
Gilbert** (German), **Guilbert**
(French), **Gilberto** (Italian,
Spanish), **Gilibeirt** (Irish),
Gilleabart (Scottish).

GILBY—Old Norse: **Gisl-
by-r.** "Pledge or hostage's
estate"; or Irish Gaelic:
Giolla-buidhe. "Yellow-haired
lad."
English variation: **Gilbey.**

GILCHRIST—Irish Gaelic:
Giolla-Chriost. "Servant of
Christ."
Foreign variation: **Gillecriosd**
(Scottish).

GILES—Old French: **Gilles.**
"Youthful; downy-bearded
one"; or Latin: **Egidius.**
"Shield-bearer." Giles Fletcher,
English dramatist (1588-1623).
Foreign variations: **Gilles,
Egide** (French), **Egidio**

(Italian), **Egidius** (German, Dutch), **Gil** (Spanish).

GILLETT—Old French: **Gilleet.** "Little Gilbert." See **Gilbert.** Gelett Burgess, American writer, illustrator; William Gillette, actor. English variations: **Gelett, Gelette, Gillette.**

GILMER—Old English: **Gisel-maere.** "Famous hostage."

GILMORE—Irish Gaelic: **Giolla-Mhuire.** "Adherent of St. Mary." English variations: **Gillmore, Gilmour.**

GILROY—Irish Gaelic: **Giolla-ruaidh.** "Servant of the red-haired youth."

GIRVIN—Irish Gaelic: **Garbhan.** "Little rough one." English variations: **Girvan, Girven.**

GLADWIN—Old English: **Glaed-wine.** "Kind, cheerful friend."

GLANVILLE—Old French: **Glande-ville.** "From the oak-tree estate."

GLENDON—Scottish Gaelic: **Glen-dun.** "From the glen-fortress, from the shady valley."

GLENN—Old Welsh: **Glyn;** Irish Gaelic: **Glaleanna.** "Dweller in a glen or valley." Glyn Philpot, English painter; Glenn Ford, Glenn Hunter, actors.

English nicknames: **Glennie, Glenny.**
English variations: **Glen, Glyn, Glynn.**

GLYNN—See **Glenn.**

GODDARD—Old German: **Gode-hard.** "Divinely firm"; or "God-firm." English variations: **Godard, Godart, Goddart.** Foreign variations: **Godard** (French), **Gotthart** (German), **Gotthard** (Dutch).

GODFREY—Old German: **Gott-fried.** "Divinely peaceful." Gottfried Leibnitz, German 17th-century mathematician; Godfrey Weitzel, Civil War leader; Godfrey Cambridge, actor. English variations: **Goeffrey, Jeffrey.** Foreign variations: **Gottfried** (German, Dutch), **Goffredo** (Italian), **Godofredo** (Spanish), **Godefroi** (French), **Gottfrid** (Swedish), **Goraidh** (Scottish), **Gothfraidh** (Irish).

GODWIN—Old English. **God-wine.** "good friend," or "friend of God." Godwin, 11th-century Earl of Wessex. English variation: **Goodwin.** Foreign variation: **Godewyn** (Dutch).

GOLDING—Old English: "Son of the golden one." Golding Bird, English physician.

GOLDWIN—Old English: **Gold-wine.** "Golden friend." Goldwin Smith, Canadian author (1823-1910).

GORDON—Old English: **Garadun.** "From the triangular or gore-shaped hill." Celebrated from the Scottish Clan Gordon. Gordon Alexander, American biologist, writer; Gordon MacRae, singer, actor.
English nicknames: **Gordie, Gordy.**
English variations: **Gordan, Gorden.**

GORMAN—Irish Gaelic: "little blue-eyed one."

GOUVERNEUR—French: "chief ruler; governor." Gouverneur Morris, American statesman (1752-1816).

GOWER—Old Welsh: **Gwyr.** "Pure one." Gower Champion, actor, dancer, director.

GRADY—Irish Gaelic: **Grada.** "Noble, illustrious."

GRAHAM—Old English: **Graeg-hamm.** "From the gray land or gray home." Graham Greene, novelist.

GRANGER—Old English: **Grangere.** "Farmer."

• **GRANT**—Middle English: **Grand.** "Great one." Grant Wood, American painter (1892–1942).

GRANTLAND—Old English: **Grand-land.** "From the great grassy plain." Grantland Rice, sportsman, film producer.

GRANVILLE—Old French: **Grande-ville.** "From the great estate or town." Granville Hall, American psychologist.

GRAYSON—Middle English: **Grayve-sone.** "Son of the reeve or bailiff." Grayson Kirk, educator.

GREELEY—Old English: **Graeg-leah.** "From the gray meadow." Horace Greeley, 19th-century journalist, founder of Republican Party.

GREGORY—Latin: **Gregorious.** "Vigilant, watchful one." St. Gregory the Great (540-604); 16 Popes were named Gregory; Gregory Peck, actor; Gregory (Pappy) Boyington, Marine ace.
English nicknames: **Greg, Gregg.**
English variations: **Gregor, Grigor.**
Foreign variations: **Gregorius** (German), **Grégoire** (French), **Gregoor** (Dutch), **Gregorio** (Italian, Spanish, Portuguese), **Griogair** (Scottish), **Greagoir, Grioghar** (Irish).

GRIFFITH—Old Welsh: **Gruff-udd.** "Fierce chief"; or Old Welsh: **Gruffin.** "Fierce lord, red-haired; ruddy one." A ferocious leader against his country's enemies.
English variation: **Griffin.**

GRISWOLD—Old German: **Gris-wald.** "From the gray forest."

GROVER—Old English: **Grafere.** "From the grove of

trees." Grover Cleveland,
22nd and 24th U.S. President.

GUNTHER—Old Norse:
Gunnr-har. "Warrior."
English and Scandinavian
variations: **Gunnar, Gun-
ner, Gunter.**

GUSTAVE—Swedish: **Gustaf.**
"Noble staff; God's staff."
Gustavus Adolphus, 16th-
century Swedish king; Gustav
Mahler, composer; Gustave
Flaubert, 19th-century French
writer.
English nicknames: **Gus,
Gussie.**
Foreign variations: **Gustav**
(German), **Gustaf** (Swe-
dish), **Gustavo** (Italian,
Spanish), **Gustave** (French),
Gustaff (Dutch).

GUTHRIE—Gaelic:
Gaothaire. "Where the wind
blows free"; or **Gund-heri.**
"War hero." Guthrie McClintic,
noted theatrical producer.

GUY—Old German: **Wido.**
"Warrior"; or Latin: **Vitus.**
"Life." Guy de Maupassant,
French writer (1850-1893).
Foreign variations: **Guido**
(German, Swedish, Italian,
Spanish), **Guy** (French).

GWYNN—Old Welsh:
Gwyn. "Fair, blond one."
Gwyn was the deity of the
underworld in Welsh myths.
English variation: **Gwyn.**
Foreign variation: **Guin**
(Gaelic).

GYLES—See **Giles.**

H

HACKETT—Old Franco-
German: **Hack-et.** "Little
hacker."

HADDEN—Old English:
Haeth-dene or **Haeth-dun.**
"From the heath-valley or
hill."
English variations: **Haddan,
Haddon.**

HADLEY—Old English:
Haeth-leah. "From the heath
meadow."
English variation: **Hadleigh.**

HADWIN—Old English:
Haetho-wine. "War-friend."

HAGEN—Irish Gaelic:
Hagan. "Little, young one."

English variations: **Hagan,
Haggan.**

HAGLEY—Old English:
Haga-leah. "From the hedged
pasture."

HAIG—Old English: **Haga.**
"Dweller at the hedged
enclosure."

HAKON—Old Norse: "of
the high or exalted race."
Hakon has been the name
of many Norwegian kings.
Foreign variations: **Haakon,
Hako** (Norse).

HALBERT—Old English:
Hale-beorht. "Brilliant hero."

HALDEN—Old Norse:

Half-Dan. "Half-Dane." A man half-Danish and half-English. Half-dan was the name of many Norwegian rulers.
English variations: **Halfdan, Haldan.**

HALE—Old English: **Haele.** "Hero in good health"; or Old English: **Heall.** "From the Hall," surname. Also: Hawaiian: **Harold.** "Army ruler." Hale Hamilton, actor.

HALEY—Irish Gaelic: **Ealad-hach.** "Ingenious, scientific."

HALFORD—Old English: **Healh-ford.** "From the hillslope-ford"; or Old English: **Heall-ford.** "From the manor house ford."

HALL—Old English: **Heall.** "Dweller at the hall or manor house."

HALLAM—Old English: **Healum.** "Dweller at the slopes."

HALLEY—Old English: **Heall-leah.** "From the manor house meadow"; or Old English: **Halig.** "Holy." Edmund Halley, English astronomer (1656-1742).

HALLIWELL—Old English: **Halig-wiella.** "Dweller by a holy spring."

HALLWARD—Old English: **Heall-weard.** "Hall warden or guardian."

HALSEY—Old English: **Hals-ig.** "From Hal's island."

Admiral "Bull" Halsey, naval hero.

HALSTEAD—Old English: **Heall-stede.** "From the manor house place."
English variation: **Halsted.**

HALTON—Old English: **Healh-tun.** "From the hillslope estate."

HAMAL—Arabic: "lamb."

HAMAR—Old Norse: **Hammar.** "Hammer." A symbol of the ingenuity of man; in Old Norse mythology, the hammer of Thor.

HAMILTON—Old English: **Hamela-tun.** "Home-lover's estate," or "wether-sheep enclosure." Place name and surname: "grassy hill." Hamilton Fish, U.S. Secretary of State (1869-1877).

HAMLET—Old Franco-German: **Hamo-elet.** "Little home." Hamlet, Prince of Denmark, famous Shakespearean character.

HAMLIN—Old Franco-German: **Hamo-elin.** "Little home-lover." Hamlin Garland, American writer.

HANFORD—Old English: **Hean-ford.** "From the high-ford."

HANLEY—Old English: **Hean-leah.** "From the high pasture," place name and surname; also Irish: "Warrior."

HANS—See **John.** Hans Christian Andersen, 19th-

century Danish writer,
Hans Holbein, Dutch painter.

HARBERT—See **Herbert**.

HARBIN—Old Franco-
German: **Hari-beorht-in**. "Lit-
tle, glorious warrior." See
Herbert.

HARCOURT—Old Franco-
German: **Hari-court**. "From
the fortified farm."

HARDEN—Old English:
Hara-dene. "From the hare-
valley." J. Harden Peterson,
U.S. Congressman.
English variation: **Hardin**.

HARDING—Old English:
Heard-ing. "Brave one's
son." Harding Lawrence,
American industrialist.

HARDWIN— Old English:
Heard-wine. "Brave friend."

HARDY—Old German:
Harti. "Bold and daring."
Hardy Kruger, actor.
English variations: **Hardey**,
Hardie.

HARFORD—Old English:
Hara-ford. "From the hare-
ford"; or Old English:
Here-ford. "Army-ford."

HARGROVE—Old En-
glish: **Hara-graf**. "From the
hare-grove."
English variation: **Hargrave**.

HARLAN—Old English:
Hari-land. "From the army-
land"; or Old English:
Hara-land. "Hare-land." Harlan Ellison, author.

HARLEY—Old English:

Hara-leah. "From the hare-
pasture." Harley Kilgore,
U.S. Senator.
English variation: **Arley**.

HARLOW—Old English:
Hari-hloew. "Army-hill; fortified hill." An army
encampment. Harlow Shapley,
astronomer.

HARMAN—See **Herman**.

HARMON—See **Herman**.

HAROLD—Old Norse:
Har-uald. "Army-ruler." Har-
old II, last Saxon king of
England (1022-1061); Harold
Arlen, composer; Harold
Lloyd, actor; Harold Macmil-
lan, British Prime Minister.
English nicknames: **Hal**,
Harry.
English variations: **Harald**,
Herold.
Foreign variations: **Harald**
(Swedish, Danish), **Araldo**
(Italian), **Herold** (Dutch),
Aralt (Irish), **Harailt**
(Scottish).

HARPER—Old English.
Hear-pere. "Harp player."
Harper Lee, author.

HARRIS—Old English:
Hanry-sone. "Son of Harry."
Harrison Ford, actor.
English variation: **Harrison**.

HARRISON—See **Harris**.

HARRY—Old English:
Hari. "Army man." See
Henry, Harold. Harry S
Truman, 33rd U.S. President;
Harry Belafonte, singer.

HART—Old English: **Heort**.

"Hart-deer." From an old shop-sign that pictured a red stag deer. Hart Crane, American poet (1899-1932).

HARTFORD—Old English: **Heort-ford.** "Stagford."

HARTLEY—Old English: **Heort-leah.** "Hart-deer pasture." Hartley Coleridge, English writer, poet (1796-1846).

HARTMAN—Old German: **Hart-mann.** "Strong, austere man"; or Old English: **Heort-man.** "Stag-deer keeper."

HARTWELL—Old English: **Heort-wiella.** Place name: "Hart-deer spring, where wild deer came to drink."

HARTWOOD—Old English: **Heort-wode.** "Hart-deer forest."

HARVEY—Old German: **Her-wig.** "Army-warrior." One who protects his country. Alternate, Old Breton French: **Hueru.** "Bitter, severe." Harvey Firestone, American industrialist; Harve Presnell, actor. English nicknames: **Harv, Harve.**
English variation: **Hervey.**

HASLETT—Old English: **Haesel-heafod.** "Hazel-tree headland." William Hazlett Upson, writer.
English variation: **Hazlett.**

HASSAN—Arabic: "handsome."

HASTINGS—Old English: **Haestingas.** "Son of the severe, violent one." Hastings was a 9th-century Scandinavian Viking leader; Hastings Keith, U.S. Congressman.

HAVELOCK—Old Norse: **Hafleik-r.** "Sea-contest." Havelock the Dane was an ancient legendary character; Havelock Ellis, English psychological writer.

HAVEN—Old English: **Haefen.** "Place of safety."

HAWLEY—Old English: **Haga-leah.** "From the hedged meadow."

HAYDEN—Old English: **Haga-dene.** "From the hedged valley."
English variation: **Haydon.**

HAYWARD—Old English: **Haga-ward.** "Hedged enclosure keeper."

HAYWOOD—Old English: **Haga-wode.** "From the high or hedged forest." Heywood Broun, literary critic (1888-1937).
English variation: **Heywood.**

HEATH—Middle English: **Hethe.** "Heath or wasteland."

HEATHCLIFF—Middle English: **Hethe-clif.** "From the heath-cliff."

HECTOR—Greek: **Hektor.** "Holds fast; steadfast." In

Greek history Hector was the bravest Trojan warrior. Foreign variations: **Ettore** (Italian), **Eachunn** (Scottish).

HELMUT—Middle French: **Healmet** "Helmet." Helmut Newton, photographer.

HENRICK—Dutch variant of Henry, "ruler of the home." Foreign variations: **Enrico** (Italian); **Hendrik, Henri** (French).

HENRY—Old German: **Heimtik**. "Ruler of a home, or private property." Henry VIII, English king; Henry Hudson, English and Dutch navigator; Henry Ward Beecher, American 19th-century clergyman; Henry Fonda, actor; Heinrich Heine, poet. English nicknames: **Harry, Hank, Hal.** English variations: **Hendrick, Henri.** Foreign variations: **Heinrich** (German), **Enrico** (Italian), **Henri** (French), **Enrique** (Spanish), **Hendrik** (Dutch, Danish), **Henrik** (Swedish), **Eanruig** (Scottish), **Hanraoi** (Irish).

HERBERT—Old German: **Heri-beraht.** "Army-brilliant; glorious warrior." Herbert Hoover, 31st U.S. President; Herbert George (H.G.) Wells, English author; Herbert Ross, director. English nicknames: **Herb, Herbie, Bert.**

English variations: **Harbert, Hebert.** Foreign variations: **Erberto** (Italian), **Heriberto** (Spanish), **Hoireabard** (Irish).

HERCULES—Greek: **Herakles.** "Glory of Hera, fame." Hercules, strongest man in mythology; Hercule Poirot, brilliant fictional detective.

HERMAN—Old German: **Heri-mann.** "Army-man; warrior"; or Latin: **Herminius.** "High-ranking person." Herman Melville, Herman Wouk, American writers. English nicknames: **Herm, Hermie.** English variations: **Ermin, Harman, Harmon.** Foreign variations: **Hermann** (German, Danish), **Armand** (French), **Armando** (Spanish), **Ermanno** (Italian).

HERNANDO—See **Ferdinand.**

HERRICK—Old German: **Heri-rik.** "Army ruler."

HERSCHEL—Hebrew: "deer." Herschel Walker, football player and sprinter. English variations: **Hershel, Hersch, Hirsch.**

HERVEY—See **Harvey.**

HEWE—See **Hugh.**

HEWETT—Old Franco-German: **Hugi-et.** "Little Hugh." See **Hugh.** English variation: **Hewitt.**

HEYWOOD—See **Haywood.**

HIATT—See **Hyatt.**

HILARY—Latin: **Hilarius.**
"Cheerful, gay one." St.
Hilary or Hilarius, Latin
writer, Bishop of Poitiers;
Hilaire Belloc, writer.
English variations: **Hillary,
Hillery.**
Foreign variations: **Hilarius**
(German, Danish, Dutch,
Swedish), **Hilaire** (French),
Ilario (Italian), **Hilario** (Spanish, Portuguese).

HILDEBRAND—Old German: **Hild-brand.** "Warsword."
Hildebrand was an ancient
legendary German hero.

HILLEL—Hebrew: "greatly
praised." Honors Rabbi Hillel,
originator of the Talmud.

HILLIARD—Old German: **Hild-hard.** "Battle-brave, war
guard." Most often from
English surname: "enclosure
on a hill."
English variations: **Hillier,
Hillyer.**

HILTON—Old English: **Hyll-tun.** "From the hill estate."
Conrad Hilton, hotel magnate.
English variation: **Hylton.**

HIRAM—Hebrew: "most
noble one." Hiram, King of
Tyre, aided King Solomon in
building his famous temple;
Hiram Johnson, U.S. Senator.
English nicknames: **Hi, Hy.**

HOBART—Old German: **Hoh-berht.** "High-brilliant";
or Old German: **Hugi-beraht.**
"Brilliant mind."

HOGAN—Irish Gaelic: **Ogan.**
"Youth."

HOLBROOK—Old English: **Hol-broc.** From the surname:
"dweller at the brook in the
hollow."

HOLCOMB—Old English: **Hol-cumb.** "Deep valley."

HOLDEN—Old English: **Hol-dene.** "From the hollow
in the valley."

HOLLIS—Old English: **Hollies.** "From the holly-tree
grove."

HOLMES—Middle English:
"from the river islands."

HOLT—Old English: "from
the forest."

HOMER—Greek: **Homeros.**
"Pledge; security." Homer,
renowned Greek poet, 9th
century B.C.; Homer Ferguson, Homer Capehart, U.S.
Senators.
Foreign variations: **Homerus**
(German, Dutch), **Homère**
(French), **Omero** (Italian).

HONORÉ—Latin: **Honoria.**
"Honor." Honoré de Balzac,
French writer.

HORACE—Latin: **Horatius.**
"Keeper of the hours; light of
the sun." Horace was an
ancient Roman poet; Horatio
Nelson, British admiral;
Horatio Alger, American
author; Horace Mann, American educator; Horace Greeley,
American journalist.
English variation: **Horatio.**
Foreign variations: **Horatius**
(German), **Horacio** (Spanish,
Portuguese), **Orazio** (Italian),
Horats (Dutch).

HORTON—Old English:
Har-tun. "From the gray
estate."

HOUGHTON—Old English:
Hoh-tun. "From the estate on
the bluff."

HOUSTON—From Scottish
surname: "Hugh's town."
Houston McTear, sprinter.

HOWARD—Old English:
Heah-weard. "Chief guard-
ian." Howard Keel, actor.
English nickname: **Howie.**

HOWE—Old German: **Hoh.**
"High; eminent one"; or
Middle English: **How.** "Hill."

HOWELL—Old Welsh:
Howel. "Little alert one."
Howell Cobb, U.S. Secretary
of the Treasury (1815-1868).

HOWLAND—Middle En-
glish: "dweller at the hilly
land."

HUBERT—Old German:
Hugi-beraht. "Brilliant mind
or spirit." St. Hubert,
7th-century French bishop;
Hubert H. Humphrey, U.S.
Vice-President.
English nicknames: **Hugh,
Hube, Bert.**
Foreign variations: **Uberto**
(Italian), **Huberto** (Spanish),
Hubert, Hugibert (German),
Hoibeard (Irish).

HUDSON—Old English:
Hod-sone. "Son of the hooded
one."

HUEY—See **Hugh.**

HUGH—Old English: **Hugi.**

"Intelligence; spirit." The
English St. Hugh of Lincoln
erected Lincoln Cathedral,
13th century; Hugh O'Brian,
actor.
English nicknames: **Huey,
Hughie, Hughy.**
Foreign variations: **Hugo**
(German, Spanish, Swedish,
Dutch, Danish), **Hugues**
(French), **Ugo** (Italian),
Aodh (Irish), **Aoidh** (Scottish).

HULBERT—Old German:
Huldi-beraht. "Graceful-
brilliant."
English variations: **Hulbard,
Hulburd, Hulburt.**

HUMBERT—Old German:
Hun-beraht. "Brilliant Hun";
or Old German: **Haim-beraht.**
"Brilliant supporter." Humbert
or Umberto I, King of Italy,
died 1900.
Foreign variation: **Umberto**
(Italian).

HUMPHREY—Old German:
Hun-frid. "Peaceful Hun"; or
Old German: **Haim-frid.**
"Peace-support." Sir Hum-
phrey Gilbert, English
explorer (1539-1583); Hum-
phrey Bogart, actor.
English nicknames: **Hump,
Humph.**
English variations: **Humfrey,
Humfry.**
Foreign variations: **Humfried**
(German, Dutch), **Onfroi**
(French), **Onofredo** (Italian),
Onofré, Hunfredo (Spanish),
Humfrid (Swedish).

HUNTER—Old English:
Huntere. "A hunter." Hunter
Thompson, journalist.

English variation: **Hunt.**

HUNTINGDON—Old English: **Huntan-dun.** "Hunter's hill."

HUNTINGTON—Old English: **Huntan-tun.** "Hunting-estate." Huntington Hartford, theatrical producer.

HUNTLEY—Old English: **Hunta-leah.** "From the hunter's meadow."

HURLBERT—Old English: **Herle-beorht.** "Army-brilliant."

HURLEY—Irish Gaelic: **Murt-huile.** "Sea-tide."

HURST—Middle English: "dweller at the forest."

English variation: **Hearst.**

HUTTON—Old English: **Hoh-tun.** "From the estate on the projecting ridge."

HUXFORD—Old English: **Huc's-ford.** "Hugh's ford."

HUXLEY—Old English: **Huc's-leah.** "Hugh's meadow."

HYATT—Old English: **Heah-yate.** "From the high gate." A. Hyatt Verrill, American explorer.

HYDE—Old English: **Hid.** "From the hide, an acreage that supported one family."

HYMAN—Hebrew: **Hhayim.** "Life." Hyman Rickover, Admiral, U.S. Navy.

I

IAN—Scottish Gaelic: **Iaian.** "God is gracious." See **John.** Ian Charleson, actor; Ian Fleming, author.

IFIELD—Anglo-Saxon: from a surname.

IGNATIUS—Latin: "fiery or ardent one." Ignace Jan Paderewski, Polish pianist (1860-1941); Ignazio Silone, Italian author.
English variations: **Ignace, Ignatz.**
Foreign variations: **Ignaz** (German), **Ignace** (French), **Ignazio** (Italian), **Ignacio** (Spanish), **Ignatius** (Dutch).

IGOR—Scandinavian, Slavic:

"hero." Igor Stravinsky, composer.
English variations: **Inge, Ingmar.**

IMMANUEL—See **Emanuel.**

INGER—Old Norse: **Ing-harr.** "A son's army." Foreign variations: **Ingar, Ingvar** (Scandinavian).

INGLEBERT—Old German: **Engel-berht.** "Angel-brilliant." English variations: **Englebert, Engelbert.**

INGMAR—Old Norse: **Inga-mar.** "Famous-son." Also: **Ingemur.** Ingemar Johansson, Swedish boxer; Ingmar

Bergman, Swedish film director.

INGRAM—English surname, based on the Old Norse: **Ing-hram.** "Ing's raven; the son's raven." The ancient Norse hero name "Ing" meant "son." The raven depicted wisdom.

INNIS—Irish Gaelic: **Inis.** "From the river-island." English variations: **Innes, Inness, Iniss.**

IRA—Hebrew: "watchful one." Ira Allen, a founder of Vermont (1751-1814); Ira Gershwin, lyricist.

IRVIN, IRVINE—See Irving.

IRVING—Old English: **Ear-wine.** "Sea friend"; or Old Welsh: **Erwyn.** "White river." Irving Stone, writer; Irving Berlin, composer; Sir Henry Irving, famous English actor. English variations: **Ervin, Irvin, Irvine, Irwin, Erwin, Irwyn.**

IRWIN, IRWYN—See Irving.

ISAAC—Hebrew: **Yitshhaq.** "He laugheth." Sir Isaac Newton, English scientist; Isaac Stern, violinist.

English nicknames: **Ike, Ikey, Ikie.**
Foreign variations: **Isaak** (German), **Isacco** (Italian), **Izaak** (Dutch).

ISHAM—Old English: **Isenham.** "From the iron-one's estate." Isham Jones, orchestra leader.

ISIDORE—Greek: **Isidoros.** "Gift of Isis." Isis, the Egyptian goddess, was wife of Osiris. Isidore Rabi, physicist. English nicknames: **Issy, Izzy.** Foreign variations: **Isidor** (German), **Isidro** (Spanish), **Isidoro** (Italian).

IVAN—See John.

IVAR—Old Norse: **Iv-har.** "Archer with a yew bow." Ivor, son of Alan, King of Brittany, A.D. 683; Ivor Novello, English actor-playwright. English variations: **Iver, Ivor.** Foreign variation: **Yvor** (Russian).

IVEN—Old French: "little yew-bow."

IVES—Old English: "archer with a yew bow; little archer." English variation: **Yves.**

J

JACINTO—Spanish, from Greek: "purple hyacinth."

JACK—French: **Jacques.** A form of **John** or **Jacob.** See **John, Jacob.**

JACKSON—Old English: **Jak-sone.** "Son of Jack."

JACOB—Hebrew: **Ya'aqob.** "The supplanter." In honor of the Biblical patriarch Jacob,

son of Abraham. See **James.**
English nicknames: **Jake,
Jakie, Jack, Cob, Cobb.**
Foreign variations: **Jayme**
(Old Spanish), **Jacobo** (Spanish), **Jacques** (French), **Jakob**
(German), **Giacobo, Giacopo,
Giacomo, Iacovo** (Italian).

JACQUES—See **Jacob.**
Jacques Cartier, discoverer of
the St. Lawrence River.

JAGGER—North English:
Jager. "Carter, teamster."

JAMAL—Arabic: "handsome
one." Also modern U.S.
name.

JAMES—Old Spanish: **Jayme**
From the Hebrew: "the
supplanter." See **Jacob.** St.
James, one of the 12 apostles;
Diego (James) Velasquez,
17th-century Spanish painter;
James Boswell, Scottish
biographer (1740–1795); James
Joyce, Irish author; James
Cagney, James Stewart,
actors.
English nicknames: **Jim,
Jimmie, Jimmy, Jamie.**
Foreign variations: **Jaime,
Diego** (Spanish), **Giacomo**
(Italian), **Seamus** (Irish).

JAN—Dutch form of **John.**
Jan Vermeer, painter; Jan
Peerce, opera star.

JARED—Hebrew: "descendant; the inheritor."

JARMAN—Old German:
Harl-man. "The German."
English variation: **Jerman.**

JARVIS—Old German: **Ger-**

hwas. "Spear-keen, or war
leader."
English variation: **Jervis.**

JASON—Greek: **Iason.**
"Healer." Jason was among
the ancient Greek Heroes.
Jason Robards, Jr., actor.

JASPER—Old French: **Jaspre.**
"Jasper stone"; or Persian:
"master of treasure"; see
Gaspar. Jasper Johns, American painter.

JAVIER—Arabic: "bright"; or
Spanish (Basque): "he has a
new home." Also: **Xavier.**

JAY—Old French: **Jaie.** "Blue
jay." Jay (Dizzy) Dean,
baseball star.

JEAN—French form of **John.**

JED—Hebrew: **Yedidiyah.**
"Beloved of the Lord." A
modern shortening of Jedediah.
Jed Harris, theatrical producer.

JEFFERSON—Old English:
Geffrey-sone. "Son of Jeffrey."
Jefferson Davis, President,
Confederate States of America, 1861–1865.

JEFFREY—Old French: **Goeffroi.** "Divinely peaceful." See
Godfrey. Actors Jeffrey
Hunter, Jeff Chandler,
Geoffrey Horne.
English nicknames: **Jeff,
Jeffy.**
English variations: **Jefferey,
Geoffrey, Godfrey.**

JENS—Scandinavian form of
John: "God is gracious."

JEREMY—Hebrew: **Yirm'yah.**

"Exalted by God." A modern form of Jeremiah. Jeremy Irons, actor.
English nickname: **Jerry**.
Foreign variations: **Jeremias** (German, Dutch), **Jéréme** (French), **Geremia** (Italian), **Jeremias** (Spanish).

JERMAINE—From a surname meaning "German." Also modern U.S. name. Jermaine Jackson, singer.

JEROME—Latin: Hieronymus. "Sacred or holy name." Jerome Kern, composer.
English nicknames: **Gerry**, **Jerry**.
English variations: **Jerrome**, **Gerome**.

JESSE—Hebrew: **Yishay**. "Wealth." Jesse Owens, track star; Jesse Jackson, American political leader.
English nicknames: **Jess**, **Jessie**.

JIM—Nickname for **James**. Also: **Jimmy, Jimmie, Jimi**. Jimi Hendrix, singer.

JOACHIM—Hebrew: "the Lord will judge."
Foreign variation: **Joaquim** (Spanish).

JOB—Hebrew: "the afflicted." The patriarch Job was a symbol of patience.

JOE—Nickname for **Joseph**. Also **Joey**.

JOEL—Hebrew: **Yoel**. "The Lord is God." Joel McCrea, actor.

JOHN—Hebrew: **Yehokhanan**.

"God is gracious." St. John the Apostle and St. John the Baptist; John F. Kennedy, 35th U.S. President; Johann Sebastian Bach, Johannes Brahms, composers; Colonel John Glenn, Jr., U.S. astronaut and U.S. Senator; actors John Gielgud, John Barrymore, John Wayne.
English nicknames: **Johnnie**, **Johnny, Jack, Jackie**.
English variations: **Jon, Jona, Jonni, Zane**.
Foreign variations: **Johann, Johannes** (German), **Jean** (French), **Juan** (Spanish), **Giovanni** (Italian), **Ivan** (Slavic), **John** (Swedish), **Eoin, Seaian, Seann, Shane** (Irish), **Iaian** (Scottish).

JONAS—Hebrew: **Yonah**. "Peace, dove." Jonas Salk, noted physician.

JONATHAN—Hebrew: **Y-honathan**. "Jehovah's gift." Jonathan was the son of Saul and the friend of David in the Bible. Jonathan Edwards, 18th-century American theologian; Jonathan Swift, English author; Jonathan Winters, comedian. Also: **Johnathan**.

JORDAN—Hebrew: **Yarden**. "Descender." The descending river of Palestine.
Foreign variations: **Jourdain** (French), **Giordano** (Italian).

JORGE—Spanish form of **George**: "farmer." Also Portuguese. Jorge Amado, Brazilian novelist.

JOSEPH—Hebrew: **Yoseph**.

...hall add." St. Joseph of ...Bible; Franz Joseph ...ydn, Giuseppe Verdi, ...mposers; Joe DiMaggio, ...baseball star; Joseph Cotten, actor. Also: **Josiah.**
English nicknames: **Joe, Joey.**
Foreign variations: **Giuseppe** (Italian), **José** (Spanish), **Iosep** (Irish), **Seosaidh** (Scottish).

JOSHUA—Hebrew: **Yehoshua.** "God of salvation." Joshua Logan, American dramatist, director, and producer.
English nickname: **Josh.**

JUDD—Hebrew: **Y-hudhah.** "Praised." A modern form of Judah.

JULIAN—Latin: **Julianus.** "Belonging to Julius." See **Julius.** Julian Lennon, singer.

JULIUS—Latin: "youthful; downy-bearded one." Jules Verne, French author; Jules Massenet, French composer; Julius Erving, athlete; Julio Iglesias, singer.
English nickname: **Jule.**
Foreign variations: **Jules** (French), **Julio** (Spanish), **Giulio** (Italian).

JUSTIN—Old French: **Justine.** "Upright, just one." From Latin: "just." The name of two 5th-century Byzantine emperors.
Foreign variations: **Giustino** (Italian), **Justino** (Spanish).

JUSTIS—Old French: **Justice.** "Justice."
English variation: **Justus.**
Foreign variations: **Giusto** (Italian), **Justo** (Spanish), **Juste** (French), **Justus** (German).

K

KALIL—Arabic: "good friend." Also: **Kahlil.** Kahlil Gibran, poet.

KANE—Irish Gaelic: **Cain.** "Tribute"; or Irish Gaelic: **Catahn.** "Little warlike one."
English variations: **Kain, Kaine, Kayne.**

KAREEM—Arabic: "noble, generous." Also: **Karim.** Kareem Abdul-Jabbar, basketball player.

KARL—See **Charles.** Karl Marx, political thinker and writer.

KARNEY—See **Kearney.**

KARR—See **Carr.**

KASPAR—See **Gaspar.**

KAVAN—See **Cavan.**

KAY—Old Welsh: **Cai.** "Rejoicer"; or Irish Gaelic: MacKay. "Fiery." Sir Kay was one of the knights of King Arthur's Round Table.

KEANE—Middle English: **Kene.** "Bold, sharp one"; or Irish Gaelic: **Caoin.** "Handsome one."

English variations: **Kean,
Keen, Keene.**

KEDAR—Arabic: **Kadar.**
"Powerful."

KEEFE—Irish Gaelic:
Caomh. "Handsome, noble,
gentle, lovable."

KEEGAN—Irish Gaelic:
Aod-hagan. "Little fiery one."

KEELAN—Irish Gaelic:
Caolan. "Little, slender one."
Seven Irish saints were
called Caolan.

KEELEY—Irish Gaelic:
Cadhla. "Handsome."
English variations: **Kealy,
Keely.**

KEENAN—Irish Gaelic:
Cianan. "Little ancient one."
Three Irish saints were
called Cianan; Keenan Wynn,
actor.
English variations: **Kienan.**

KEITH—Irish Gaelic: **Caith.**
"From the battle place"; or
Old Welsh: **Coed.** "From
the forest." Keith Hernandez,
baseball player; Keith
Baxter, actor.

KELL—Old Norse: **Kelda.**
"From the spring."

KELLER—Irish Gaelic:
Ceil-eachan. "Little companion."

KELLY—Irish Gaelic:
Ceallach. "Warrior."
English variation: **Kelley.**

KELSEY—Old Norse:
Kiolls-ig. "Dweller at
ship-island."

KELVIN—Irish:
Caol-abhuinn. "...
narrow river."
English variations: ...
Kelven.

KEMP—Middle English:
Kempe. "Warrior, champ..."

KENDALL—Old English:
Cain-dale. "From the clear-
river valley or bright
valley."
English variations: **Kendal,
Kendell.**

KENDRICK—Irish Gaelic:
Mac-Eanraic. "Son of Henry";
or Old English: **Cyne-ric.**
"Royal ruler."

KENLEY—Old English:
Cyne-leah. "Dweller at the
royal meadow."

KENN—Old Welsh: **Cain.**
"Clear, bright water."

KENNARD—Old English:
Cene-hard. "Bold, strong."

KENNEDY—Irish Gaelic:
Cin-neididh. "Helmeted head;
Helmeted chief." An old
Scottish and Irish clan name.

KENNETH—Irish Gaelic:
Coin-neach. "Handsome one";
Old English: **Cyne-ath.**
"Royal oath." Kenneth
MacAlpin, Scottish king,
A.D. 843-858; Kenneth Keating,
U.S. Senator.
English nicknames: **Ken,
Kenney, Kenny.**

KENRICK—Old English:
Cene-ric. "Bold ruler"; or Old
English: **Cyne-ric.** "Royal
ruler."

...lsh: **Cant.**
..."

...Old English:
..."From the royal

...WARD—Old English:
...e-ward. "Bold guardian";
Old English: **Cyne-ward.**
Royal guardian."

KENWAY—Old English:
Cene-wig. "Bold warrior"; or
Old English: **Cyne-wig.**
"Royal warrior."

KENYON—Irish Gaelic:
Ceann-fhionn. "White-headed."
Also from an English place
name. Kenyon Nicholson,
American dramatist.

KERMIT—Irish Gaelic:
Diar-maid. "Free man."
Kermit Roosevelt, son of
U.S. President Theodore
Roosevelt.

KERN—Irish Gaelic: **Ceirin.**
"Little dark one."

KERR—Irish Gaelic: **Carra.**
"Spear." See **Carr.** Alternate,
Irish Gaelic: **Ciar.** "Dark
one."

KERRY—Irish Gaelic:
Ciarda. "Son of the dark
one"; or English: "ship
captain."

KERWIN—Irish Gaelic:
Ciar-dubhan. "Little, jet-
black one."
English variations: **Kerwen,
Kirwin.**

KESTER—Old English:
Caster. "From the Roman

army camp." Also from a
Dutch place name.

KEVIN—Irish Gaelic:
Caoim-hin. "Gentle, lov-
able." Kevin McCarthy,
Kevin Kline, actors.
English variations: **Kevan,
Keven.**

KEY—Irish Gaelic: **MacAoidh.**
"Son of the fiery one."

KIERAN—Irish Gaelic:
Ciaran. "Little dark-
complexioned one."

KILLIAN—Irish Gaelic:
Cillin. "Little warlike one."

KIM—Old English: **Cyne.**
"Chief, ruler."

KIMBALL—Old Welsh:
Cyn-bel. "Warrior chief"; or
Old English: **Cyne-bold.**
"Royal and bold."
English variations: **Kimble,
Kimbell.**

KING—Old English: **Cyning.**
"Ruler." King Vidor. motion
picture director.

KINGSLEY—Old English:
Cinges-leah. "From the king's
meadow."
English variation: **Kinsley.**

KINGSTON—Old English:
Cingestun. "Dweller at the
king's estate."

KINGSWELL—Old En-
glish: **Cinges-wiella.** "Dweller
at the king's spring."

KINNARD—Irish Gaelic:
Cinn-ard. "From the high
hill."

KINNELL—Irish Gaelic:

Cinn-fhail. "From the head of the cliff."

KINSEY—Old English: Cyne-sige. "Royal, victorious one."

KIPP—North English: Kip. "Dweller at the pointed hill."

KIRBY—Old Norse: Kirkja-byr. "From the church village."
English variation: Kerby.

KIRK—Old Norse: Kirkja. "Dweller at the church." Kirk Douglas, actor.

KIRKLEY—Old North English: Circe-leah. "Church-meadow."

KIRKWOOD—Old North English: Circe-wode. "From the church forest."

KIRWIN—

KNIGHT—M. Kniht. "Soldier.

KNOX—Old Englr. "From the hills."

KNUT—See Canute.

KONANE—Hawaiian: "br. moonlight."

KONRAD—See Conrad.

KOSEY—African: "lion." Also; Kosse.

KRISHNA—Hindi: "de-lightful." Also: Krisha, Krishnah.

KURT—See Conrad.

KYLE—Irish Gaelic: Caol. "From the strait."

KYNE—Old English: Cyne. "Royal one."

L

LACH—Old English: Laec. "Dweller by the water."
English variation: Lache.

LACHLAN—Scottish Gaelic: Laochail-an. "Warlike one"; or Scottish Gaelic: Loch-lainn. "From the water."

LACY—Latin: Latiacum. "From Latius' estate."

LADD—Middle English: Ladde. "Lad or attendant."

LAIBROOK—Old English: Lad-brooc. "Path by the brook."

LAIDLEY—Old English: Lad-leah. "From the water-course meadow."

LAIRD—Scottish: "Landed proprietor."

LAMAR—Old German: Land-mari. "Land-famous."

LAMBERT—Old German: Land-bercht. "Land-brilliant, his country's light."
English nicknames: Bert, Bertie.
Foreign variations: Landbert (German), Lamberto (Italian).

...rse: **Log-**
...lawyer."
...ıs: **Lamond,**

...ld French:
... "Attendant, he
...ves." A modern
...form of the old English
...ncelot."

...ANDER—Middle English: **Launder.** "Launderer";
or Middle English: **Landere.**
"Owner of a grassy plain."
English variations: **Landor,
Landers.**

LANDON—See **Langdon.**

LANE—Middle English:
Lane. "From the narrow
road." The old English
Hundred Rolls of A.D. 1273
list Cecil "In the Lane."

LANG—Old Norse: **Lang-r.**
"Long or tall man." Andrew
Lang, English writer
(1844-1912).

LANGDON—Old English:
Lang-dun. "Dweller at the
long hill."
English variation: **Landon.**

LANGFORD—Old English: **Lang-ford.** "Dweller at
the long ford."

LANGLEY—Old English:
Lang-leah. "From the long
meadow or wood." Samuel
P. Langley, U.S. astronomer
(1834-1906).

LANGSTON—Old English:
Langs-tun. "Tall man's estate
or town." Langston Hughes,
poet.

LANGWORTH—Old English: **Lang-worth.** "From the
long enclosure."

LARS—Scandinavian form
of **Lawrence.**

LARSON—Scandinavian:
Lars-son. "Son of Lars." See
Lawrence.

LATHAM—Old Norse:
Hlathum. "From the barns."

LATHROP—Old English:
Lath-throp. "From the
barn-farmstead."

LATIMER—Middle English: **Latimer.** "Interpreter."

LAURENCE—See **Lawrence.**

LAVAL—Modern U.S.
name. Laval Wilson, superintendent of Schools, Boston.

LAWFORD—Old English:
Hloew-ford. "From the ford
at the hill."

LAWLER—Irish Gaelic:
Leath-labhra. "Mumbler,
half-speaker."

LAWLEY—Old English:
Hloew-leah. "From the
hill-meadow."

LAWRENCE—Latin:
Laurens. "Laurel-crowned
one." St. Laurence, celebrated 3rd-century martyr;
Lorenzo de' Medici, 15th-century Florentine ruler;
Lawrence Wien, philanthropist; Lawrence Welk, orchestra leader, Sir Laurence
Olivier, Laurence Harvey,
English actors.
English nicknames: **Larry,**

Lauren, Laurie, Lawry, Loren, Lorin, Lon, Lonnie. English variations: Laurence, Larrance, Lawrance. Foreign variations: Lorenz, Laurenz (German), Laurent (French), Lorenzo (Italian, Spanish), Lorenz, Lauritz (Danish), Lars (Swedish), Laurens (Dutch), Labhras (Irish), Labhruinn (Scottish).

LAWSON—Old English: Lawe-sone. "Son of Lawrence."

LAWTON—Old English: Hloew-tun. "From the hill-town or estate."

LAZARUS—Hebrew: El'azar. "God will help." Lazaro Cardenas, Mexican statesman. Foreign variations: Lazaro (Italian, Spanish), Lazare (French).

LEAL—Middle English: Lele. "Loyal; faithful."

LEANDER—Greek: Leiandros. "Lion-man." Leander was famous in Greek myths. Foreign variations: Léandre (French), Leandro (Italian, Spanish).

LEE—Old English: Leah. "From the pasture meadow"; or Irish Gaelic: Laoidheach. "Poetic." Lee Iacocca, author-industrialist; actor Lee J. Cobb. English variation: Leigh.

LEGGETT—Old French: Legat. "Envoy or delegate." English variations: Leggitt, Liggett.

LEIF—Old Norse: Leif. "Beloved one." Leif Erickson, famous Norse explorer.

LEIGH—See Lee.

LEIGHTON—Old English: Leah-tun. "Dweller at the meadow farm."

LEITH—Scottish Gaelic: Leathan. "Broad, wide river."

LELAND—Old English: Leah-land. "From the meadow-land." Leland Hayward, film producer.

LEMUEL—Hebrew: "consecrated to God." English nicknames: Lem, Lemmie.

LENARD—See Leonard.

LENNON—Irish Gaelic: Leannan. "Little cloak." John Lennon of the Beatles.

LENNOX—Scottish Gaelic: Leamhnach. "Abounding in elm trees."

LEO—Latin: "lion." Thirteen popes were named Leo; Leo Tolstoy, Russian novelist; Leo Durocher, baseball manager.

LEON—French: "lion-like." Léon Blum, French statesman (1872-1950); Leon Bakst, artist and designer.

LEONARD—Old Frankish: Leon-hard. "Lion-brave." Leonardo da Vinci, Italian painter, sculptor, architect; Leonard Bernstein, composer-conductor.

English nicknames: **Len, Lennie, Lenny.**
English variations: **Leonerd, Lennard.**
Foreign variations: **Leonardo** (Italian, Spanish), **Léonard** (French), **Leonhard** (German), **Leonid** (Russian).

LEOPOLD—Old German: **Leut-pald.** "Bold for the people." Leopold I, II, III, Kings of Belgium; Leopold Stokowski, noted orchestra conductor.
Foreign variations: **Léopold** (French), **Luitpold, Leupold** (German), **Leopoldo** (Italian, Spanish).

LEROY—Old French: "king." A person who was given the title of king for his royal bearing, or for the part he played in a religious pageant. LeRoi Jones, poet.
English nicknames: **Lee, Roy.**

LESLIE—Scottish Gaelic: **Lios-liath.** "Dweller at the gray fortress." Leslie Howard, actor.

LESTER—Latin: **Ligera-castra.** "Chosen camp; legion camp." Lester B. Pearson, Canadian statesman.
English nickname: **Les.**

LEVERETT—Old French: **Leveret.** "Young rabbit." Leverett Saltonstall, U.S. Senator.
English nickname: **Lev.**

LEVERTON—Old English: **Laefer-tun.** "From the rush-farm."

English nickname: **Lev.**

LEVI—Hebrew: **Lewi.** "Joined; united." Levi in the Bible was a son of Jacob and Leah.

LEWIS—See **Louis.**

LINCOLN—Old English: **Lin-colne.** "From the colony by the pool." Abraham Lincoln, 16th U.S. President, was the famous prototype of this name; Lincoln Steffens, writer, lecturer.
English nickname: **Linc.**

LIND—Old English: "Dweller at the linden or lime tree."
English variation: **Linden.**

LINDBERG—Old German: **Linde-berg.** "Linden tree hill." Charles A. Lindbergh, famous flier.
English nickname: **Lindy.**

LINDELL—Old English: **Lind-dael.** "Dweller at the linden tree valley."

LINDLEY—Old English: **Lind-leah.** "At the linden tree meadow." Lindley Bickworth, U.S. Congressman.

LINDON—See **Lyndon.**

LINDSEY—Old English: **Lindes-ig.** "Pool-island."
English variations: **Lindsay, Linsay, Linsey.**

LINFORD—Old English: **Lind-ford.** "From the linden tree ford."

LINK—Old English: **Hlinc.** "From the bank or ridge."

LINLEY—Old English:

Lin-leah. "From the flax field."

LINN—See **Lynn.**

LINTON—Old English: **Lin-tun.** "From the flax enclosure."

LINUS—Greek: **Linos.** "Flax-colored hair." Linus Pauling, scientist.

LIONEL—Old French: "young lion." Lionel Barrymore, actor, Lionel Richie, singer.
Foreign variation: **Lionello** (Italian).

LITTON—Old English: **Hlith-tun.** "Hillside town or estate."

LLEWELLYN—Old Welsh: **Llyw-eilun.** "Like a ruler, or lightning or lionlike." Llewellyn the Great was a 13th-century Welsh ruler.

LLOYD—Old Welsh: **Llwyd.** "Gray-haired one." Lloyd George, English statesman; Lloyd Nolan, Lloyd Bridges, actors.
English variation: **Floyd.**

LOCKE—Old English: **Loc.** "Dweller by the stronghold or enclosure."

LOGAN—Scottish Gaelic: **Lagan.** "Little hollow." Logan is a famed Scottish clan name.

LOMBARD—Latin: **Longobard.** "Long bearded one."

LON—Irish Gaelic: **Lonn.**
"Strong, fierce." See **Law**
Lon Chaney, Lon Chaney, Jr., actors.

LORANT—Hungarian, from Latin, "laurel, victory."

LOREN—See **Lawrence.** Also: **Lorin, Lorne.** Lorin Hollander, pianist.

LORIMER—Middle English: **Lorimer.** "Saddle, spur and bit maker."

LORING—Old German: **Lotharing.** "Son of famous-in-war." Son of the leader of a victorious army. Loring "Red" Nichols, orchestra leader.

LOUIS—Old German: **Hlut-wig.** "Famous warrior, or warrior prince." Honoring St. Louis, 13th-century king of France; Louis Joliet, 17th-century French explorer; Ludwig van Beethoven, German composer; Luigi Pirandello, Italian playwright; Louis Pasteur, French chemist; Louis Jourdan, actor.
English nicknames: **Lon, Lew, Louie.**
English variation: **Lewis**
Foreign variations: **Ludwig** (German), **Luigi, Lodovico** (Italian), **Luis** (Spanish), **Lodewijk** (Dutch), **Ludvig, Ludvik** (Swedish), **Lugaidh** (Irish), **Luthais** (Scottish).

LOVELL—Old English: **Leof-el.** "Little beloved one"; or Old French: **Louvel.** "Little wolf." Lowell Thomas, commentator, writer.

variation: **Lowell.**

...**ELL**—See Lovell.

...**AL**—Old French: **Loial.** ...ue, faithful, unswerving."

...**LUCAS**—See **Luke.**

LUCIAN—Latin: **Lucius.** "Light." A name sometimes given to a child born at dawn. See **Luke.** Foreign variations: **Luciano** (Italian), **Lucien** (French).

LUCK, LUCKY—See **Luke.**

LUDLOW—Old English: **Leod-hloew.** "Dweller at the prince's hill."

LUDWIG—See **Louis.**

LUKE—Latin: **Lucius.** "Light; bringer of light or knowledge." Primary usage commemorates St. Luke the Evangelist. Lucius Beebe, columnist, publisher. English variations: **Lucas, Lucian, Lucius, Luck, Lucky.** Foreign variations: **Lucas** (German, Dutch, Danish, Irish) **Luc, Lucien** (French), **Luca** (Italian), **Lucio** (Spanish), **Lukas** (Swedish), **Lucais** (Scottish).

LUNDY—French: **Lundi.** "Born on Monday"; or Scottish: **Lundie.** "Island grove."

LUNN—Irish Gaelic: **Lonn.** "Strong, fierce."

LUNT—Old Norse: **Lund-r.** "From the grove."

LUTHER—Old German: **Hlut-heri.** "Famous warrior." Luther Adler, actor; Luther Burbank, horticulturist. Foreign variations: **Lothaire** (French), **Lotario** (Italian), **Lutero** (Spanish).

LYLE—Old French: **Del isle.** "From the isle." English variation: **Lyell.**

LYMAN—Middle English: **Leyman.** "Meadow-man." Lyman Hall, doctor and Georgia statesman.

LYNDON—Old English: **Linddun.** "Dweller at the lime tree or linden tree hill." Lyndon B. Johnson, 36th U.S. President. English variation: **Lindon.**

LYNN—Old Welsh: **Llyn.** "From the pool or waterfall." English variation: **Lyn.**

M

MACADAM—Scottish Gaelic: **MacAdhamh.** "Son of Adam." A descendant of the "man of the red earth." See **Adam.**

MACDONALD—Scottish Gaelic: **MacDomhnall.** "Son of world-mighty." Macdonald Carey, actor.

MACDOUGAL—Scottish Gaelic: MacDubhghall. "Son of the dark stranger."

MACKINLEY—Irish Gaelic: MacCinfhaolaidh. "Learned or skillful leader." William McKinley, 25th U.S. President.

MACMURRAY—Irish Gaelic: MacMaureadhaigh. "Son of the mariner." Fred MacMurray, actor.

MACY—Old French: Macey. "From Mathew's estate."

MADDOCK—Old Welsh: Madawc. "Good and beneficient." Madoc was a renowned 12th-century Welsh ruler. English variations: Madoc, Madock, Madog.

MADDOX—Old Anglo-Welsh: Maddock-son. "The benefactor's son." See Maddock.

MADISON—Old English: Mahhild-son. "Son of war-mighty, Heir of the valiant warrior. James Madison, 4th U.S. President.

MAGEE—Irish Gaelic: MacAodha. "Son of the fiery one.

MAGNUS—Latin: "great one." Magnus was the name of many important Norwegian kings.

MAITLAND—Old English: Maed-land. "Dweller at the meadowland."

MAJOR—Latin: "greater."

MAL-
Meal-c
Columba.
(Malcolm II, Scottish king; Campbell, racing ist; Malcolm Forbe, publisher.

MALIN—Old English: Mahhild-in. "Little war-mighty one."

MALLORY—Old German: Madel-hari. "Council-army; army counselor"; or Old French: Mail-hair-et. "Unfortunate-strong."

MALONEY—Irish Gaelic: MaoIdhomhnaigh. "Devoted to Sunday worship."

MALVIN—Irish Gaelic: Maol-min. "Polished chief"; or Old English: Maethel-wine. "Council-friend." See Melvin. English nickname: Mal.

MANDEL—German: "almond." English nickname: Manny.

MANFRED—Old English: Mann-frith. "Peaceful man, peaceful hero."

MANLEY—Old English: Mann-leah. "From the man's or hero's meadow."

MANNING—Old English: Mann-ing. "Son of the hero."

MANSFIELD—Old English: Maun-feld. "From the field by the small river." Mike Mansfield, U.S. Senator; Richard Mansfield, American actor.

...sh form of
...d be with us."

...—Old French:
...le. "From the great

...RCEL—Latin: **Marcellus**,
...ittle hammer, little warlike
one." Marcel Proust,
French novelist (1871-1922);
Marcel Marceau, actor and
mime.
Foreign variations: **Marcellus**
(French), **Marcello** (Italian),
Marcelo (Spanish).

MARCUS—See Mark.

MARDEN—Old English:
Mere-dene. "From the
pool-valley."

MARIO—Latin: **Marius.**
"Martial one." Mario Pei,
author, linguist; Mario
Lanza, noted singer; Mario
Puzo, novelist.

MARION—Old French:
Marion. "Little Mary." A
French masculine form of
Mary.
Foreign variation: **Mariano**
(Spanish).

MARK—Latin: **Marcus.**
"Warlike one." Celebrated
from Marco Polo, Italian
traveler (1254-1324); Mark
Twain, writer (1835-1910).
Main usage from St. Mark the
Evangelist.
English variation: **Marcus.**
Foreign variations: **Marc**

(French), **Marco** (Italian),
Markus (German, Swedish,
Dutch, Danish), **Marco**,
Marcos (Spanish).

MARLAND—Old English:
Mere-land. "From the lake
land."

MARLEY—Old English:
Mere-leah. "From the lake
meadow."

MARLON—Old French:
Esmerillon. "Little falcon or
hawk." Marlon Brando,
actor.
English variation: **Marlin.**

MARLOW—Old English:
Mere-hloew. "From the hill
by the lake." Christopher
Marlowe, 16th-century En-
glish dramatist.
English variation: **Marlowe.**

MARMION—Old French:
Mer-meion. "Very small one."
Marmion was the medieval
hero of Sir Walter Scott's
balladic poem *Marmion*.

MARSDEN—Old English:
Mersc-dene. "Dweller at the
marshy valley."
English variation: **Marsdon.**

MARSH—Old English:
Mersc. "From the marshy
place."

MARSHALL—Middle En-
glish: **Marschal.** "Steward;
horse-keeper." Marshall
Field III, publisher, philanthropist (1893-1956); Marshall McLuhan, media critic;
Marshall Mason, director.

MARSTON—Old English:

MARTIN—Latin: Martinus. "Warlike one." A name taken from Mars, the Roman war god, from whom the planet was named. Martin Luther, German religious reformer (1483-1546); Martin Van Buren, 8th U.S. President; Martin Johnson, famed African explorer.
English nicknames: Martie, Marty, Mart.
English variations: Marten, Marton.
Foreign variations: Martino (Italian, Spanish), Martin (Spanish), Martijn (Dutch), Martain (Scottish).

MARVIN—Old English: Maer-wine. "Famous friend"; or Old English: Mere-wine. "Sea-friend." Marvin Hagler, boxing champion.
English nickname: Marv.

MARWOOD—Old English: Mere-wode. "From the lake-forest."

MASLIN—Old French: Masselin. "Little Thomas."
English variation: Maslen.

MASON—Old French— Masson. "Stone-worker." Also from the English family name: James Mason, actor.

MATHER—Old English: Maeth-here. "Powerful-army." Cotton Mather, American theologian, writer (1663-1728).

MATTHEW—Hebrew: Mattithyah. "Gift of Jehovah." St. M[atthew], one of the 12 Apos[tles]; 19th-centu[ry] photographer Mathew Brad[y].
English nicknames: Matt, Mattie, Matty.
English variations: Mathias, Mattias.
Foreign variations: Mathieu (French), Matthäus (German), Matteo (Italian), Mateo (Spanish), Mattheus (Swedish, Dutch), Matthaeus (Danish), Mata (Scottish).

MAURICE—Late Latin: Mauricius. "Dark-complexioned one." Maurice Maeterlinck, Belgian writer; Maurice Evans, Maurice Chevalier, actors.
English nicknames: Maurie, Maury, Morrie.
English variations: Morris, Morrell, Morrill.
Foreign variations: Maurizio (Italian), Moritz (German), Mauricio (Spanish), Maurits (Dutch), Maolmuire (Scottish).

MAXIMILIAN—Latin: Maximilianus. "Greatest in excellence." Maximilian, Holy Roman Emperor (1459-1519); Maximilian, Emperor of Mexico (1864-1867); Maximilian Schell, actor; Maxim Gorki, Russian novelist.
English nicknames: Max, Maxie, Maxy, Maxim.
Foreign variations: Maximilien (French), Maximo, Maximiliano (Spanish), Massimiliano (Italian), Maximilianus (Dutch).

Meres-tun. "Dweller at the lake-farm."

n:
le-
ng," or
xwell
wright; Max
eatrical pro-
Beerbohm,
author; Maxwell
.s, famous editor.
glish nicknames: **Max,**
Maxie, Maxy.

MAYER—Latin: **Major.**
"Greater one." Also, Germanic: "farmer or overseer." See **Meyer.**

MAYFIELD—Old English:
Maga-feld. "From the warrior's field."

MAYHEW—Old French:
Mahieu. "Gift of Jehovah. A variation of **Matthew.**

MAYNARD—Old German:
Megin-hard. "Powerful, brave."
Maynard Dixon, Western painter.
Foreign variation: **Menard**
(French).

MAYO—Irish Gaelic: **Magheo.**
"From the plain of the yew trees."

MEAD—Old English:
Maed. "From the meadow."

MEDWIN—Old English:
Maeth-wine. "Powerful friend."

MELBOURNE—Old English: **Myln-burne.** "From the mill-stream."
English variations: **Melburn,**
Milburn.

MELDON—Old English:

Myln-dun. "Dweller at the mill-hill."

MELDRICK—Old English:
Myln-ric. "Powerful mill."
Meldrick Taylor, Olympic boxer.

MELVILLE—Old French:
Amal-ville. "From the industrious-one's estate."
Melville Fuller, Chief Justice of the U.S. (1888-1910).

MELVIN—Old English:
Mael-wine. "Sword-friend or speech-friend"; or Irish Gaelic: **Maol-min.** "Polished chief." Melvyn Douglas, actor.
English nickname: **Mel.**
English variations: **Malvin,**
Melvyn.

MENDEL—East Semitic:
Min'da. "Knowledge, wisdom." L. Mendel Rivers, U.S. Congressman.

MERCER—Middle English: "merchant, storekeeper." Also: **Merce.**
Merce Cunningham, choreographer.

MEREDITH—Old Welsh:
Meredydd. "Guardian from the sea." Meredith Willson, composer, conductor.

MERLE—French:
"blackbird."

MERLIN—Middle English:
Merlion. "Falcon or hawk."
Merlin was a famous 5th-century adviser and magician.

MERRILL—Old French:
Mer-el. "Little famous one."

MERRITT—Old English: **Maeret.** "Little famous one."

MERTON—Old English: **Mere-tun.** "From an estate or town by a lake or the sea."

MERVIN—Old English: **Maere-wine.** "Famous friend"; or Scottish Gaelic: **Muir-finn.** "Beautiful sea." Mervyn Le Roy, noted motion picture producer, director. English variations: **Merwin, Merwyn.**

MEYER—German: **Meier.** "Steward; farmer"; or Hebrew: "bringer of light." English variations: **Meir, Meier, Myer, Mayeer, Mayer, Mayor.**

MICHAEL—Hebrew: **Mikhael.** "Who is like God." Honoring the archangel St. Michael. Michael Arlen, writer; Mickey Mantle, baseball star; Mickey Rooney, actor; Mike Todd, motion picture producer; Michael Jackson, singer. English nicknames: **Mike, Mickie, Micky.** English variation: **Mitchell.** Foreign variations: **Michel** (French). **Michele** (Italian). **Miguel** (Spanish), **Mikael** (Swedish), **Micheil** (Scottish), **Mikhail, Mischa, Misha** (Slavic).

MILES—Late Latin: "soldier, warrior." Miles Standish, leader in the founding of New England. Miles Davis, jazz musician. English variation: **Myles.**

MILL—**Myln-fo.** mill-ford.

MILLARD—**Emille-hard.** "F... winning and strong Millard Filmore, 13t... President.

MILLER—Middle English. **Millere.** "Grain-grinder; flour-miller."

MILO—Latin: **Milon.** "Miller." Milo O'Shea, actor.

MILTON—Old English: **Myln-tun.** "Dweller at the mill-town." Milton Berle, comedian, actor.

MILWARD—Old English: **Myln-weard.** "Mill-keeper."

MINER—Old French: **Mineor.** "A miner"; or Latin: **Minor.** "Young person." English variation: **Minor.**

MISCHA—See **Michael.** Mischa Baryshnikov, ballet dancer-choreographer.

MITCHELL—Middle English: **Michell.** "Who is like God." See **Michael.** Mitch Miller, musician, entertainer; Mitch Gaylord, gymnast. English nickname: **Mitch.**

MODRED—Old English: **Mod-raed.** "Courageous counsellor."

MOHAMMED—Arabic: **Muhammed.** "A praiseworthy man." The 6th-century prophet of Islam. Also: **Mohammad, Muhammed.**

...et

...aelic:
...rom the red
... Monroe,
...esident.
...ariations: **Monro,**
, Munroe.

...**NTAGUE**—French: **Mont-**
..gu. "Dweller at the pointed
hill.
English nicknames: **Monte,**
Monty.

MONTGOMERY—Old
French: **Mont-gomeric.** "From
the wealthy-one's hill or
hill-castle." Montgomery Clift,
actor; Monty Hall, television personality.
English nicknames: **Monte,**
Monty.

MOORE—Old French:
More. "Dark-complexioned."
A dark and handsome man
like Shakespeare's Moor in
Othello. Alternate, Middle
English: **More.** "From the
moor."

MORELAND—Old En-
glish: **Mor-land.** "From the
moor-land."

MORGAN—Old Welsh:
Mor-can. "White sea, dweller."
Morgan Beatty, commentator.
English variation: **Morgen.**

MORLEY—Old English:
More-leah. "From the moor
meadow, wood by a
marsh." Morley Safer,
newscaster.

MORRIS—See **Maurice.**

MORRISON—Old English:
More-sone. "Son of Maurice."
See **Maurice.** Morrison
Waite, Chief Justice of the
United States, 1874–1888.

MORSE—Old English:
More-s. "Son of the dark-
complexioned one."

MORTIMER—Old French:
Morte-mer. "From the still
water"; or Irish Gaelic:
Muircheartaigh. "Sea-director."
English nicknames: **Mort,**
Mortie.

MORTON—Old English:
Mor-tun. "From the moor
estate or town." Morton
Gould, composer, conductor;
Mort Sahl, comedian.
English nicknames: **Mort,**
Mortie.

MORVEN—Irish Gaelic:
Mor-finn. "Great, fair-
complexioned one."
English variation: **Morfin.**

MOSES—Hebrew: **Mosheh.**
"Taken out of the water"; or
Egyptian: **Mesu.** "Child."
Honoring the great Hebrew
prophet, lawgiver and
Israelite leader. Moses
Malone, basketball player.
English nicknames: **Mose,**
Mosie, Moe, Moshe, Moss.
Foreign variations: **Moise**
(French, Italian), **Moisés**
(Spanish), **Mozes** (Dutch).

MUIR—Scottish Gaelic:
"from the moor or wasteland."
John Muir, Scottish-
American naturalist.

MUNROE—See **Monroe.**

MURDOCK—Scottish Gaelic: Muireadhach. "Prosperous from the sea."

MURPHY—Irish Gaelic: Murchadh. "Sea warrior."

MURRAY—Scottish Gaelic: Mor... warrior; Morag; "..."

MYLES—Se...

MYRON—Greek. ointment, sweet oil.

N

NAIRN—Scottish Gaelic: Am-huinn. "Dweller at the alder-tree river."

NALDO—See Reginald.

NATHAN—Hebrew: "a gift," or "given of God." Endowed with the gift of prophecy, Nathan saved Solomon's kingdom. Nathan Hale, American Revolutionary War patriot; Nathan Milstein, violinist. English nicknames: Nat, Nate.

NATHANIEL—Hebrew: Nethan-el. "Gift of God." A gifted disciple of Christ in the Bible. Nathaniel Hawthorne, 19th-century American writer; Nat King Cole, singer. English nicknames: Nat, Nate. Foreign variations: Natanael, Nataniel (Spanish).

NEAL—Irish Gaelic: Niall. "Champion." Niall of the Nine Hostages, who died in A.D. 919, famous Irish ruler, was founder of the celebrated clan O'Neill. English variations: Nial, Neall, Neale, Neil, Neill, Neel, Niels, Niles. Foreign variations: Nels, Niels, Nils (Scandinavian), Niall (Scottish).

NEHEMIAH—Hebrew: "the Lord's compassion." Nehemiah Persoff, actor.

NELSON—English: Neilson. "Champion's-son." Nelson Rockefeller, New York governor; Nelson Doubleday, publisher; Nelson Eddy, singer, actor. English variations: Nealson, Nilson.

NEMO—Greek: Nemos. "From the glen or glade." Famed from Captain Nemo, Jules Verne character in Twenty Thousand Leagues under the Sea and Mysterious Island.

NESTOR—Greek: "departer or traveler." Figurative meaning, "wisdom." A ruler of ancient Pylos who aided the Greek victory in the Trojan War by giving wise advice.

NEVILLE—Old French: Neuve-ville. "From the new town." Neville Chamber-

vil,

Gaelic:
n. "Worshipper
'; or Old German:
Nephew." Ethel-
Nevin, composer.
glish variation: **Niven.**

NEWELL—Old English:
Niew-heall. "From the new
Hall or manor house"; or
Old French: **Nouel.** "A
kernel."
English variation: **Newall.**

NEWLAND—Old English:
Niew-land. "Dweller on
reclaimed land."

NEWLIN—Old Welsh:
Newydd-llyn. "Dweller at the
new pool."
English variation: **Newlyn.**

NEWMAN—Old English:
Niew-man. "Newcomer."
John Henry Cardinal
Newman, English prelate
(1801-1890).

NEWTON—Old English:
Niew-tun. "From the new
estate or new town."
Newton Baker, Secretary of
War under President
Woodrow Wilson.

NIAL—See **Neal.**

NICHOLAS—Greek:
Nikolaos. "Victorious army;
victorious people." St.
Nicholas, the wonder worker,
was a 4th-century bishop of
Myra, the patron of children.

Nikolaus Copernicus, 16th-
century Polish astronomer;
Nicholas Murray Butler,
educator; Nicholas Longworth,
U.S. statesman.
English nicknames: **Nick,
Nicky, Nik, Nikki, Nichol,
Nicol, Cole, Claus.**
Foreign variations: **Nicolas**
(French), **Nicolo, Nicola,
Niccolo** (Italian), **Nicolas**
(Spanish), **Nikolaus** (Ger-
man), **Neacail** (Scottish),
Nicolaas (Dutch), **Nicolai,
Nikolai** (Slavic).

NIGEL—Latin: **Nigellus.**
"Dark one." Nigel Patrick,
Nigel Bruce, English actors.

NILES—See **Neal.**

NIXON—Old English: **Nicson.**
"Son of Nicholas." See
Nicholas.

NOAH—Hebrew: "rest;
comfort." A descendant of
Adam; at God's command
Noah built the Ark that saved
his family from the flood.
Noah Webster, lexicographer
(1758-1843); Noah Beery,
actor.
Foreign variations: **Noé**
(French, Spanish), **Noach**
(Dutch), **Noak** (Swedish).

NOBLE—Latin: **Nobilis.**
"Well-known and noble."
Noble Johnson, U.S.
Congressman.

NOEL—French, from Latin.
"born at Christmas." Noel
Coward, English play-
wright, actor, producer.
English variation: **Nowell.**

Foreign variations: **Natale** (Italian), **Natal** (Spanish).

NOLAN—Irish Gaelic: **Nuallan.** "Famous, noble."

NORBERT—Old German: **Nor-beraht.** "Brilliant hero"; or Old Norse: **Njorth-r-biart-r.** "Brilliance of Njord." Njord was the ancient Norse deity of the winds and of seafarers.

NORMAN—Old French: **Normand.** "A Northman." Norman Rockwell, artist, Norman Thomas, U.S. Socialist; Norman Vincent Peale, clergyman, author. English nicknames: **Norm, Normie, Normy.**

NORRIS—Old French: **Noreis.** "Northerner."

NORTHCLIFF—Old English: **North-clif.** "From the north cliff." Lord Northcliffe was publisher of the *London Times* until his death in 1922.

NORTHROP—Old English: **North-thorp.** "From the north farm." English variation: **Northrup.**

N... **Nort**... estate o.

NORVILL... French: **North**... the north estate. English variations: . **Norvil.**

NORVIN—Old English: **North-wine.** "Friend from t. north." English variations: **Norwin, Norwyn.**

NORWARD—Old English: **North-weard.** "Northern guardian."

NORWELL—Old English: **North-wiella.** "From the north spring."

NORWOOD—Old English: **North-wode.** "From the north forest."

NOWELL—See **Noel.**

NURI—Hebrew: "fire." Also, Arabic. English variations: **Nur, Nuriel, Nuris.**

NYE—Middle English: **At-then-eye.** "Dweller at the island."

O

OAKES—Middle English: **Okes.** "Dweller at the oak trees."

OAKLEY—Old English: **Ac-leah.** "From the oak meadow."

OBERT—Old German: **Od-bert.** "Wealthy, brilliant one."

OCTAVIUS—Latin: "eighth-born child." Octavius was a Roman imperial name.

...vus.

...lo-French:
...althy one"; or
...sh: **Wode-hull.**
...orested hill."

...f—Old German:
...wulf. "Wealthy wolf." The
...me "wolf" was applied to
men of courage in the Middle
Ages.

OGDEN—Old English:
Oke-dene. "From the oak
valley." Ogden Mills, U.S.
Secretary of the Treasury;
Ogden Reid, U.S. Con-
gressman; Ogden Nash,
writer. Also: **Ogdon.**

OGILVIE—Pictish-Scottish:
Ogil-binn. "From the high
peak."

OGLESBY—Old English:
Oegels-by. "Awe-inspiring."

OLAF—Old Norse: **Oleif-r.**
"Ancestral relic." See **Oliver.**
Five Norwegian kings were
named Olaf, the first in A.D.
995.
Foreign variations: **Olav**
(Norse), **Amblaoibh** (Irish).

OLIN—A variation of **Olaf.**
Olin Johnston, U.S. Senator.

OLIVER—Old Norse:
Olvaerr. "Kind, affectionate
one"; or Old French: "olive
tree." Named from the olive
tree that was a symbol of
peace. Oliver Cromwell,
17th-century English ruler;
Oliver Wendell Holmes, U.S.

Supreme Court Justice,
1902–1932.
English nicknames: **Ollie,
Olley, Olly.**
Foreign variations: **Olivier**
(French), **Oliviero** (Italian),
Oliverio (Spanish), **Olaf,**
(Norwegian).

OLNEY—Old English:
Ollan-eg. "Olla's island."

OMAR—Arabic: "most
high; richness; first son;
follower of the Prophet."
There are diverse Arabic
meanings for **Omar.** Omar
Khayyam, 12th-century Persian
poet; Omar Bradley, U.S.
Army general.

ONSLOW—Old English:
Ondes-hloew. "Zealous one's
hill."

ORAM—Old English: **Ora-
hamm.** "From the riverbank
enclosure."

ORAN—Irish Gaelic: **Odhran.**
"Pale-complexioned one."
English variations: **Oren,
Orin, Orran, Orren, Orrin.**

OREN—Hebrew: "the
pine." Also: **Oran, Orin,
Orren, Orrin.** Oren Long,
U.S. Senator.

ORESTES—Greek: **Oreias.**
"Mountaineer." In the myths
Orestes was the son of the
hero Agamemnon.

ORFORD—Old English:
Orf-ford. "Dweller at the
cattle-ford."

ORION—Greek: "son of
fire," or "son of light." A

hunter in Greek myths, who was slain by Artemis and became the giant constellation of Orion.

ORLAN—Old English: Ord-land. "From the pointed land."
English variation: **Orland**.

ORLANDO—Italian, Spanish: "from the famous land." See **Roland**.

ORMAN—Old English: Ord-man. "Spear-man."; or Old English: **Orme-man**. "Ship-man."

ORMOND—Old English: Ord-mund. "Spear-protector"; or Old English: **Orme-mund**. "Ship-protector." Irish place name. Also: **Ormand**.

ORO—Spanish: "golden one."

ORRICK—Old English: Har-ac. "Dweller at the ancient oak tree." Where the tree in silent dignity guarded the valley.

ORRIN—See **Oran**.

ORSON—Old English: Ord-sone. "Spear-man's son"; or Old French: **Ourson**. "Little bear." Orson Welles, Orson Bean, actors.
English variation: **Urson**.

ORTON—Old English: Ora-tun. "From the shore-farmstead or town."

ORVAL—Old English: Ord-wald. "Spear-mighty."

ORVILLE—Old French:

Au.
estate
Wright,
(1871-194

ORVIN—Old
wine. "Spear-fri

OSBERT—Old En
Os-beorht. "Divinely
liant." Sir Osbert Sitweh, English poet.

OSBORN—Old English: Os-beorn. "Divine warrior"; or Old Norse: **As-biorn**. "Divine bear."

OSCAR—Old Norse: Oskar. "Divine spear; divine spear-man." Also: **Oskar**. Swedish kings Oscar I and Oscar II; Oscar Dystel, eminent publisher and executive; Oscar Hammerstein, II, librettist, producer.

OSGOOD—Old Norse: Asgaut. "Divine Goth." Osgood Perkins, actor.

OSMAR—Old English: Os-maer. "Divinely glorious."

OSMOND—Old English: Os-mund. "Divine protector." English variations: **Osmund**, **Osmont**.

OSRED—Old English: Os-raed. "Divine counselor."

OSRIC—Old English: "divine ruler."

OSWALD—Old English: Os-weald. "Divinely powerful." Oswald Spengler, German philosophical writer (1880-1936); Ozzie Nelson, actor.

man (1815-1898); Otto
Kruger, actor.

OWEN—Old Welsh: **Owein.**
"Well-born one; young
warrior." Owen Roberts,
U.S. Supreme Court Justice;
Owen Wister, American
author.
English variation: **Evan.**

OXFORD—Old English:
Oxna-ford. "From the oxen
ford."

OXTON—Old English:
Oxna-tun. "From the ox-
enclosure."

ـ‌ ‌:
‌ous

ـOtos.
‌n of hearing"; or
‌‌an: **Otho.**
‌‌y." Otis Skinner,
(1858-1942); Otis Pike.
‌. Congressman.

OTTO—Old German: **Otto,
Otho.** "Prosperous, wealthy
one." Prince Otto Bismarck-
Schonhausen, German states-

P

PABLO—Spanish form of
Paul: "little one." Pablo
Picasso, artist; Pablo Casals,
musician.

PADDY—See **Patrick.**

PADGETT—French: **Paget.**
"Young attendant."
English variations: **Padget,
Paget.**

PAGE—French: "attendant,
youthful attendant." Also:
Paige. Page Belcher, U.S.
Congressman.

PALMER—Old English:
Palmere. "Palm-bearing pilgrim, crusader."

PARK—Old English: **Pearroc.**
"Dweller at the enclosed land
or park." Parke Godwin,
author.
English variation: **Parke.**

PARKER—Middle English:

"park keeper or guardian."
From the surname.

PARKIN—Old English:
Perekin. "Little Peter."

PARLE—Old French:
Pierrel. "Little Peter."

PARNELL—Old French:
Pernel. "Little Peter." Also:
Pernell.

PARR—Old English: **Pearr.**
"Dweller at the cattle
enclosure."

PARRISH—Middle En-
glish: **Parisch.** "From the
church area."

PARRY—Old Welsh: **Ap-
Harry.** "Son of Harry."
Edward Parry, English
Arctic explorer.

PASCAL—Italian: **Pascale;
Pasquale.** "Born at Easter."

A child born at the Jewish Passover or Christian Easter. St. Paschal was a 9th-century pope. Also: **Pascual.**

PATRICK—Latin: **Patricius.** "Noble one." Honoring St. Patrick, 5th-century missionary, patron saint of Ireland. Patrick Henry, American statesman; Patrick O'Neal, Pat Boone, actors. English nicknames: **Pat, Paddy.**
Foreign variations: **Patrizius** (German), **Patrice** (French), **Patrizio** (Italian), **Patricio** (Spanish), **Padruig** (Scottish), **Padraic, Padraig** (Irish).

PATTON—Old English: **Beadu-tun.** "From the warrior's estate."
English variations: **Patten, Pattin, Paton.**

PAUL—Latin: **Paulus.** "Little." Paul was an early missionary of Christianity. Paul Cézanne, French painter; actors Paul Muni, Paul Newman, Paul Henreid. Foreign variations: **Paolo** (Italian), **Pablo,** (Spanish), **Paavo** (Scandinavian), **Pavel** (Slavic).

PAXTON—Old English: **Paeccs-tun.** "Peace-town." English nickname: **Pax.**

PAYAT—North American Indian: "he is coming." Also: **Pay, Payatt.**

PAYNE—Latin: **Paganus.** "Villager; one from the country." Payne Stewart, golfer.

PAYTON—Old English: **Paegas-tun.** "Dweller at the fighter's estate." Peyton Randolph, President of the 1st American Congress (1723-1775).
English variation: **Peyton.**

PAZ—Spanish: "peace."

PEDRO—See **Peter.**

PELL—Old English: **Paella.** "Mantle or scarf."

PELTON—Old English: **Pell-tun.** "From an estate by a pool."

PEMBROKE—Welsh place name: "headland."

PENLEY—Old English. **Penn-leah.** "Enclosed pasture-meadow."

PENN—Old German: **Bannan.** "Commander"; or Old English: **Penn.** "Enclosure" William Penn, English Quaker, founded Pennsylvania.

PENROD—Old German: **Bann-ruod.** "Famous commander." Popularized from Booth Tarkington's stories of Penrod
English nicknames: **Pen, Rod, Roddy.**

PEPIN—Old German: **Peppi.** "Petitioner" or "perseverant one." Pepin the Short, 8th-century king of the Franks, was the father of the Emperor Charlemagne. English nicknames: **Pepi, Peppi.**

PERCIVAL—Old French:

Perce-val. "Valley-piercer." A knight of King Arthur's court who sought the holy grail. Percy Bysshe Shelley, English poet.
English nicknames: **Perce, Percy, Perc.**
English variations: **Parsefal, Parsifal, Perceval.**

PERKIN—Old English: **Perekin.** "Little Peter." A son of the Fisherman of Galilee. Sir William Perkin, English chemist (1838–1907).

PERNELL—See **Parnell.** Pernell Roberts, actor.

PERRIN—Old French: **Perin.** "Little Peter."

PERRY—Middle English: **Perye.** "From the pear tree"; or Old Anglo-French: **Pierrey.** "Little Peter." Perry Como, singer, entertainer.

PERTH—Pictish-Celtic: **Pert.** "Thorn-bush thicket." A Scottish county and town and an Australian city are called Perth.

PETER—Latin: **Petrus.** "Rock or stone." Honors St. Peter, acclaimed as the first Pope of the Catholic Church. Peter the Great, Russian Emperor; Pierre Curie, French chemist; Peter O'Toole, Peter Ustinov, actors.
English nicknames: **Pete, Petie, Petey.**
Foreign variations: **Pietro, Pedro, Pero, Piero** (Italian), **Pedro** (Spanish), **Peadair**

(Scottish), **Pierre** (French), **Petrus** (German), **Peadar** (Irish), **Pieter** (Dutch), **Peder** (Scandinavian), **Pjotr, Pyotr** (Slavic).

PEVERELL—Old French: **Piperel.** "Piper or whistler." Famous from the novel *Peveril of the Peak* by Sir Walter Scott.
English variations: **Peverel, Peveril.**

PEYTON—See **Payton.**

PHELAN—Irish Gaelic: **Faolan.** "Little wolf." "Wolf" was a complimentary name for courage.

PHELPS—West English: **Phelips.** "Son of Philip."

PHILIP—Greek: **Philippos.** "Lover of horses." St. Philip was one of the 12 Apostles. Philip Barry, American dramatist; Prince Philip, husband of England's Queen Elizabeth II; Phil Silvers, comic actor; Phil Harris, orchestra leader.
English nickname: **Phil.**
Foreign variations: **Filippo** (Italian), **Felipe** (Spanish), **Philippe** (French), **Philipp** (German), **Pilib, Filib** (Irish), **Filip** (Swedish).

PHILLIPS—Old English: **Philips.** "Son of Philip." Phillips Brooks, clergyman, author of "O Little Town of Bethlehem."

PHILO—Greek: "loving; friendly." Judaeus Philo was a 1st-century Jewish philosopher; Philo Vance, fictional detective created by S. S. Van Dine.

PHINEAS—Greek: **Phinees.** "Mouth of brass." Phineas T. Barnum, famous showman.

PICKFORD—Old English: **Pic-ford.** "From the ford at the peak."

PICKWORTH—Old English: **Pica-worth.** "From the woodcutter's estate."

PIERCE—Old Anglo-French: **Piers.** "Rock or stone." A man named from an old stone landmark where he lived. An early variation of **Peter.** Pierce Butler, U.S. Supreme Court Justice, 1922-1939; Pierce Brosnan, actor.

PIERRE—See **Peter.**

PITNEY—Old English: **Bitan-ig.** "Persevering one's island."

PITT—Old English: **Pyt.** "From the hollow or pit"; or Old German: **Bittan.** "Desire; longing."

PLATO—Greek: **Platos.** "Broad one; broad-shouldered." Plato, world famous Greek philosopher, 427-347 B.C.

PLATT—Old French: **Plat.** "From the flat land."

POLLOCK—Old English: **Pauloc.** "Little Paul." Sir Frederick Pollock, English author (1845-1937).

POMEROY—Old French:

Pommeraie. "From the apple orchard."

PORTER—French, from Latin: **Portier.** "Gatekeeper"; or **Porteur.** "Porter."

POWELL—Old Welsh: **Ap-Howell.** "Son of Howell." See **Howell.**

PRENTICE—Middle English: "A learner or apprentice." Also: **Prentiss.**

PRESCOTT—Old English: **Preost-cot.** Place name: "from the priest's dwelling." W. H. Prescott, historian (1796-1859).

PRESLEY—Old English: **Preost-leah.** "Dweller at the priest's meadow." J. B. Priestley, English author and playwright. English variations: **Pressley, Priestley.**

PRESTON—Old English: **Preost-tun.** "Dweller at the priest's place." Preston Foster, actor.

PREWITT—Old French: **Preuet.** "Little valiant one." English variation: **Pruitt.**

PRICE—Old Welsh: **Ap rhys.** "Son of the ardent one."

PRIMO—Italian: "first child born to a family." Primo de Rivera, Spanish statesman; Primo Levi, author.

PROCTOR—Latin: **Procurator.** "Administrator." English variations: **Procter, Prockter.**

R—Old French:
..ar. "Head of a
..ory."
..glish variation: **Prior.**

PUTNAM—Old English:
Put-tan-ham. "From the
commander's estate or
pit-dweller's estate."

Q

QUENNEL—Old French:
Quesnel. "Dweller at the little
oak tree."

QUENTIN—See **Quinton.**

QUIGLEY—Irish Gaelic:
Coig-leach. "Distaff."

QUILLAN—Irish Gaelic:
Cuilean. "Cub."

QUIMBY—Old Norse:
Kuan-by-r. "Dweller at the
woman's estate."
English variations: **Quinby,
Quenby.**

QUINCY—Old French:

Quincey. "Dweller at the fifth
son's estate." Celebrated
from John Quincy Adams, 6th
U.S. President.

QUINLAN—Irish Gaelic:
Caoinleain. "Well-shaped
one."

QUINN—Irish Gaelic:
Cuinn. "Wise; intelligent."

QUINTON—Latin: **Quinctus.**
"Fifth child"; or Old English:
Cwen-tun. "From the
queen's estate or town." St.
Quentin, martyred in A.D.
287 in France; Quentin
Burdick, U.S. Senator.

R

RAD—Old English: **Raed.**
"Counselor."

RADBERT—Old English:
Raed-beorht. "Brilliant
counselor."

RADBORNE—Old En-
glish: **Read-burne.** "From the
red stream."

RADCLIFF—Old English:
Read-cliff. "Dweller at
the red cliff."

RADFORD—Old English:
Read-ford. "From the red
ford."

RADLEY—Old English:
Read-leah. "Red pasture-
meadow."

RADNOR—Old English:
Readan-oran. "At the red
shore."

RADOLF—Old English:
Raed-wulf. "Swift wolf;
counsel wolf."

RAFAEL—See **Raphael.**

RAFER—Variant of **Raphael:**
"healed by God." Rafer
Johnson, Olympic decathlon
champion.

RAFFERTY—Irish Gaelic: **Rab-hartach.** "Prosperous and rich."

RAGNAR—Norwegian, Swedish: "mighty army." English variations: **Ragnor, Rainer, Rayner, Raynor, Rainier.**

RALEIGH—Old English: **Ra-leah.** "Dweller at the roe-deer meadow." Sir Walter Raleigh, English explorer (1552-1618). English variation: **Rawley.**

RALPH—Old English: **Raed-wulf.** "Swift wolf or counsel wolf." Ralph Waldo Emerson, philosopher, poet (1803-1882); Ralph Bunche, United Nations official; Ralph Bellamy, actor. English variations: **Ralf, Raff, Rolf, Rolph.** Foreign variation: **Raoul** (French).

RALSTON—Old English: **Raed-wulf-tun.** "Dweller at Ralph's estate or town."

RAMBERT—Old German: **Regin-beraht.** "Mighty-brilliant." St. Rambert, 7th century.

RAMON— See Raymond.

RAMSDEN—Old English: **Ramm-dene.** "Ram's valley."

RAMSEY—Old English: **Hraem's-eg.** "Raven's island"; or Old English: **Ram-eg.** "Ram's island." English variation: **Ramsay.**

RANDALL—See Randolph.

RANDOLPH—Old English; **Rand-wulf.** "Shield-wolf." Randolph Scott, actor. English nicknames: **Rand, Randy.** English variations: **Randolf, Randall, Randell.**

RANGER—Old French: "forest keeper." English variation: **Rainger.**

RANKIN—Old English: **Randkin.** "Little shield."

RANON—Hebrew: "to be joyful." English variations: **Ranen, Raman.**

RANSFORD—Old English: **Hraefn-ford.** "From the raven's ford." In ancient days the raven symbolized great bravery.

RANSLEY—Old English: **Hraefn-leah.** "From the raven's meadow."

RANSOM—Old English: **Rand-son.** "Son of shield."

RAOUL—French form of Ralph, Randolph.

RAPHAEL—Hebrew: **R'phael.** "Healed by God." Raphael, Italian "old master" painter; Rafael Sabatini, novelist. Foreign variations: **Rafaelle, Rafaello** (Italian), **Rafael** (Spanish).

RASHID—Popular modern U.S. name, perhaps of African origin.

RAWLINS—Old Anglo-

French: **Raoulin-sone.** "Son of little counsel-wolf."

RAWSON—Old English: **Raed-wulf-sone.** "Son of little counsel-wolf."

RAY—Old French: an honored title given to a sovereign. Ray Bolger, actor, dancer; Ray Milland, actor;

RAYBURN—Old English: **Ra-burne.** "From the roe-deer brook."

RAYMOND—Old German: **Ragin-mund.** "Mighty or wise protector." Raymond Massey, actor; Ramón Magsaysay, Philippine statesman.
English nickname: **Ray.**
Foreign variations: **Ramon, Raimundo** (Spanish), **Raimondo** (Italian), **Raimund** (German), **Reamonn** (Irish).

RAYNOR—Old Norse: **Ragnar.** "Mighty army."
Foreign variation: **Rainer** (German).

READ—Old English: **Read.** "Red-haired or red-complexioned."
English variations: **Reid, Reed.**

READING—Old English: **Reading.** "Son of the red-haired one." Rufus Reading, Chief Justice of England (1860-1935).
English variation: **Redding.**

REDFORD—**Read-ford.** "From the red ford."

REDLEY—Old English:

Read-leah. "Dweller at the red meadow."

REDMAN—Old English: **Raed-man.** "Counsel-man"; or Old English: **Raede-man.** "Horseman."

REDMOND—Old English: **Raed-mund.** "Counsel, protector."
English variations: **Redmund, Radmund.**

REDWALD—Old English: **Raed-weald.** "Counsel-mighty."

REECE—Old Welsh: **Rhys.** "Ardent one."
English variations: **Reese, Rees, Rice.**

REED—See **Read.**

REEVE—Middle English: **Reve.** "Steward, bailiff."
English variations: **Reave, Reeves.**

REGAN—Irish Gaelic: **Riagan.** "Little king."
English variations: **Reagan, Reagen, Regen.**

REGINALD—Old English: **Regen-weald.** "Mighty and powerful." Reginald Denny, Reginald Gardiner, actors.
English nicknames: **Reg, Reggie, Reggy, Rene.**
English variations: **Reynold, Reynolds, Ronald.**
Foreign variations: **Reinwald, Reinald** (German), **Regnauld, Renault, René** (French), **Rinaldo** (Italian), **Reinaldo, Reinaldos, Renato, Naldo** (Spanish), **Reinold** (Dutch), **Reinhold** (Swedish, Danish), **Raghnall** (Irish).

REID—See Read.

REMINGTON—Old English: **Hremm-ing-tun.** "From the raven-family estate."

REMUS—Latin: "speedy motion; fast rower of a boat." Remus and Romulus were the legendary founders of the city of Rome.

RENAULT—See Reginald.

RENE—See Reginald.

RENFRED—Old English: **Regen-frithu.** "Mighty and peaceful."

RENFREW—Old Welsh: **Rhin-ffrew.** "From the still river or channel."

RENNY—Irish Gaelic: **Raighne.** "Little, mighty, and powerful."

RENSHAW—Old English: **Hraefn-scaga.** "From the raven forest."

RENTON—Old English: **Ran-tun.** "Roebuck-deer estate."

REUBEN—Hebrew: **R'ubhen.** "Behold a son." Rube Goldberg, cartoonist; Rubén Dario, noted Nicaraguan poet. English nickname: **Rube.** Foreign variation: **Rubén** (Spanish).

REX—Latin: "king, all-powerful in his majesty." Rex Harrison, Rex Robbins, actors. Foreign variations: **Rey** (Spanish), **Roi** (French).

REXFORD—Old English:

Rex-ford. "Dweller at the king's ford." Rexford Tugwell, political writer.

REYNARD—Old German: **Regin-hard.** "Mighty-brave." English variations: **Renard, Rennard, Raynard.** Foreign variations: **Reinhard** (German), **Renard, Renaud** (French).

REYNOLD—See Reginald.

RHODES—Middle English: **Rodes.** "Dweller at the crucifixes"; or Greek: **Rhodeos.** "Place of the roses."

RICH—Old English: **Rice.** "Powerful, wealthy one." See **Richard.**

RICHARD—Old German: **Rich-hart.** "Powerful ruler"; or Old English: **Ric-hard.** "Powerful-brave." Famous from the 12th-century English King Richard the Lion-Hearted; Richard Wagner, German composer; Richard Nixon, 37th U.S. President; Richard E. Byrd, explorer; actors Richard Widmark, Ricardo Montalban, Ricky Nelson. English nicknames: **Dick, Dicky, Rick, Ricky, Richie, Ritchie, Rich, Ritch.** English variations: **Ricard, Richerd, Rickert.** Foreign variations: **Riccardo** (Italian), **Ricardo** (Spanish), **Richart** (Dutch), **Riocard** (Irish).

RICHMAN—Old English: **Ric-man.** "Powerful man."

RICHMOND—Old German: **Rich-mund.** "Powerful protector."

RICKER—Old English: **Ric-here.** "Powerful army."

RICKWARD—Old English: **Ric-weard.** "Powerful guardian."
English variation: **Rickwood.**

RICO—Spanish, Italian form of **Enrico**, Teutonic Henry: "ruler of the home."

RIDDOCK—Irish Gaelic: **Reidh-achadh.** "From the smooth field."

RIDER—Old English: **Ridere:** "Knight or horseman."
English variation: **Ryder.**

RIDGE—Old English: **Hrycg.** "From the ridge."

RIDGEWAY—Old English: **Hrycg-weg.** "From the ridge road."

RIDGLEY—Old English: **Hrych-leah.** "Dweller at the ridge meadow."

RIDLEY—Old English: **Read-leah.** "From the red meadow."

RIDPATH—Old English: **Read-paeth.** "Dweller on the red path."

RIGBY—Old English: **Rica-dene.** "Ruler's valley."

RIGG—Old English: **Hrycg.** "From the ridge."

RILEY—Irish Gaelic: **Rag-hallach.** "Valiant, warlike one."

English variations: **Reilly, Ryley.**

RING—Old English: **Hring.** "A ring." Ring Lardner, writer.

RIORDAN—Irish Gaelic: **Rioghbhardan.** "Royal poet or bard."

RIPLEY—Old English: **Hrypan-leah.** "Dweller at the shouter's meadow." Rip Torn, actor.
English nickname: **Rip.**

RISLEY—Old English: **Hrisleah.** "From the brush-wood meadow."

RISTON—Old English: **Hris-tun.** "From the brush-wood estate or town."

RITCHIE—See **Richard.**

RITTER—North German: **Ritter.** "A knight." John Ritter, actor.

ROALD—Old German: **Hrodo-wald.** "Famous ruler." Roald Amundsen, Norwegian polar explorer (1872-1928).

ROAN—North English: **Rowan.** "Dweller by the rowan-tree"; or Spanish: **Roano.** "Reddish-brown-colored."

ROARKE—Irish Gaelic: **Ruarc;** Old Norse: **Hroth-rekr.** "Famous ruler." Robert Ruark, novelist.
English variations: **Ruark, Rourke, Rorke.**

ROBERT—Old English: **Hroth-beorht.** "Bright or

deer forest." Also an English place name. Roscoe Drummond, columnist; Roscoe Lee Browne, actor.

ROSLIN—Old French: **Ros-elin.** "Little red-haired one." English variations: **Rosselin, Rosslyn.**

ROSS—Scottish Gaelic: **Ros.** "From the peninsula." The Scottish clan Ross are famous in history. Ross Rizley, U.S. Congressman; Ross Hunter, motion picture producer.

ROSWALD—Old German: **Ros-walt.** "Horse-mighty," or "mighty with a horse." English variation: **Roswell.**

ROSWELL—See **Roswald.**

ROTHWELL—Old Norse: **Rauth-uell.** "From the red spring."

ROURKE—See **Roarke.**

ROVER—Middle English: **Rovere.** "Wanderer, rambler."

ROWAN—Irish Gaelic: **Ruad-han.** "Red-haired." English variations: **Rowen, Rowe.**

ROWE—See **Rowan.**

ROWELL—Old English: **Ra-wiella.** "From the roe-deer spring."

ROWLAND—See **Roland.**

ROWLEY—Old English: **Ruh-leah.** "Dweller at the rough meadow."

ROWSON—Anglo-Irish: **Ruadh-son.** "Son of the red-haired one."

ROXBURY—Old English: **Hroces-burh.** "From Rook's fortress."

ROY—French: **Roi.** "King"; or Celtic: "red-haired." Roy Woodruff, U.S. Congressman; Roy West, U.S. Secretary of the Interior; Roy Campanella, baseball star; actor Roy Rogers. Foreign variations: **Roi** (French), **Rey** (Spanish).

ROYAL—Old French: **Roial.** "Regal one."

ROYCE—Old English: **Royse.** "Son of the king." Josiah Royce, educator, philosopher (1855-1916).

ROYD—Old Norse: **Riodh-r.** "From the clearing in the forest."

ROYDON—Old English: **Ryge-dun.** "Dweller at the rye-hill."

RUBEN—See **Reuben.**

RUCK—Old English: **Hroc.** "Rook-bird."

RUDD—Old English: **Reod.** "Ruddy-complexioned."

RUDOLPH—Old German: **Ruod-wolf.** "Famous wolf." A complimentary name for great daring. Famous from Rudolf of Hapsburg, 13th-century Holy Roman Emperor; Rudolf Friml, composer; Rudolph Valentino, silent screen actor.

English nicknames: **Rudie, Rudy, Rolf, Rolph, Rollo, Dolf.**

English variations: **Rodolf, Rodolph, Rudolf.**

Foreign variations: **Rodolphe, Raoul** (French), **Rodolfo** (Italian, Spanish), **Rudolf** (German, Danish, Swedish, Dutch).

RUDYARD—Old English: **Rudu-geard.** "From the red enclosure." Rudyard Kipling, English author (1865-1936).

RUFF—French: **Ruffe.** "Red-haired."

RUFFORD—Old English: **Ruh-ford.** "From the rough ford."

RUFUS—Latin: "red-haired one." Famous from William Rufus, King of England, 1087-1100. Rufus Peckham, U.S. Supreme Court Justice, 1895–1910; Rufus King, author.

English nicknames: **Rufe, Ruff.**

RUGBY—Old English: **Hroc-by.** "Rook-estate."

RULE—Latin: **Regulus.** "Ruler." Saint Richard de Rule or Regulus, famous for bringing relics of St. Andrew to Scotland in the 4th century. Alternate origin Old French: **Ruelle.** "Famous wolf." Variation: **Reule,** which may also be from the Hebrew: "God is his friend."

RUMFORD—Old English:

Rum-ford. "From the wide ford."

RUPERT—See **Robert.** Rupert Brooke, English poet.

RURIK—See **Roderick, Rory.** "Rurik, 9th-century Scandinavian leader, founded the Russian Empire.

RUSH—French: **Rousse.** "Red-haired."

RUSHFORD—Old English: **Rysc-ford.** "From the rush-ford."

RUSKIN—Franco-German: **Rousse-kin.** "Little red-head." John Ruskin, 19th-century English author.

RUSSELL—Old French: **Roussel.** "Red-haired one." Russell Sage, financier (1816-1906).

English nicknames: **Rus, Russ, Rusty.**

RUST—Old French: **Rousset.** "Red-haired."

English nickname: **Rusty.**

RUTHERFORD—Old English: **Hryther-ford.** "From the cattle-ford." Rutherford Hayes, 19th U.S. President.

RUTLAND—Old Norse: **Rot-land.** "From the root or stump land."

RUTLEDGE—Old English: **Reod-laec.** "From the red pool."

RUTLEY—Old English: **Rote-leah.** "From the root or stump meadow."

RYAN—Irish Gaelic: **Ri-an.** "Little king." Robert Ryan, Ryan O'Neal, actors.

RYCROFT—Old English: **Ryge-croft.** "From the rye field."

RYDER—See **Rider.**

RYE—Old French: **Rie.** "From the riverbank."

RYLAND—Old English:

Ryge-land. "Dweller at the rye land." English variation: **Ryland.**

RYLE—Old English: **Ryge-hyll.** "From the rye hill."

RYLEY—See **Riley.**

RYMAN—Old English: **Ryge-man.** "Rye seller."

RYTON—Old English: **Ryge-tun.** "From the rye enclosure."

S

SABER—French: "a sword."

SABIN—Latin: **Sabinus.** "A man of the Sabine people." Sabinus, planter of vines, gave his name to the ancient Sabini people, conquered by the Romans in 290 B.C.

SAFFORD—Old English: **Salh-ford.** "From the willow ford."

SAHEN—Indian: "falcon."

SALIM—Arabic: "peace." Also: **Saleem, Salem.**

SALTON—Old English: **Sael-tun.** "From the manor-hall town"; or Old English: **Salh-tun.** "From the willow enclosure."

SALVADOR—Spanish: "savior." Salvador Dali, Spanish painter; Sal Mineo, actor. English nickname: **Sal.** Foreign variations: **Sauveur** (French), **Salvatore** (Italian), **Xavier, Salvador** (Spanish).

SAM—Hebrew: **Shama.** "To hear." See **Samuel, Sampson.** Sam Rayburn, U.S. Speaker of House of Representatives.

SAMPSON—Hebrew: **Shimshon.** "Sun's man or splendid man." Samson of the Bible was an Israelite judge noted for his great strength. English nicknames: **Sam, Sammie, Sammy.** English variations: **Samson, Sansom.** Foreign variations: **Sansón** (Spanish), **Sansone** (Italian), **Samson** (French, Danish, Dutch, Swedish).

SAMUEL—Hebrew: **Shemuel.** "His name is God," or "heard or asked of God." A famous Biblical judge and prophet. Samuel Adams, American patriot; Samuel Johnson, English writer (1709-1784); Samuel Goldwyn, pioneer film producer.

English nicknames: **Sammie,
Sammy, Sam.**
Foreign variations: **Samuele**
(Italian), **Samuel** (French,
German, Spanish), **Somhairle**
(Irish).

SANBORN—Old English:
Sand-burne. "Dweller at the
sandy brook."

SANCHO—Spanish, from
Latin: **Sanctius.** "Sanctified;
truthful, sincere." Sancho
Panza, famous character in
Cervantes' *Don Quixote*.

SANDERS—Middle En-
glish: **Sander-sone.** "Son of
Alexander." George San-
ders, actor.
English nicknames: **Sandie,
Sandy.**
English variations: **Sanderson,
Saunders, Saunderson.**

SANDOR—Slavic, Hungarian
form of Greek: **Alexander.**
"He helps people." Also:
Sander.
English nickname: **Sandy.**

SANFORD—Old English:
Sand-ford. "Dweller at the
sandy ford."

SANSOM—See **Sampson.**

SANTO—Italian, Spanish:
"saintly; holy; sacred." Famil-
iar Spanish usage: Santo
Domingo (St. Dominic), Santo
Tomas (St. Thomas),
Espiritu-Santo (Holy Spirit).
Santo Loquasto, stage
designer.

SANTON—Old English:
Sand-tun. "Sandy enclosure or
town."

SARGENT—Old French:
Sergent. "Officer, attendant."
"A sergeant of the law, war
(wary) and wyse (wise)."
—Chaucer, 13th century.
John Singer Sargent, noted
portrait painter (1856–1925):
Sargent Shriver, politician,
head of Peace Corps.
English nicknames: **Sarge,
Sargie.**
English variations: **Sergeant,
Sergent.**

SAUL—Hebrew: **Sha'ul.**
"Asked for." Biblical Saul was
King of Israel and father of
Jonathan. "Saul of Tarsus,"
the original name of the
Apostle St. Paul. Saul Bellow,
novelist.
English nicknames: **Sol, Solly.**

SAVILLE—North French:
Sau-ville. "Willow estate."
Saville is a noted English
family name, often used as a
given name.

SAWYER—Middle English:
Sawyere. "A sawer of wood."
Famed from Tom Sawyer,
Mark Twain's youthful hero of
his novel.

SAXE—See **Saxon.**

SAXON—Old English:
Saxan. "Of the Saxons or
sword-people." Saxon was
the designation used by the
Roman conquerors for
Germans who used short
swords in war. John Saxon,
actor.

SAYER—Welsh; Cornish:
Saer. "Carpenter." Saer Bude

is listed in the English Hundred Rolls, A.D. 1273. English variations: **Sayre, Sayers, Sayres.**

SCANLON—Irish Gaelic: **Scan-nalan.** "A little scandal or snarer." English and Irish variation: **Scanlan.**

SCHUYLER—Dutch: **Schuyler.** "Shield," or "scholar, teacher." Schuyler Bland, U.S. Congressman; Schuyler Colfax, 17th U.S. Vice-President. English variations: **Sky, Skylar.**

SCOTT—Old English: **Scottas.** "From Scotland." The source of "scot" is the Early Irish word Scothaim meaning "tattooed," referring to the appearance of the ancient Pictish-Scottish people. Scott Carpenter, astronaut. English nicknames: **Scottie, Scotty.** Foreign variation: **Scotti** (Italian).

SCOVILLE—Old French: **Escot-ville.** "From the Scotsman's estate" (meaning doubtful).

SCULLY—Irish Gaelic: **Scolaighe.** "Town crier or herald." Scolaighe or Scully was the grandson of the ancient Irish King Aedhacan of Dartry.

SEABERT—Old English: **Sae-beorht.** "Sea-glorious." English variations: **Seabright, Sebert.**

SEABROOK—Old English: **Sae-broc.** "From the brook by the sea."

SEAMUS—See **James.**

SEAN—See **John:** "God is gracious." Popular modern U.S. variant. Also: **Shawn, Shane.** Sean O'Casey, playwright; Sean O'Faolain, writer; Sean Connery, actor.

SEARLE—Old German: **Saerle.** "Armor; armed one."

SEATON—Old Anglo-French: **Sai-tun.** "From Sai's estate or town." The Norman French Baron Saher de Sai entered England with William the Conqueror in 1066; he later founded a town called Seaton in southern Scotland. English variations: **Seton, Seeton, Seetin.**

SEBASTIAN—Latin: **Sebastianus.** "August one; reverenced one." St. Sebastian was a renowned 3rd-century Roman martyr; Sebastian Cabot, actor. Foreign variations: **Sébastien** (French), **Sebastiano** (Italian).

SEDGLEY—Old English: **Secg-leah.** "From the sword-grass meadow or swords-man's meadow."

SEDGWICK—Old English: **Secg-wic.** "Dweller at the sword-grass place."

SEELEY—Old English: **Saelig.** "Happy; blessed." Sir John Seeley, 19th-century English historian.

English variations: **Seelye,
Sealey.**

SEGER—Old English:
Sae-gar. "Sea-spear; sea-
warrior"; or Old English:
Sige-here. "Victorious army."
Sigehere was a 7th-century
king of the East Saxons in
England.
English variations: **Seager,
Segar.**

SELBY—Old English:
Sele-by. "From the manor-
house or village."
English variation: **Shelby.**

SELDEN—Old English:
Salh-dene. "From the willow-
tree valley."

SELIG—Old German:
Saelec. "Blessed, happy one."
Also: **Zelig.**

SELWYN—Old English:
Sele-wine. "Manor-house
friend"; or Old English:
Sel-wine. "Good friend."
Selwyn Lloyd, English
diplomat.
English variation: **Selwin.**

SENIOR—Old French:
Seignour. "Lord of the manor
or estate."

SENNETT—French: **Senet.**
"Old, wise one."

SEPTIMUS—Latin: "seventh
son."

SERENO—Latin: **Serenus.**
"Calm, tranquil one."

SERGE—Latin: **Sergius.**
"The attendant." St. Sergius
was a pope in the 7th

century; Sergei Rachmaninoff,
pianist, composer.
English variation: **Sergei.**

SERGEANT—See **Sargent.**

SETH—Hebrew: **Sheth.**
"Appointed." Seth was the
third son of Adam.

SETON—See **Seaton.**

SEVERN—Old English:
Saefren. "Boundary." The
River Severn flows from
north Wales to the Atlantic
through southwest England.

SEWARD—Old English:
Sae-weard. "Sea-guardian."
William H. Seward, Ameri-
can statesman (1801-1872).

SEWELL—Old English:
Sae-wald. "Sea-powerful."
English variations: **Sewald,
Sewall.**

SEXTON—Middle English:
Sex-tein. "Church official or
sacristan."

SEXTUS—Latin: "sixth
son." Sextus Empiricus,
3rd-century philosopher.

SEYMOUR—Old French:
St. Maur. "From the town of
St. Maur, Normandy,
France." Seymour Chassler,
publisher; Seymour Harris,
noted educator.

SHADWELL—Old En-
glish: **Schad-wiella.** "From the
shed-spring of arbor-spring."

SHAMUS—An Irish form of
James. Also: **Seamus.**

SHANAHAN—Irish Gaelic:

Seanachan. "Wise, sagacious one."

SHANDY—Old English: **Scandy.** "Little boisterous one."

SHANE—An Irish form of **Sean.** See **John.**

SHANLEY—Irish Gaelic: **Sean-laoch.** "Old hero."

SHANNON—Irish Gaelic: **Sea-nan.** "Little old wise one."

SHARIF—Arabic: "honest."

SHATTUCK—Middle English: **Schaddoc.** "Little shad-fish."

SHAW—Old English: **Scaga.** "Dweller at a grove of trees."

SHAWN—Popular U.S. variant of **John:** "God is gracious." Also: **Sean, Shane.**

SHEA—Irish Gaelic: **Seaghda.** "Majestic, courteous, scientific, ingenious one."

SHEEHAN—Irish Gaelic: **Siodhachan.** "Little peaceful one."

SHEFFIELD—Old English: **Scaffeld.** "From the crooked field."

SHELBY—Old English: **Scelf-by.** "From the ledge estate." Isaac Shelby, American frontiersman (1750-1826).

SHELDON—Old English: **Scelf-dun.** "From the ledge-hill." Sheldon Cheney,

writer; Shelley Berman, comedian.
English nickname: **Shelley.**

SHELLEY—Old English: **Scelf-leah.** "Dweller at the ledge-meadow."

SHELTON—Old English: **Scelf-tun.** "From the ledge farm or town." Shelton of Tibet, noted American missionary.

SHEPHERD—Old English: **Sceap-hierde.** "Shepherd." Shepperd Strudwick, actor.
English nicknames: **Shep, Shepp, Sheppy.**
English variations: **Shepard, Sheppard, Shepperd.**

SHEPLEY—Old English: **Sceap-leah.** "From the sheep meadow."

SHERBORNE—Old English: **Scir-burne.** "From the clear brook."
English variations: **Sherbourn, Sherbourne, Sherburne.**

SHERIDAN—Irish Gaelic: **Seireadan.** "Wild man or satyr." Sheridan Downey, U.S. Senator.

SHERLOCK—Old English: **Scir-locc.** "Fair or white-haired." Famous from Sherlock Holmes, detective in Sir Arthur Conan Doyle's stories.

SHERMAN—Old English: **Sceran-man.** "Wool cutter." Sherman Minton, U.S. Supreme Court Justice, 1949-1956; Sherman Adams, New Hampshire governor.

SHERWIN—Middle English: **Sherwynd**. "Swift runner"; or Old English: **Scir-wine**. "Splendid friend."

SHERWOOD—Old English: **Scir-wode**. "Bright forest." Sherwood Forest was the home of Robin Hood in old England. Robert Sherwood, American dramatist.

SHIPLEY—Old English: **Sceap-leah**. "Dweller at the sheep meadow."

SHIPTON—Old English: **Sceap-tun**. "Dweller at the sheep estate."

SHOLTO—Irish Gaelic: **Siolta**. "Teal or merganser duck."

SIDDELL—Old English: **Sid-dael**. "From the wide valley."

SIDNEY—Old English: **Sydney**, from Old French: **Saint-Denis**. "From St. Denis"; or Phoenician: **Sidon**. "From the city of Sidon." Sid Caesar, comedian, actor; Sidney Sheldon, author. English nickname: **Sid**. English variations: **Sydney, Cid**.

SIEGFRIED—Old German: **Sigi-frith**. "Victorious, peaceful." The hero of the Nibelungenlied, old German legends, a prince of the lower Rhine Valley who captured a treasure, killed a dragon, and won Brunhild for King Gunther. Foreign variations: **Sigfrid**

(German), **Siffre** (French), **Sigvard** (Norwegian).

SIGMUND—Old German: **Sigi-mund**. "Victorious protector." In Norse myths Siegmund was the father of Siegfried. Sigmund Freud, writer and psychologist; Sigmund Romberg, composer; Foreign variations: **Sigismond** (French), **Sigismondo** (Italian), **Sigismundo** (Spanish), **Sigmund, Sigismund** (German), **Sigismundus** (Dutch).

SIGURD—Old Norse: **Sigurdhr**. "Victorious guardian." In Norse myths Sigurd was the son of Sigmund.

SIGWALD—Old German: **Sigi-wald**. "Victorious ruler or governor."

SILAS—See **Silvanus**. Silas was a companion of St. Paul in the Bible.

SILVANUS—Latin: "forest dweller." There are over 14 Saints Silvanus; Silvanus Morley, Yucatan achaeologist. English variations: **Sylvanus, Silas**. Foreign variations: **Silvain** (French), **Silvano, Silvio Sylvio** (Italian, Spanish).

SILVESTER—Latin: "from the forest." St. Silvester was a pope from A.D. 314 to 335. English variations: **Sylvester**. Foreign variations: **Silvestre** (French, Spanish), **Silvestro** (Italian), **Sailbheastar** (Irish). English nickname: **Sly**.

SIMEON—See **Simon**.

SIMON—Hebrew: **Shim'on.**
"Hearing; one who hears." St.
Simeon, the son of
Cleophas, was crucified in
A.D. 107; Simón Bolivar,
South American liberator
(1783-1830).
English variation: **Simeon.**
Foreign variations: **Siméon**
(French), **Simone** (Italian),
Siomonn (Irish), **Sim** (Scottish).

SINCLAIR—French: **St.
Clair.** "From the town of St.
Clair, Normandy." An
English dialectical contraction
of St. Clair. Sinclair Lewis,
American novelist (1885–1951).

SKEET—Middle English:
Skete. "Swift one."
English variations: **Skeat,
Skeets, Skeeter.**

SKELLY—Irish Gaelic:
Sgeulaiche. "Historian, story-
teller."

SKELTON—Old English:
Scelf-tun. "From the estate or
town on the ledge." Red
Skelton, noted comedian,
actor.

SKERRY—Old Norse: **Sker-
eye.** "From the rocky island."

SKIPP—Old Norse: **Skip.**
"Ship owner."
English nicknames: **Skip,
Skippy.**

SKIPPER—Middle English:
Skippere. "Ship-master."
English nicknames: **Skip,
Skippy.**

SKIPTON—Old English:
Scip-tun. "From the sheep-
estate."

SLADE—Old English:
Slaed. "Dweller in the valley.

SLATON—Modern U.S.
From a family name.

SLEVIN—Irish Gaelic:
Sliabhin. "Mountaineer."
English variations: **Slavin,
Slaven, Sleven.**

SLOAN—Irish Gaelic:
Sluaghan. "Warrior." Sloan
Wilson, American novelist.
English variation: **Sloane.**

SMEDLEY—Old English:
Smethe-leah. "From the flat
meadow." Smedley D.
Butler, U.S. Marine Corps
general.

SMITH—Old English:
"blacksmith; worker with a
hammer." Smith Thomp-
son, U.S. Secretary of the
Navy under President
Monroe.
English nickname: **Smitty.**

SNOWDEN—Old English:
Snaw-dun. "From the snowy
hill."

SOL—Latin: "the sun."
Also a diminutive of **Solomon.**

SOLOMON—Hebrew:
Shelomon. "Peaceful." King
Solomon of Israel was
famous for his wisdom.
English nicknames: **Sol,
Sollie, Solly.**
English variations: **Solaman,
Soloman, Salomon.**
Foreign variations: **Salomon**
(French), **Salomone** (Italian),
Salomón (Spanish), **Salomo**
(German, Dutch), **Solamh**
(Irish).

SOLON—Greek: "wise man." Solon was a 6th-century B.C. Athenian Greek lawgiver noted for his wisdom.

SOMERSET—Old English: **Sumer-saete.** "From the place of the summer settlers." Somerset Maugham, English novelist.

SOMERTON—Old English: **Sumer-tun.** "From the summer estate." Somerton in the English country of Somerset was the summer home of the Saxon kings.

SOMERVILLE—Old Franco-German: **Sumar-ville.** "From the summer estate."

SORRELL—Old French: **Sorel.** "Reddish-brown hair."

SOUTHWELL—Old English: **Suth-wiella.** "From the south spring." Robert Southwell, 16th-century English poet.

SPALDING—Old English: **Speld-ing.** "From the split meadow." A field divided by a river, fence, or hedge. Spaulding Gray, actor and writer.
English variation: **Spaulding.**

SPANGLER—South German: **Spengler.** "Tinsmith."

SPARK—Middle English: **Sparke.** "Gay, gallant one."

SPEAR—Old English: **Spere.** "Spear-man."

SPEED—Old English: **Sped.** "Success, prosperity."

James Speed, American statesman (1812-1887).

SPENCER—Middle English: "dispenser of provisions." H. Spender Lewis, historian, archaeologist; Spencer Tracy, actor.

SPROULE—Middle English: **Sproul.** "Energetic, active one."
English variation: **Sprowle.**

SQUIRE—Middle English: **Squier.** "Knight's attendant; shield-bearer." Sir Squire Bancroft, English actor.

STACEY—Middle Latin: **Stacius.** "Stable; prosperous."

STAFFORD—Old English: **Staeth-ford.** "From the landing-place ford."

STAMFORD—Old English: **Stan-ford.** "From the stony-ford."

STANBURY—Old English: **Stan-burh.** "From the stone fortress."
English variation: **Stanberry.**

STANCLIFF—Old English: **Stan-clif.** "From the rocky cliff."

STANDISH—Old English: **Stan-edisc.** "From the rocky park or enclosure." Celebrated from Miles Standish, New England founding settler.

STANFIELD—Old English: **Stan-feld.** "From the rocky field."

STANFORD—Old English:

"from the rocky ford."
Stanford White, famous
American architect (1853-1906).

STANHOPE—Old English:
Stan-hop. "From the rocky
hollow."

STANISLAUS—Slavic:
Stanislav. "Stand of glory;
glorious position." St.
Stanislaus was the patron of
Poland.
English nickname: **Stan.**
Foreign variations: **Stanislav**
(German), **Stanislas** (French),
Aineislis (Irish).

STANLEY—Old English:
Stan-leah. "Dweller at the
rocky meadow." Stanley
Matthews, U.S. Supreme
Court Justice, 1881–1889;
Stanley Kramer, motion
picture producer; Stanley
Holloway, actor.
English nicknames: **Stan,**
Stannie.
English variations: **Stanleigh,**
Stanly.

STANMORE—Old English:
Stan-mere. "From the rocky
lake."

STANTON—Old English:
Stan-tun. "From the stony
estate." Edwin M. Stanton,
U.S. Secretary of War under
President Abraham Lincoln.
English variation: **Staunton.**

STANWAY—Old English:
Stan-weg. "Dweller on the
paved stone road."

STANWICK—Old English:
Stan-wic. "Dweller at the
rocky village."

STANWOOD—Old En-
glish: **Stan-wode.** "Dweller at
the rocky forest."

STARLING—Old English:
Staer-ling. "Starling-bird."

STARR—Middle English:
Sterre. "Star."

STEDMAN—Old English:
Stede-man. "Farmstead
owner."

STEIN—German: "stone."

STEPHEN—Greek:
Stephanos. "Crowned one."
Honoring St. Stephen, the
first Christian martyr and St.
Stephen, 10th-century King
of Hungary. Stephen Decatur,
U.S. Naval Commodore
(1779-1820); Stephen Vincent
Bénet; writer, Stephen
Foster, composer; actors
Steve Allen, Steve McQueen,
Stephen Boyd.
English nicknames: **Steve,**
Stevie.
English variations: **Steven,**
Stevenson, Stephenson.
Foreign variations: **Etienne**
(French), **Estevan, Esteban**
(Spanish), **Stefan** (German,
Danish), **Stefano** (Italian),
Stephanus (Swedish), **Steaphan**
(Scottish).

STERLING—Middle En-
glish: a nickname from an old
English coin; or Old Welsh:
Ystrefelyn. "From the yellow
house." Sterling Holloway,
Sterling Hayden, actors.
English variation: **Stirling.**

STERNE—Middle English:
"austere one."

English variations: **Stern, Stearn, Stearne.**

STEVEN—See **Stephen.**

STEWART—Old English: **Sti-ward.** "Bailiff or steward of a manorial estate." Stewart or Stuart was the surname of a long line of Scottish and English rulers. Stuart Chase, writer; Stewart Alsop, journalist; actors Stewart Granger, Stuart Whitman. English nicknames: **Stu, Stew.** English variations: **Stuart, Steward.**

STILLMAN—Old English: **Stille-man.** "Quiet man."

STINSON—Old English: **Staen-sone.** "Son of stone."

STIRLING—See **Sterling.**

STOCKLEY—Old English: **Stoc-leah.** "From the tree-stump meadow."

STOCKTON—Old English: **Stoc-tun.** "From the tree-stump estate or town." Frank Stockton, American writer (1834-1902).

STOCKWELL—Old English: **Stoc-wiella.** "From the tree-stump spring."

STODDARD—Old English: **Stod-hierde.** "Horse-keeper."

STOKE—Middle English: "village."

STORM—Old English: "tempest; storm."

STORR—Old Norse: **Stor-r.** "Great one."

STOWE—Old English: **Stowe.** "From the place."

STRAHAN—Irish Gaelic: **Sruth-an.** "Poet, wise man."

STRATFORD—Old English: **Straet-ford.** "River-ford on the street." Famous from Shakespeare's birthplace, Stratford-on-Avon, in Warwickshire.

STREPHON—Greek: "one who turns." Made familiar by Gilbert and Sullivan in *Iolanthe.* English variations: **Strep, Strephonn.**

STRONG—Old English: **Strang.** "Powerful one."

STROUD—Old English: **Strod.** "From the thicket."

STRUTHERS—Irish Gaelic: **Sruthair.** "From the stream."

STUART—See **Stewart.**

STYLES—Old English: **Stigols.** "Dweller by the stiles." An old enclosure or stockade. Styles Bridges, U.S. Senator.

SUFFIELD—Old English: **Suth-feld.** "From the south field."

SULLIVAN—Irish Gaelic: **Suileabhan.** "Black-eyed one." Sir Arthur Sullivan, English composer (1842-1900). English nicknames: **Sullie, Sully.**

SULLY—Old English: **Suth-leah.** "From the south meadow." See **Sullivan.**

SUMNER—Middle English: **Sumenor.** "Summoner; church legal officer." Sumner Welles, U.S. statesman; Sumner Whittier, U.S. Veterans Administrater.

SUTCLIFF—Old English: **Suth-clif.** "From the south cliff."

SUTHERLAND—Old Norse: **Suthrland.** "From the southern land." In the time of the Vikings this was a name for the Shetland Islands and north Scotland.

SUTTON—Old English: **Suth-tun.** "From the south estate."

SWAIN—Middle English:

Swayn. "Herdsman; knight's attendant." King Sweyn Forkbeard of Denmark, died A.D. 1014, was the father of England's famous King Canute.
English variations: **Swayne.**

SWEENEY—Irish Gaelic: **Suidhne.** "Little hero."

SWINTON—Old English: **Swin-tun.** "Dweller at the swine-farm."

SYDNEY—See **Sidney.**

SYLVESTER—See **Silvester.** Sylvester Stallone, actor.

SYMINGTON—Old English: **Symon-tun.** "Dweller at Simon's estate." Stuart Symington, U.S. Senator.

T

TAB—Old German: **Tabbert.** "Brilliant among the people"; or Middle English: **Taburer.** "Drummer." Tab Hunter, actor.
English nickname: **Tabby.**

TAD—Old Welsh: "father." English variation: **Tadd.**

TAFFY—Old Welsh: "beloved one." A Welsh form of **David.**

TAGGART—Irish Gaelic: **Mac-an-T-sagairt.** "Son of the prelate."

TAJ—Urdu: "exalted." Popular modern U.S. name. Taj Mahal, singer.

TALBOT—Old French: **Talebot.** "Pillager"; or Old English: **Talbot.** An extinct type of dog, the ancestor of the bloodhound. Talebotus Talebot is recorded in Lancashire, England, in A.D. 1284.

TANNER—Old English: **Tannere.** "Leather maker."

TANTON—Old English: **Tam-tun.** "From the quiet-river estate or town."

TARLETON—Old English **Thorald-tun.** "Thunder-r~ estate."

TARRANT—Old W **Taran.** "Thunder."

TATE—Middle English: Tayt. "Cheerful one." English variation: **Tait**.

TAVIS—Scottish Gaelic. Tamnais. "Twin." A Scottish form of **Thomas**. English variations: **Tavish**, **Tevis**.

TAYLOR—Middle English: Taylour. "A tailor." English variation. **Tailor**.

TEAGUE—Irish Gaelic: Taidhg; Tadhg. "Poet."

TEARLE—Old English: Thearl. "Stern, severe one."

TED—Short form of **Edward** or **Theodore**. Ted Williams, baseball great.

TEDMOND—Old English: Theod-mund. "National protector."

TELFORD—Old French: Tail-lefer. "Iron-hewer or cutter." An ancient French occupational title for a miner or metalworker. English variations: **Telfer**, **Telfor**, **Telfour**.

TEMPLETON—Old English: Tempel-tun. "Temple or religious edifice-town."

TENNESSEE—American Indian (Cherokee): a place name. Tennessee Williams, playwright; Tennessee Ernie Ford, country singer.

TENNYSON—Middle English: Tennyson. "Son of Dennis. See **Dennis**. Tennyson, 19th-century English poet laureate.

TERENCE, TERRANCE—Latin: **Terentius**. "Smooth, polished one"; or Irish Gaelic: **Toirdealbhach**. "Shaped like the god Thor." Terence Rattigan, English dramatist. English nickname: **Terry**. Foreign variation: **Terencio** (Spanish).

TERRELL—Old English: Tirell. "Thunder ruler." A man compared to Thor, the old Norse god. Tyrrell Biggs, Olympic boxer. English variations: **Terrill**, **Tirrell**, **Tyrrell**.

TERRIS—Old English: Terry-sone. "Son of Terrell or Terence."

TEVIS—See **Tavis**.

THADDEUS—Latin: "praiser"; or Greek: **Thaddaios**. "Stout-hearted, courageous." Thaddeus was one of the 12 Apostles. Thaddeus Kosciusko, Polish military leader (1746-1817); Thaddeus Stevens, American statesman. English nicknames: **Thad**, **Tad**, **Taddy**. Foreign variations: **Thaddäus** (German). **Taddeo** (Italian), **Tadeo** (Spanish), **Tadhg** (Irish).

THAINE—See **Thane**.

THANE—Old English: Thegn. "Follower or warrior attendant."

English variations: **Thaine,**
Thayne.

THATCHER—Middle English: **Thackere.** "roof-
thatcher."
English nickname: **Thatch.**

THAW—Old English:
Thawian. "Ice thaw."

THAYER—Old Frankish:
Thiad-here. "National army."

THAYNE—See **Thane.**

THEOBALD—Old German: **Theudo-bald.** "Boldest
of the people." Theodbald
was a 7th-century brother of
Athelfrith, English king of
Northumbria.
English variation: **Tybalt.**
Foreign variations: **Thebault,**
Thibaut, Thibaud (French),
Dietbold, Tibold (German),
Teobaldo (Spanish, Italian),
Tiebout (Dutch), **Tioboid**
(Irish).

THEODORE—Greek: **Theo-**
doros. "Gift of God."
Theodore Roosevelt, 26th
U.S. President; Theodore
Dreiser, novelist (1871-1945).
English nicknames: **Ted,**
Teddie, Teddy.
Foreign variations: **Théodore**
(French), **Teodoro** (Spanish,
Italian), **Theodor** (German,
Danish, Swedish), **Theodorus**
(Dutch), **Feodor** (Slavic).

THEODORIC—Old German: **Theudo-ric.** "Ruler of
the people."
English nicknames: **Ted,**
Teddie, Teddy, Rick,
Derek, Derk, Derrick.

Foreign variations: **Dietrich**
(German), **Teodorico** (Spanish).

THEON—Greek: "godly."

THERON—Greek: "a
hunter."

THOMAS—Greek: **Thomas;**
Aramaic: **Teoma.** "A twin."
St. Thomas was one of the
12 Apostles. Thomas Jefferson, 3rd U.S. President;
Thomas A. Edison, American
inventor; Thomas Wolfe,
Thomas Carlyle, writers;
Thomas Dewey, U.S.
statesman.
English nicknames: **Tom,**
Tommie, Tommy, Tam,
Tammy, Massey.
Foreign variations: **Tomaso**
(Italian), **Tomás** (Spanish),
Tomas (Irish).

THOR—Old Norse: **Thor-i-r.**
"Thunder." Thor was the
ancient Norse god of
thunder. This name became
well established in England.
Thor Heyerdahl, Norwegian
author, explorer.
English and Scandinavian
variation: **Tor.**

THORALD—Old Norse:
Thor-uald-r. "Thor-ruler;
thunder-ruler."
English variations: **Torald,**
Thorold, Terrell, Tyrell.

THORBERT—Old Norse:
Thor-biart-r. "Brilliance of
Thor or thunder-glorious."
English variation: **Torbert.**

THORBURN—Old Norse:
Thor-biorn "Thor's bear
thunder-bear."

THORLEY—Old English: **Thur-leah.** "Thor's meadow." English variation: **Torley.**

THORMOND—Old English: **Thur-mund.** "Thor's protection."
English variations: **Thormund, Thurmond.**

THORNDYKE—Old English: **Thorn-dic.** "From the thorny dike or embankment."

THORNE—Old English: **Thorn.** "Dweller by a thorn tree." A common English place name.

THORNLEY—Old English: **Thornig-leah.** "From the thorny meadow."

THORNTON—Old English: **Thorn-tun.** "From the thorny estate." Thornton Wilder, writer.

THORPE—Old English: **Thorp.** "From the village."

THURLOW—Old English: **Thur-hloew.** "From Thor's hill."

THURSTON—Old English: **Thur-stan.** "Thor's stone or jewel." This name was introduced in England by the Danes before the Norman conquest in 1066. Also: **Thurstan.** Thurstan Clarke, American writer.

TIERNAN—Irish Gaelic: **Tighearnan.** "Lord or master."

⸱ERNEY—Irish Gaelic: **⸱earnach.** "Lordly one."

⸱⸱N—Old English:

Tila-dene. "From the good, liberal one's valley."

TILFORD—Old English: **Tila-ford.** "From the good, liberal one's ford."

TILTON—Old English: **Tila-tun.** "From the good, liberal one's estate."

TIMON—Greek: **Timun.** "Honor, reward, value." Timon of Athens, vitalized by Shakespeare's play of that name, was a Greek skeptic philosopher.

TIMOTHY—Greek: **Timotheos.** "Honoring God." St. Timothy was a colleague of St. Paul.
English nicknames: **Tim, Timmie, Timmy.**
Foreign variations: **Timothée** (French), **Timoteo** (Italian, Spanish), **Timotheus** (German), **Tiomoid** (Irish).

TIRRELL—See **Terrell.**

TITUS—Greek: **Titos.** "Of the giants." Titus was a giant slain by Apollo in Greek myths.
Foreign variations: **Tite** (French), **Tito** (Italian, Spanish).

TOBIAS—Hebrew: **Tobhiyah.** "The Lord is good." Tobias Asser, Dutch Nobel Peace Prize winner.
English nicknames: **Tobe, Toby.**
Foreign variations: **Tobie** (French), **Tobia** (Italian), **Tobias** (Spanish), **Tioboid** (Irish).

TODD—North-English: **Tod.** "A fox." Robert Todd Lincoln, son of President Abraham Lincoln; Todd Rundgren, musician.

TOFT—Old English: "a small farm."

TOLAND—Old English: **Toll-land.** "Owner of taxed land."

TOMKIN—Old English: "little Tom." Named for his father Thomas. English variation: **Tomlin.**

TORBERT—See **Thorbert.**

TORLEY—See **Thorley.**

TORMEY—Irish Gaelic: **Tor-maigh;** Old German: **Thor-mod.** "Thor or thunder spirit."

TORR—Old English: "from the tower."

TORRANCE—Anglo-Irish: **Tor-rans.** "From the knolls." From a place of little hills. English nicknames: **Torey, Torrey, Torry.**

TOWNLEY—Old English: **Tun-leah.** "From the town-meadow."

TOWNSEND—Old English: **Tunes-ende.** "From the end of town."

TRACY—Latin: **Thrasius.** "Bold, courageous one"; or Irish Gaelic: **Treasach.** "Battler."

TRAHERN—Old Welsh: **Trahayarn.** "Super-iron, super-strength."

TRAVERS—Old French: **Traverse.** "From the crossroads." English variation: **Travis.**

TREDWAY—Old English: **Thryth-wig.** "Mighty warrior."

TREMAYNE—Old Cornish: **Tre-men.** "Dweller in the house at the rock."

TRENT—Latin: **Torrentem;** Welsh: **Trent.** "Torrent, rapid stream."

TREVELYAN—Old Cornish: **Trev-elian.** "From Elian's homestead."

TREVOR—Irish Gaelic: **Treabhar.** "Prudent, discreet, wise." Trevor Howard, actor.

TRIGG—Old Norse: **Trygg-r.** "True, trusty one."

TRIPP—Old English: **Trip.** "Traveler."

TRISTAN—Old Welsh: **Trys-tan.** "Noisy one." Tristan, whose name was confused with Tristram, was a famous knight of King Arthur's Round Table in old English legends.

TRISTRAM—Latin-Welsh: **Tris-tram.** "Sorrowful labor." Tristram Speaker, baseball star.

TROWBRIDGE—Old English: **Treow-brycg.** "Dweller by the tree-bridge."

TROY—Old French: **Troyes.** "At the place of the

curly-haired people." Troy
Donahue, actor.

TRUE—Old English: **Treowe.**
"Faithful, loyal, true one."

TRUESDALE—Old English: **Truite-stall.** "From the beloved one's farmstead."

TRUMAN—Old English: **Treowe-man.** "Faithful one's adherent." Harry S. Truman, 33rd U.S. President; Truman Capote, author.

TRUMBLE—Old English: **Trum-bald.** "Strong, bold one."

TUCKER—Middle English: **Toukere.** "A tucker or fuller of cloth." See **Fuller.**

TUDOR—Old Welsh: **Tewdwr.** A Welsh variation of **Theodore.**

TULLY—Irish Gaelic: **Tuathal; Maoltuile; Taithleach.** "People-mighty," or "Devoted to the will of God," or "quiet, peaceful one." Tully Marshall, silent screen actor.

TUPPER—Old English: **Tup-pere.** "Ram raiser."

TURNER—Middle English: **Tournour.** "Latheworker."

TURPIN—Old Norse: **Thorfinn.** "Thunder-Finn." This man from Finland was named for Thor, the god of

thunder. A Turpin was Archbishop of Rheims, France, in the 10th century.

TUXFORD—Old Norse-English: **Thiod-geir-ford.** "Ford of the national spear-man."

TWAIN—Middle English: **Twein.** "Cut apart or cut in two." An heir named for his divided estate or farm that was in two parts.

TWITCHELL—Old English: "dweller on a narrow passage."

TWYFORD—Old English: **Twi-ford.** "From the double river-ford."

TYE—Old English: **Tyg.** "From the enclosure"; or Middle English: **Teyen.** "Tied or bound."

TYLER—Middle English: **Tylere.** "Tile maker and roofer." Ty Hardin, actor. English nickname: **Ty.**

TYNAN—Irish Gaelic: **Teimhnean.** "Dark or gray."

TYRONE—Greek: **Turannos.** "Sovereign." Also, an Irish place name: "Eogham's land." Famous from Tyrone Power, actor.

TYSON—Old French: **Tyeis;** English: **Son.** "Son of the Teuton or German."

U

UDELL—Old English: **Iw-dael.** "From the yew-tree valley." English variations: **Udale, Udall.**

UDOLF—Old English: **Od-wulf.** "Prosperous wolf." The wolf depicted courage.

ULFRED—Old English: **Wulf-frith.** "Wolf-peace."

ULGER—Old English: **Wulf-gar.** "Wolf-spear."

ULLOCK—Old English: **Ulve-laik.** "Wolf-sport."

ULMER—Old Norse: **Ulf-macrr.** "Wolf-famous." English variation: **Ulmar.**

ULRIC—Old German: **Wolf-rik.** "Wolf-ruler"; or Old German: **Alh-rik.** "All-ruler."

ULYSSES—Greek: **Odysseus.** "Hater." Ulysses is a Latin form of the Greek hero-name Odysseus. Ulysses S. Grant, 18th U.S. President. Foreign variations: **Ulises** (Spanish), **Uillioc** (Irish).

UNWIN—Old English: **Un-wine.** "Not a friend."

UPTON—Old English: **Up-tun.** "Upper estate or town." Upton Sinclair, author.

UPWOOD—Old English: **Up-wode.** "From the upper forest."

URBAN—Latin: **Urbanus.** "From the city." Eight Popes of the Roman Catholic Church were named Urban. Foreign variations: **Urbano** (Spanish, Italian), **Urbanus** (German), **Urbaine** (French).

URIAH—Hebrew: **Uriyah.** "Flame of Jehovah: My Light is Jehovah." Foreign variation: **Yuri** (Russian).

URSON—See **Orson.**

V

VACHEL—Old French: "little cow." Vachel Lindsay, poet.

VAIL—Middle English: **Vale.** "Valley dweller." English variation: **Vale.**

VAL—Latin: **Valentis.** "Strong." See **Valentine.**

VALDEMAR—Old German: **Waldo-mar.** "Famous ruler."

VALENTINE—Latin: **Valentinus.** "Strong, valorous, healthy." St. Valentine was a famous Roman martyr; his feast day is celebrated in

many countries on February 14.
Foreign variations: **Valentín** (Spanish), **Valentin** (French, German, Danish, Swedish), **Valentijn** (Dutch), **Valentino** (Italian), **Bailintin** (Irish).

VALERIAN—Late Latin: **Valerianus**. "Strong, healthy, powerful." Valerian was a 3rd-century A.D. Roman emperor; St. Valerianus, Bishop of Auxerre, 4th century. Valery Borzov, Valery Brumel, Russian track stars.
English variation: **Valery**.

VALLIS—Old French: **Vallois**. "Welshman."

VAN—Dutch: "from or of." A nickname from many Dutch surnames, used as a given name. Van Cliburn, concert pianist; actors Van Johnson, Van Heflin.

VANCE—Middle English: **Vannes**. "Resident at the grain-winnowing fans."

VARDEN—Old French: **Verddun**. "From the green hill."
English variations: **Vardon**, **Verdon**.

VARIAN—Latin: **Variantia**. "Variable."

VASILIS—Greek: "knightly, magnificent."

VASSILY—Russian: "unwavering protector."
English variations: **Vassi**, **Vasya**, **Vas**.

VAUGHN—Old Welsh: **Vychan**. "Small one." Also: **Vaughan**. Vaughn Monroe, orchestra leader; Vaughn Taylor, actor.

VERGE—Anglo-French: "owner of a quarter-acre."

VERNE—Latin: **Vernus**. "Springlike, youthful."

VERNER—See **Werner**.

VERNEY—Old French: **Vernay**. "From the alder grove."

VERNON—Latin: **Vernum**. "Springlike, youthful"; or Old French: "little alder grove." A name given boys born in the spring. Vernon Castle, dancer; Vernon Duke, composer.

VERRILL—Old French: **Verel**. "True one"; or Teutonic: "manly."
English variations: **Verrall**, **Verrell**, **Veryl**.

VICK—Old French: **Vicq**. "From the village." See **Victor**.

VICTOR—Latin: "conqueror." Victor Hugo, French author (1802–1885); Victor Herbert, composer (1859–1924); Victor Borge, musician, entertainer; Victor McLaglen, Victor Mature, actors.
English nicknames: **Vic**, **Vick**.
Foreign variations: **Vittorio** (Italian), **Vitorio** (Spanish), **Buadhach** (Irish).

VINCENT—Latin: **Vincentius**. "Conquering one." Honoring

St. Vincent de Paul, French priest (1576–1660). Vincent Price, actor; Vincent Van Gogh, artist.
English nicknames: **Vin, Vince**.
Foreign variations: **Vincente** (Italian), **Vincenz** (German), **Vincentius** (Dutch), **Vicente** (Spanish), **Uinsionn** (Irish).

VINSON—Old English: **Vin-sone**. "Son of Vincent."

VIRGIL—Latin: **Virgula**. "Rod or staff bearer." The staff was used to designate authority or an official. Virgil Chapman, U.S. Senator; Virgil Grissom, U.S. astronaut.
English nickname: **Virge**.

Foreign variation: **Virgilio** (Spanish, Italian).

VITO—Latin: **Vitus**. "Live; living; alive." Vito Marcantonio, U.S. Congressman; Vito "Vic" Damone, singer, actor.
Foreign variation: **Witold** (Polish).

VLADIMIR—Old Slavic: **Vladimiru**. "Royally peaceful or famous." St. Vladimir, Russian prince, died A.D. 1018; Vladimir Horowitz, pianist.

VLADISLAV—Old Slavic: **Vladi-slava**. "Glorious ruler, royal glory."

VOLNEY—Old German: **Voll-my**. "People's or national spirit."

W

WADE—Old English: **Wada**. "The advancer"; or Old English: **Waed**. "Dweller at the river crossing."

WADLEY—Old English: **Wada-leah**. "The advancer's meadow."

WADSWORTH—Old English: **Wades-weorth**. "From the advancer's estate." Henry Wadsworth Longfellow, American poet.
English nicknames: **Waddie, Waddy**.

WAGNER—German: **Wagner**. "A wagoner or wagon-maker."

WAINWRIGHT—Old English: **Waen-wryhta**. "Wagon-maker."

WAITE—Middle English: **Wayte**. "Guard, watchman."

WAKE—Old English: **Wacian**. "Alert, watchful one."

WAKEFIELD—Old English: **Wac-feld**. "Dweller at the wet field." Charles Wakefield Cadman, American composer.

WAKELEY—Old English: **Wac-leah**. "From the wet meadow."

WAKEMAN—Old English: **Wacu-man**. "Watchman."

WALBY—Old English: **Wal-by.** "From the walled-dwellings", or "home by an ancient Roman wall in England."

WALCOTT—Old English: **Weall-cot.** "Dweller at the wall-enclosed cottage."

WALDEMAR—Old German: **Waldo-mar.** "Famous ruler"; or Old English: **Weald-maer.** "Powerful, famous." Waldemar the Great was a 12th-century Danish king. Waldemar Cierpinski, Olympic marathon champion. English and Scandinavian variation: **Valdemar.**

WALDEN—Old English: **Weal-dene.** "From the forest valley"; or Old German: **Walten.** "Ruler."

WALDO—Old German: "ruler"; or Old English: **Weald.** "Mighty." Ralph Waldo Emerson, author.

WALDRON—Old German: **Wald-hramn.** "Ruling raven." The raven depicted strength and authority.

WALFORD—Old English: **Weala-ford.** "From the Welshman's ford."

WALFRED—Old German: **Waldi-frid.** "Peaceful ruler."

WALKER—Middle English: **Walkere.** "Thickener of cloth, or 'fuller.'" Walker Percy, author.

WALLACE—Old English: **Waleis.** "Man from Wales; Welshman." Sir William Wallace, famous Scottish hero, died 1305; Wally Cox, entertainer; Wallace Stevens, poet.
English nicknames: **Wallie, Wally.**
English variations: **Wallis, Walsh, Welch, Welsh.**
Foreign variation: **Wallache** (German).

WALLER—Old English: **Weallere.** "Wall-builder; mason"; or Old German: **Walt-hari.** "Army ruler."

WALLIS—See **Wallace.**

WALMOND—Old German: **Wald-munt.** "Mighty or ruling protector."

WALSH—See **Wallace.**

WALTER—Old German: **Walt-hari.** "Powerful warrior, army ruler." Sir Walter Raleigh, 16th-century English navigator; Sir Walter Scott, author; Walt Whitman, poet; Walt Disney, motion picture producer; Walt Frazier, basketball player.
English nicknames: **Walt, Wat.**
Foreign variations: **Gauthier, Gautier** (French), **Gualtiero** (Italian), **Gualterio** (Spanish), **Walther** (German), **Ualtar** (Irish), **Bhaltair** (Scottish).

WALTON—Old English: **Weall-tun.** "Dweller at the town near a ruined Roman wall"; or Old English: **Wald-tun.** "Dweller at the forest town."

WALWORTH—Old English: **Weala-worth**. "From the Welsh-man's farm."

WALWYN—Old English: **Wealh-wine**. "Welsh friend."

WARBURTON—Old English: **Warburh-tun**. "From the enduring castle town."

WARD—Old English: **Weard**. "Watchman, guardian." Ward Hunt, U.S. Supreme Court Justice, 1873–1882; Ward Bond, actor.
English variations: **Warde, Warden, Worden**.

WARDELL—Old English: **Weard-hyll**. "From the watch-hill."

WARDEN—See **Ward**.

WARDLEY—Old English: **Weard-leah**. "From the guardian's meadow."

WARE—Old English: **Waer**. "Wary, astute, prudent one"; or Old German: "defender."

WARFIELD—Middle English: **Ware-feld**. "Dweller at the weir-field."

WARFORD—Middle English: **Ware-ford**. "From the weir-ford."

WARING—See **Warren**.

WARLEY—Middle English: **Ware-ley**. "From the weir-meadow."

WARMOND—Old English: **Waer-mund**. "True protector."

WARNER—Old German:

Waren-hari. "Defending army or warrior." Warner Baxter, actor.
Foreign variation: **Werner** (German).

WARREN—Old German: **Waren**. "Watchman, defender or true-man"; or Middle English: **Wareine**. "Game-preserve keeper." Warin or Guarin was among the heroes of the medieval ballad, *Chanson de Roland*, the story of the nephew of the Emperor Charlemagne. Warren G. Harding, 29th U.S. President; actor Warren Beatty.

WARTON—Old English: **Ware-tun**. "From the weir-dam town or estate."

WARWICK—Old English: **Waeringawicum**. "Fortress of the defender's family."
English variation: **Warrick**.

WASHBURN—Old English: **Waesc-burne**. "Dweller at the flooding-brook."

WASHINGTON—Old English: **Hwaesinga-tun**. "From the estate of the keen-one's family." George Washington, 1st U.S. President; Washington Irving, American writer (1783–1859); Washington Allston, painter (1779–1843).

WATFORD—Old English: **Watel-ford**. "From the hurdle-ford."

WATKINS—Old English:

Watte-kin-sone. "Son of Walter."

WATSON—Old English: **Watte-sone.** "Son of Walter."

WAVERLY—Old English: **Waefre-leah.** "Quaking-aspen tree meadow."

WAYLAND—Old English: **Weg-land.** "From the pathway land or property."

WAYNE—Old English: **Waen-man.** "Wagoner or wagon-maker." Wayne Morse, U.S. Senator; Wayne Rogers, actor.

WEBB—Old English: Webbe. "A weaver."

WEBER—German: "a weaver."

WEBLEY—Old English: **Webbe-leah.** "From the weaver's meadow."

WEBSTER—Old English: **Webbestre.** "A weaver."

WEDDELL—Old English: **Wadan-hyll.** "Dweller at the advancer's hill."

WELBORNE—Old English: **Wiella-burna.** "Dweller at the spring-brook."

WELBY—Old English: **Wiella-by.** "Dweller at the spring-farm."

WELDON—Old English: **Wiella-dun.** "From the spring-hill."

WELFORD—Old English: **Wiella-ford.** "From the spring-ford."

WELLINGTON—Old English: **Weolingtun.** "From the prosperous one's family estate."

WELLS—Old English: **Wiellas.** "From the springs."

WELSH—See **Wallace.**

WELTON—Old English: **Wiella-tun.** "Dweller at the spring-town or estate."

WENCESLAUS—Old Slavic: **Wenceslava.** "Wreath or garland of glory." St. Wenceslaus was a 10th-century King of Bohemia.

WENDELL—Old German: **Wendel.** "Wanderer"; or Old English: **Wend-el.** "Boundary-dweller." Wendell Willkie, U.S. attorney, statesman; Wendell Corey, actor.

WENTWORTH—Old English: **Wintan-weorth.** "White one's estate."

WERNER—Old German: **Warin-hari.** "Defending warrior or army." Wernher Von Braun, U.S. space engineer.

WESLEY—Old English: **West-leah.** "From the west meadow."
English variation: **Westleigh.**

WEST—Old English: "man from the west." Directional names were popular in medieval England.

WESTBROOK—Old English: **West-broc.** "From the west-brook." Westbrook Pegler, journalist, columnist.

WESTBY—Old English: **West-by.** "From the west-farmstead."

WESTCOTT—Old English: **West-cot.** "From the west cottage."

WESTON—Old English: **West-tun.** "From the west estate."

WETHERBY—Old English: **Wethr-by.** "From the wether-sheep farm."

WETHERELL—Old English: **Wethr-healh.** "From the wether-sheep corner."

WETHERLY—Old English: **Wethr-leah.** "Dweller at the wether-sheep meadow."

WHARTON—Old English: **Hwer-tun.** "Estate at the hollow, or embankment."

WHEATLEY—Old English: **Hwaete-leah.** "Wheat meadow."

WHEATON—Old English: **Hwaete-tun.** "Wheat estate or town."

WHEELER—Old English: **Hweol-ere.** "Wheel-maker."

WHISTLER—Old English: **Hwistlere.** "Whistler or piper." James McNeill Whistler, painter (1834–1903).

WHITBY—Old English: **Hwit-by.** "From the white farmstead."

WHITCOMB—Old English: **Hwit-cumb.** "From the white hollow." James

Whitcomb Riley, poet (1853–1916).

WHITELAW—Old English: **Hwit-hloew.** "From the white hill." Whitelaw Reid, journalist, diplomat (1837–1912).

WHITFIELD—Old English: **Hwit-feld.** "From the white field."

WHITFORD—Old English: **Hwit-ford.** "From the white ford."

WHITLEY—Old English: **Hwit-leah.** "From the white meadow."

WHITLOCK—Old English: **Hwit-locc.** "Man with a white lock of hair"; or Old English: **Hwit-loc.** "From the white stronghold."

WHITMAN—Old English: **Hwit-man.** "White-haired man."

WHITMORE—Old English: **Hwit-mor.** "From the white moor."

WHITNEY—Old English: **Hwitan-ig.** From a place name: "from the white-haired one's island."

WHITTAKER—Old English: **Hwit-acer.** "Dweller at the white field."

WICKHAM—Old English: **Wic-hamm.** "From the village meadow or enclosure."

WICKLEY—Old English: **Wic-leah.** "Village meadow

WILBUR—Old German:
Willa-perht. "Resolute-brilliant
one"; or Old English:
Willa-burh. "From the firm
fortress." Wilbur Wright,
aviation pioneer (1867–1912).
English variations: **Wilbert,
Wilburt.**

WILEY—See **William.**
Wiley Post, aviator (1900–
1935).

WILFORD—Old English:
Wylig-ford. "Dweller at the
willow-ford."

WILFRED—Old German:
Willi-frid. "Resolute, peaceful
one, determined peace-
maker." St. Wilfrid, 8th-
century English prelate;
Wilfrid Sheed, author.
English variation: **Wilfrid,
Wilfried.**

WILL—Old English: **Willa.**
"Determined, firm, resolute."
See **William.**

WILLARD—Old English:
Will-hard. "Resolute and
brave." Willard F. Libby,
U.S. atomic scientist; Willard
Parker, actor.

WILLIAM—Old German:
Willi-helm. "Resolute protector." William the Con-
queror, Norman subjugator of
England in 1066; William
Randolph Hearst, publisher;
William Shakespeare, dra-
matist; William C. Men-
ninger, psychiatrist; William
Beebe, scientist; Willie Mays,
baseball star; Will Rogers,
r.

English nicknames: **Will,
Willie, Willi, Willy, Bill,
Billy.**
English variations: **Wiley,
Wilkie, Wilkes, Wilson,
Williamson, Willis.**
Foreign variations: **Wilhelm**
(German), **Guillaume** (French),
Guglielmo (Italian), **Guillermo**
(Spanish), **Vihelm** (Swe-
dish), **Willem, Wim** (Dutch),
Uilleam (Scottish), **Uilliam**
(Irish).

WILLOUGHBY—Old En-
glish: **Wylig-by.** "From the
willow farm."

WILMER—Old German:
Willa-mar. "Resolute, famous
one."

WILMOT—Old German:
Willi-mod. "Resolute spirit or
mind."

WILSON—Old English:
Wille-sone. "Son of William
or Will." See **William.**
Wilson Bissel, U.S. Postmaster General (1893–1894).

WILTON—Old English:
Wyll-tun. "From the spring
farm."

WINCHELL—Old English:
Wincel. "From a corner or
bend in a piece of land or a
road." Walter Winchell,
columnist, commentator;
Winchell Smith, American
playwright.

WINDSOR—Old English:
Wendles-ora. "Boundary
bank."

WINFIELD—Old English:

Wine-feld. "From the friend's field"; or Teutonic: "friend of the soil." Winfield Scott, U.S. Army general (1786–1866).

WINFRED—Old English: **Wine-frith.** "Peaceful friend." English variation: **Winifred.**

WINGATE—Old English: **Wine-god.** "Divine protection"; or Old English: **Windan-geat.** "From the winding-gate," a gate on a turnscrew.

WINSLOW—Old English: **Wines-hloew.** "From the friend's hill." Winslow Homer, American painter (1836–1910).

WINSTON—Old English: **Windes-tun.** Place name and surname: "from the friend's estate or town." Winston Churchill, English statesman; Winston Graham, Winston Groom, authors.

WINTER—Old English: "born in the wintertime."

WINTHROP—Old English: **Wine-torp.** "Dweller at the friend's estate." Winthrop Rockefeller, business executive; Winthrop Ames, American theatrical producer.

WINTON—Old English: **Wine-tun.** "From the friend's estate."

WINWARD—Old English: **Wine-wode.** "Friend's forest"; or Old English: **Wine-weard.** "Friend-guardian."

WITT—Old English: **Witta.** "Wise man."

WITTER—Old English: **Witta-here.** "Wise warrior." Witter Bynner, poet.

WITTON—Old English: **Witta-tun.** "From the wise man's estate."

WOLCOTT—Old English: **Wulf-cot.** "From Wolf's cottage." Wolf names were only applied to men of outstanding courage and bravery.

WOLFE—Old English: **Wulf.** "A wolf."

WOLFGANG—Old German: **Wolf-gang.** "Advancing wolf." Wolfgang Mozart, composer; Johann Wolfgang Goethe, German author.

WOODROW—Old English: **Wudo-roew.** "Dweller at the hedge by the forest." Woodrow Wilson, 28th U.S. President.

WOODRUFF—Old English: **Wudo-raefa.** "Forest-warden or bailiff."

WOODWARD—Old English: **Wudo-weard.** "Forest-warden; forester."

WOODY—Modern U.S., from a nickname, also used alone. Woody Allen, actor and director; Woody Guthrie, folk balladeer.

WOOLSEY—Old English: **Wulf-sige.** "Victorious wolf." Cardinal Woolsey, famous

English prelate under King
Henry VIII.

WORCESTER—Old English: **Wire-ceaster.** "Alder-forest army camp."

WORDSWORTH—Old English: **Wulfweards-weorth.** "Wolf-guardian's farm." William Wordsworth, famous English poet.

WORRELL—Old English: **Waer-heall.** "Dweller at the true-man's manor."

WORTH—Old English: **Weorth.** "Farmstead."

WORTON—Old English: **Wyrt-tun.** "Dweller at the vegetable enclosure."

WRAY—Old Norse: **Ura.** "From the corner property."

WREN—Old Welsh: **Ren.** "Chief or ruler"; or Old English: **Wrenna.** "Wren-bird." Christopher Wren, architect of St. Paul's Cathedral, London (1632–1723).

WRIGHT—Old English:

Wryhta. "Carpenter." Wright Patman, U.S. Congressman.

WYATT—Old French: **Guyot.** "Little warrior." Wyatt Earp, famous American lawman, frontiersman.

WYBORN—Old Norse: **Uig-biorn.** "War-bear."

WYCLIFF—Old English: **Hwit-clif.** "From the white cliff."

WYMAN—Old English: **Wig-man.** "Warrior."

WYMER—Old English: **Wig-maere.** "Famous in battle."

WYNDHAM—Old English: **Windham.** "From the enclosure with the winding path."

WYNN—Old Welsh: **Wyn.** "Fair; white one." English variation: **Winn.**

WYTHE—Middle English: **Wyth.** "Dweller by a willow-tree." George Wythe, a signer of the Declaration of Independence (1726–1806).

X

XAVIER—Spanish Basque: **Javerri; Xaver.** "Owner of the new house"; or Arabic: "bright." Honoring St. Francis de Xavier of Javier, born at his family's castle of Javier in Navarra, Spain; he was a missionary known as the

"Apostle of the Indies." Xavier Cugat, bandleader. Foreign variations: **Javier, Xever** (Spanish).

XENOS—Greek: **Xenos.** "Stranger or guest."

XERXES—Persian: **Ksathra.**

"Ruler; royal prince." Xerxes, King of Persia, B.C. 486–465, known in the Bible as Ahasuerus, was the husband of Esther in the Book of Esther.

XYLON—Greek: "from the forest."

Y

YALE—Old English: **Healh.** "From the slope or corner of land." Elihu Yale, founder of Yale University (1648–1721).

YANCY—American Indian: **Yankee.** "Englishman." 17th-century New England Indians distorted "English" to "Yankee," it is stated.

YATES—Middle English: "dweller at the gates."

YEHUDI—Hebrew: **Jehujidah.** "The praise of the Lord." Yehudi Menuhin, violinist.

YEOMAN—Middle English: **Yoman.** "Retainer."

YORK –Old English: **Eoforwic.** "Boar-estate"; or Old Celtic: **Eburacon.** "Yew-tree estate."

YULE—Old English: **Geol.** "Born at Christmas." Also: **Yul.** Yul Brynner, actor.

YURI—See **Uriah.**

YVES—See **Ives.** St. Yves or Yvo Helory, 13th-century Breton, is patron saint of lawyers. Yves Montand, actor, Yves St. Laurent, fashion designer.

Z

ZACHARY—Hebrew: **Zekharyah.** "Jehovah hath remembered." The modern form of Zachariah, from the Bible. St. Zachary, a Pope, died in 752; Zachary Taylor, 12th U.S. President; Zachary Scott, actor. Foreign variations: **Zacharias** (German), **Zacarías** (Spanish), **Zacharie** (French), **Zakarias** (Swedish), **Zaccaria** (Italian), **Zakarij** (South Slavic).

ZADOK—Hebrew: **Tsadhoq.** "Just, righteous one." Foreign variation: **Zadoc.** (French).

ZALE—Greek: "power of the sea."

ZANE—See **John.** Zane Grey, American author.

ZARED—Hebrew: "ambush."

ZEBULON—Hebrew: "dwelling place." Zebulon was one of Jacob's sons in the

Bible. Zebulon Weaver, U.S. Congressman; Zebulon Pike, U.S. Army officer and explorer.

ZEDEKIAH—Hebrew: **Tsidhqiyah.** "Justice of the Lord."

ZEEMAN—Dutch: "seaman." Peter Zeeman, Dutch physicist.

ZELOTES—Greek: "zealous one." A person diligent and enthused with life and responsibilities.

ZENAS—Greek: "living." English variation: **Zeno.**

ZEPHANIAH—Hebrew: "treasured by the Lord." English variations: **Zeph, Zephan.**

ZERO—Arabic: "the empty." Zero Mostel, actor.

ZEUS—Greek: "living one," or "father of gods and men." Zeus was the ancient Greek ruler of heaven.

ZIV—Old Slavic: **Zivu.** "Living one."

ZURIEL—Hebrew: **Zuriyel.** "God; my stone or rock."